HANDBOOK OF

Medical Device Regulatory Affairs in Asia

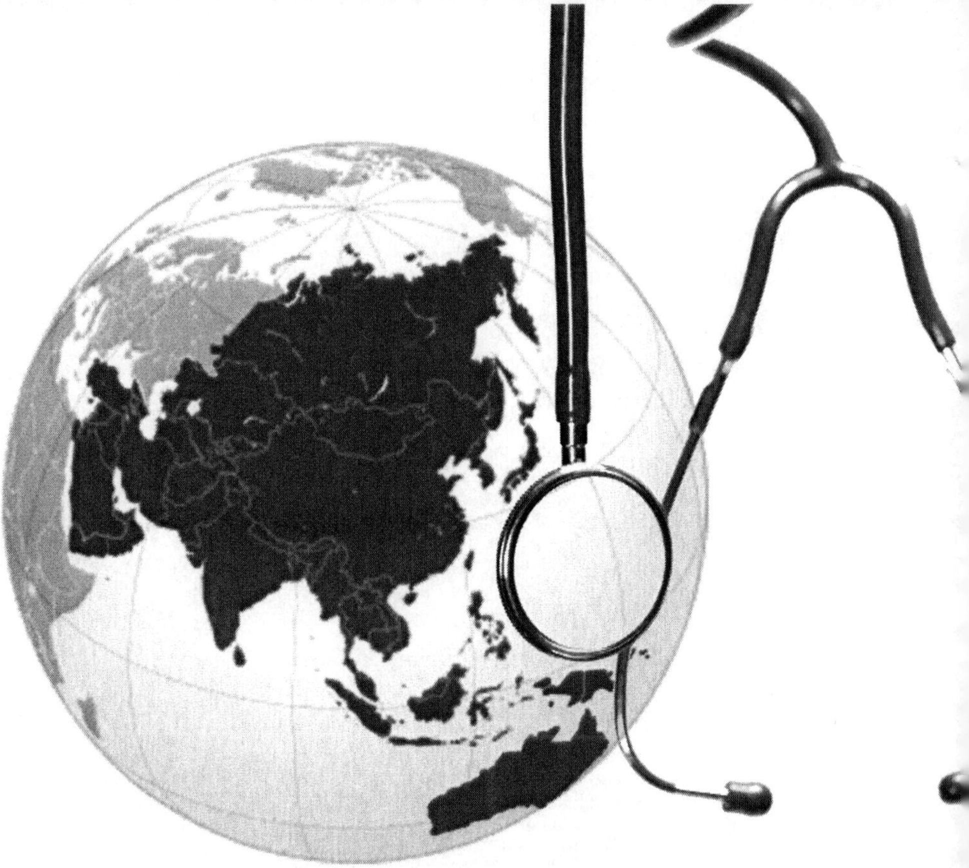

HANDBOOK OF

Medical Device Regulatory Affairs in Asia

Jack Wong

Raymond K.Y. Tong

PAN STANFORD PUBLISHING

Published by

Pan Stanford Publishing Pte. Ltd.
Penthouse Level, Suntec Tower 3
8 Temasek Boulevard
Singapore 038988

Email: editorial@panstanford.com
Web: www.panstanford.com

British Library Cataloguing-in-Publication Data
A catalogue record for this book is available from the British Library.

Handbook of Medical Device Regulatory Affairs in Asia

Disclaimer

The regulatory information contained in this book is intended for academic learning and market planning and is subject to change frequently. Translations of laws and regulations are unofficial.

ISBN 978-981-4411-21-9 (Hardcover)
ISBN 978-981-4411-22-6 (eBook)

Printed in the USA

Contents

Preface

Medical device regulation in Asian markets has become important. Governments and regulatory bodies of countries across the region have placed new regulatory systems or refined the existing ones. Regulatory affairs (RA) is a science of how to get a medical product registered with different countries' health authorities. A registered product would demand a lot of technical documentation to prove its efficacy, safety, and quality. To successfully and smoothly register a product, many soft skills are required for dealing with various key stakeholders in governments, testing centers, hospitals, and medical doctors.

The handbook is the first to cover medical device regulatory affairs in Asia. It is enriched by contributions by authors working with several regulatory bodies, including the US Food and Drug Administration (FDA), UK Medicines and Healthcare Products Regulatory Agency (MHRA), Japan Pharmaceuticals and Medical Devices Agency (PMDA), Saudi Food and Drug Authority (SFDA), Korea Testing Laboratory (KTL), Taiwan FDA, World Health Organization (WHO), Asian Harmonization Working Party (AHWP), Regulatory Affairs Professionals Society (RAPS), and British Standards Institution (BSI). Each chapter provides substantial background materials relevant to a particular area to provide the reader a better understanding of regulatory affairs. The text also presents in-depth discussion on requirements for medical device registration in China and India.

Government bodies will find this book useful to understand the global regulatory environment to help enhance their regulatory systems. The medical device industry can use it to better understand and access the Asian market. Academics and students will find this book very important for their careers in biomedical engineering and medical device–related fields. In research and development, with the help of this book, companies can plan their projects and ensure that the developed medical devices adhere to the global regulatory environment.

The chapters have been grouped into five main parts as follows:

- Part 1 explains what RA is, how to be a good RA professional, how a RA professional works with other team members, and some associated soft skills.
- Part 2 focuses on medical device fundamentals, such as history, labeling requirement, clinical trial requirement, how to do classification, and two important standards for medical device regulatory (ISO 13485 and ISO 14971).
- Part 3 introduces key global (WHO, APEC, RAPS) and regional (AHWP, ASEAN) organizations.
- Part 4 discusses the US and EU regulatory systems in detail. We also invite two experts from the US FDA and the UK MHRA to share their experience on combinational product regulatory. Their experience will be very helpful for Asia.
- Part 5 is the core of this book. It describes the regulatory system in the Asia-Pacific market, with contributions from regulatory authorities, testing laboratories, and industries.

This book would not have been possible without contributions from outstanding experts in various topics discussed in it. We wish to express our gratitude to all of them for their precious efforts and strong support.

Fifty percent of the revenue from this book will be donated to the Asia Regulatory Professional Association and the remaining 50% to the Interdisciplinary Division of Biomedical Engineering in Hong Kong Polytechnic University for future regulatory professionals' development.

Finally, many thanks to our families (Jack Wong's mother, Cheung Shim Kuen, wife, Sherry Kwan Suet Sum, and son, Jay Wong Yat; Raymond Tong's wife, Wai-nga Lam, and daughter and sons, Lok-ching, Lok-tin, and Lok-ting), for their support, encouragement, and patience. They have been our driving forces.

Jack Wong
Asia Regulatory Professional Association

Raymond Kai-yu Tong
Professor, The Hong Kong Polytechnic University
Hong Kong Academy Chair, Asia Regulatory Professional Association

Asia Regulatory Professional Association

The Asia Regulatory Professional Association (ARPA) is an organization of Healthcare Regulatory Affairs professionals in Asia. ARPA aims to raise the standard and social recognition of Regulatory Professionals as part of healthcare team.

We are working with different regulatory expertise globally to achieve the above objectives. ARPA created this first Regulatory textbook in Asia and arranged a number of Regulatory Certificate courses in order to raise the standard of Regulatory Professionals.

You will also get awareness from key regulatory bodies, including the US Food and Drug Administration, the Japan Pharmaceuticals and Medical Devices Agency, Korea Testing Laboratory, and Taiwan FDA, and regulatory organizations, including the World Health Organization, Regulatory Affairs Professionals Society, and British Standards Institution, which support this book and endorse the importance of Regulatory Professional development.

The ARPA membership is free. Anyone who is interested in the Asia regulatory affairs can join ARPA. For more details, visit http://www.healthcare.org.hk/Health2.aspx?id=1&Cid=0.

Jack Wong
General Manager
Asia Regulatory Professional Association
speedxquality@yahoo.com

Chapter 1

How to Train University Students in Regulatory Affairs

Raymond K. Y. Tong
Hong Kong Polytechnic University, Hung Hom, Hong Kong
Asia Regulatory Professional Association (ARPA)
k.y.tong@polyu.edu.hk

This chapter focuses on how to design a regulatory course to train university students in regulatory affairs.

1.1 Introduction

Medical device regulations are coming up in many Asian markets. The course should be suitable for students who are studying biomedical engineering, healthcare, or medical device engineering. These students should have some experience in a health- or engineering-related field and should wish to start working in the growing field of regulatory affairs. The course in regulatory affairs aims to give both factual and practical knowledge of what is regulatory requirement and how to handle future regulatory tasks.

Handbook of Medical Device Regulatory Affairs in Asia
Edited by Jack Wong and Raymond K. Y. Tong

ISBN 978-981-4411-21-9 (Hardcover), 978-981-4411-22-6 (eBook)
www.panstanford.com

On completion of the course, students will be able to demonstrate their understanding of how to meet the standards and regulatory requirements, and they will be able to handle regulatory tasks, including classification, risk management, ISO standard, product registration, and commercial materials review.

Students will be trained to understand the global, regional, and local medical device regulatory requirements and trends. Besides conducting lectures, students will be arranged into a small group to work on a medical device and practice preparing a medical device registration submission to a competent authority. The competent authority is a body that has authority to act on behalf of the government to ensure that the requirements of the medical device directives are transposed into the national law and are applied. Guest lecturers with regulatory experience and network will be invited to share their experience. Students who finish the course will be eligible for attending related medical device regulatory examination conducted by external bodies, such as notified bodies and the Asia Regulatory Professional Association.

1.2 A Sample of Regulatory Affairs Exercises for Students

1.2.1 Background

Consider this case. You have just been recruited by a manufacturing company, Poly Technologies Corporation (PTC), as project manager under its newly found business section for medical and healthcare products. The company has little, if any, experience in designing and manufacturing medical devices. Your primary duty is to provide internal consultancy to the top management of the company on new business development analysis and management of medical device design and manufacturing projects.

Last month your company's top management signed a business agreement to collaborate with an overseas client, which is a global distributor of medical products. Under this collaboration agreement, your client and PTC will co-develop a series of medical devices for global markets. Your client has proposed to start a project with the sterile disposable hypodermic syringes with needles — for single-dose hypodermic injection (Fig. 1.1).

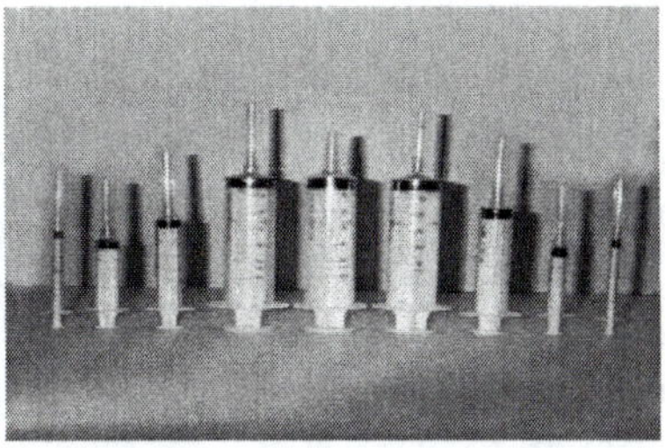

Figure 1.1 Various sizes of hypodermic syringes.

To begin with, your client has suggested designing and manufacturing the products for the US and EU markets and, if possible, extend the market to China in future.

Task 1: Classification

Your first task is to brief your management about the product classifications of the device. For more details, see Chapter 11, "Medical Device Classification Guide."

Target market	Device classification	What are the US FDA regulation numbers	Classification rules applied to the product under EU medical device directive	Notified body involvement for CE marking?
EU				
US				
China				

Task 2: Risk Analysis

(For more details, see Chapter 13 on ISO14971.)
During the design phase of the device, suggest hazards for the product that the product design team has to include in the design input considerations.

Suggest the severity and occurrence for the suggested hazards. Ensure that you have provided your own table and definition of different levels of severity and occurrence.

Task 3: Risk Evaluation and Risk Control

(For more details, see Chapter 13 on ISO14971.)

You have to develop a risk graph (group for risk regions and decide the risk acceptability) and risk matrix (put all the above risks in your device)

Implement risk control measures for all of your hazards. After all risk control measures have been implemented and verified, the manufacturer shall decide whether the overall residual risk posed by the medical device is acceptable using the criteria defined in the risk management plan.

Task 4: Medical Device Registration Submission

Prepare a medical device registration submission to your competent authority.

References

1. ISO 13485 (Medical devices — Quality management systems — Requirements for regulatory purposes).
2. ISO 14971 (Medical devices — Application of risk management to medical devices).
3. EU Directive 93/42/EEC regarding medical devices.
4. MDCO, http://www.mdco.gov.hk/eindex.html.
5. AHWP, http://www.ahwp.info/.
6. GHTF, http://www.ghtf.org/.
7. Asia Regulatory Professional Association (ARPA) http://www.healthcare.org.hk/E_Doctors/Health2.aspx?id=1&Cid=0.
8. International Organization for Standardization, http://www.iso.ch/iso/.

Part 1

Introduction

Chapter 2

The Evolution of the Regulatory Professional: Perspectives on the Skill Sets and Capabilities That Will Define the Next Generation of Regulatory Professionals

David Martin and Neil Lesser

Deloitte Consulting LLP

davidmartin@deloitte.com, nlesser@deloitte.com

2.1 Introduction

Historically, the role of the regulatory affairs function within companies that develop and sell medical devices has been more tactical than strategic. While this tactical focus has served the industry well in the past, regulatory authorities around the world are raising the bar for market access. Regulatory reforms as well as the increased availability of real-world safety and efficacy data continue to alter the path to approval and the underlying investment case for medical devices. Globalization will also play a key role in shifting regulatory requirements — New regulatory frameworks are evolving and regional partnerships will be the main driver of harmonization going forward, especially in the Asia-Pacific market area.

Handbook of Medical Device Regulatory Affairs in Asia
Edited by Jack Wong and Raymond K. Y. Tong

ISBN 978-981-4411-21-9 (Hardcover), 978-981-4411-22-6 (eBook)
www.panstanford.com

In response, manufacturers are seeking a new type of regulatory professional that can continuously adapt to this more complex regulatory environment. The new regulatory professional will continue to execute tactical requirements and will also own strategic relationships with regulators and thought leaders that can help shape future policies. Guiding the regulatory professional will be a fluent understanding of the organization's strategy and active participation in product development and commercialization, making them a more robust business partner to the clinical and commercial functions.

2.2 Drivers of Change

The regulatory environment in the global medical device industry is and will continue to undergo major shifts. In December 2011, the Asia-Pacific Economic Cooperation group announced a new plan to harmonize regulations for medical devices by 2020. The proposal is based on the Global Harmonization Task Force (GHTF) — recently re-formed into the **International Medical Devices Regulators' Forum** (IMDRF) — and intends to create a predicable regulatory framework for device manufacturers. This large-scale initiative will require an unprecedented level of cooperation across national health authorities. If successful, the harmonization will eliminate some of the unknowns in the regulatory environment, but getting there will challenge manufacturers that must reconcile the harmonized promise of tomorrow against the fragmented regulatory landscape of the near term. In addition, regulations have a history of lagging behind the rate of product innovation, meaning there will be a continued need for sophistication in the regulatory affairs function to navigate the evolution of the national, regional, and global regulatory environment. Regulatory professionals in the medical device and diagnostics industry must become aware of the three main influencers to the environment: rapid change, harmonization on a global scale, and increased safety and effectiveness requirements.

First, the regulatory environment is changing rapidly and professionals must be able to gauge how new developments will affect the future environment. New regulations with far-reaching ramifications have emerged in only the last few months; in January of 2012, Chinese officials issued a set of rules to deal with the conflict of interest of healthcare government officials in connection with pharmaceutical and device manufacturers,[1] and released a new Five Year Plan for the pharmaceutical and medical device industries.[2]

Second, as firms increasingly develop a global footprint, the comparative global regulatory frameworks must be taken into account. These regulatory frameworks are embarking on a period of standardization, led predominantly by the Global Harmonization Task Force, founded in 1992 with the stated goal of achieving greater uniformity between national medical device regulatory systems. This agency is playing a key role in driving standardization and continues to leverage existing international organizations (such as the Association of Southeast Asian Nations (ASEAN)) to achieve greater coordination. For example, the Malaysian Medical Device Control Division has drafted guidelines for the *in vitro* diagnostics sector which are based on recommendations from GHTF and ASEAN guidelines.[3] In addition, these regulatory frameworks are also currently going through a period of change. The GHTF itself has recently announced a successor organization, the International Medical Devices Regulatory Forum (IMDRF) which will continue the goal of acceleration of harmonization, but will also assemble ad hoc working groups comprised of various stakeholders to discuss key issues.[4]

Third, there has been an increased emphasis placed on safety and effectiveness in the data required for clinical trials. Several developing nations are incorporating adverse event reporting capabilities and requirements into their regulatory frameworks, including India and China.[5] Singapore is also planning to introduce regulations for medical device clinical trials in 2012.[6] This trend is of increased importance, as clinical data will become more crucial for pre-market decisions due to the greater overall emphasis placed on patient safety recently. However, this trend will need to be monitored closely across the region as China has actually begun to relax clinical trial regulations for specific medical device classes.[7]

2.3 Historical Role and Skill Set of a Regulatory Professional

Historically, the regulatory professional has served an important operational role within a life sciences organization. The role could be described as process oriented in nature: managing the submission process, communicating to stakeholders and ensuring compliance with rules and policies to secure the smooth delivery of a product submission (see Fig. 2.1 below for an example of a job description for a traditional regulatory position).

- Compile and format departmental documentation for inclusion in regulatory submissions (IDE, 510(k), International Registrations).
- Participate in the complaint management process and ensure timely completion of adverse event reporting as required by the FDA and international regulatory agencies.
- Work closely with the Sr. Director of Regulatory and related departments in order to support Regulatory submission activities.
- Coordinate and consult with other departments, including Engineering, Manufacturing, Marketing and Quality, in order to support the collection of documentation, review and assembly of regulatory submissions.
- Ensure the quality, content and format of regulatory submissions to state, federal and international agencies.
- Ensure consistency, completeness and adherence of standards for all submissions. Submissions will include IDEs, 510(k)s, federal and state establishment licensing applications, international regulatory device licensing applications, etc.

Figure 2.1 Sample job description for a traditional regulatory professional role.[8]

The primary skill sets necessary for the completion of the above tasks are excellent organizational and managerial skills as well as a thorough understanding of standards and regulations. The requirements for this position are more focused on adherence to regulations and curating the appropriate compliance documentation, with less emphasis on analyzing the larger regulatory-industry environment to understand its far reaching implications.

While these process and organizational skills will remain essential, tectonic shifts in the environment have manufacturers seeking to unlock the strategic value of the regulatory function. They are looking for their regulatory leaders to contribute outside of their functional vertical and leverage their expertise across the organization. This enhanced position requires a broader skill set and leading manufacturers have already begun hiring for this evolved regulatory role as evidenced in the job description below (Fig. 2.2).

- Independently lead global regulatory strategy development, planning, and implementation for multiple complex programs and platforms. Participate in identification of risk areas and develop alternative courses of action including anticipation of regulators responses through scenario planning and development of contingency plans.
- Guide and influence technical groups in areas of product development and lifecycle enhancement. Participate in potential and established third part efforts (i.e. due diligence activities, joint ventures, etc.).
- Initiate and maintain appropriate communication within the RA function and represent Regulatory Affairs with business units and other functions. Implement policies to ensure ongoing compliance of regulatory requirements.
- Develop and implement regulatory strategy aligned with business strategy. Assess impact of new regulations and implement appropriate changes as well as lead development of company policy and positions on draft regulation and guidance.
- Responsible for negotiating and decision making with regulators and stakeholders with complex and high-risk projects.
- Provide direct supervision of individuals including mentoring, performance management and staffing decisions.
- Represent company externally at appropriate industry associations. May act as primary contact with regulatory authorities including the planning and leadership of meetings. May participate in management of budgets.

Figure 2.2 Example job description for the changing regulatory professional role.[9]

2.4 Changing Role and Skill Set of the Regulatory Professional

In light of the aforementioned shifts in the regulatory environment, it is clear that an expansion of capabilities will be required in the future within regulatory departments. These capabilities will go beyond the traditional realm of regulatory affairs and move the function closer to "heart of the business" issues that shape the strategic direction of the organization. Regulatory professionals that are able to make this leap will become trusted partners and contributors as they will have found ways to unlock value in the regulatory process. Described below are a few of the next-generation capabilities that will empower the regulatory professional.

2.5 Develop as a Center of Intelligence

To adjust to the dynamic regulatory environment found in both the Asia-Pacific region and the broader global environment, the regulatory function should strive to operate as a center of intelligence for the organization — proactively sensing signals of change in the external environment and disseminating the insights to the organization. Such a role requires that the professional be capable of synthesizing data and trends from a variety of sources and developing a recommendation that considers complex points of view. To do this successfully requires that regulatory professionals are able to capture intelligence from a variety of sources and detect signals from extraneous noise.

Regulatory intelligence is available from myriad sources: interactions with health authorities, conversations with key opinion leaders (KOLs), in the presentations of academics, through networking at conferences and summits, and from the outcome of product submissions. The efficiency and certainty of signal detection will improve with the collective experience of the regulatory professional and the level of rigor used to assess and document regulatory trends. In summary, the regulatory professional will need to develop a process to collect data, perform trend analysis, develop summary insights, and possess the ability to communicate the findings to various stakeholders within the organization.

2.6 Advance Toward Strategic Relationship Management

As the fundamental gatekeeper to market access, health authorities/regulatory agencies play a "make or break" role in the success of a product. For this reason, it is paramount that manufacturers consider means to maximize the value of interactions with key figures from a regulatory body. One such way to maximize value is to implement a more thoughtful approach to interacting with key figures in the approval process and those external stakeholders (e.g.,

KOLs) that might influence it. By formulating a clear understanding of its goals and needs, a manufacturer can align its outreach efforts to effect more purposeful and productive conversations with external figures. By cultivating advanced communication and negotiation skills the organization can help shape the dialogue around reforms and regulatory findings rather than being blocked from the conversation. While not necessarily a cure-all or a quick fix, an organization with a deep understanding of the landscape of influencers and a network to match is more prepared to respond in times of crisis or more able to pick up the phone and get an answer to a burning question.

2.7 Develop as a Strategic Business Partner

Foundational to the aforementioned capabilities will be the expansion of the regulatory professional as a strategic minded individual. With primary access to regulators and a keen understanding of the levers that guide their review and lines of inquiry, the regulatory professional is in a unique position to add value to the organization. By understanding where the key interests and points of debate are for a health authority (e.g., efficacy, safety, cost) the regulatory professional can help guide the direction of a clinical program or a commercial campaign toward those areas most likely to satisfy a regulators priorities while still serving the organization's needs. Part of this role will include actively participating in the strategic business planning process to lend a perspective on feasibility and any prior precedent. It will be critical for the internal expert to communicate across the organization into both commercial and clinical functions and serve as a strategic business partner that can help decipher the "noise" to guide informed decision making for commercial and clinical investment. Delivering in this expanded role will require flexible strategic thinking, complex stakeholder management and a firm understanding of the organization's goals and plans.

2.8 Conclusion: What Will It Take to Get There?

Having laid out a few of the capabilities and skills that the regulatory professional of the future will need, what follows is a discussion of how one can attain the skills and experiences to best position themselves for future success.

Primarily, one must gain the foundational strategic, analytical and communication skills that will be required. This is best accomplished through coursework in Strategy, Operations and Communications. Further coursework in the fields of Negotiation and Marketing would provide the necessary "big picture" view required of the new regulatory role, a skill set in synthesizing information and an understanding of how to manage multiple shareholders and their diverse incentives.

To complement this coursework, one should pursue opportunities to network with a wide array of students and professionals from across life sciences, health care, and the government in order to enrich one's understanding of the needs and motivations of various stakeholders in the system. Memberships in professional societies and industry groups and attending summits and conferences should be at the forefront of any career development strategy, but in this case these associations are particularly important in order to gain a viewpoint on the changing environment of regulation and develop a network of colleagues throughout the industry.

Further, a rotational role within a life sciences organization would be especially valuable. Such a role would provide exposure to a broad spectrum of functions and stakeholders and their diverse incentives and viewpoints. This position represents an ideal experience for a professional in this industry seeking to become fluent in the internal workings of an organization and competent in a strategic partner role.

Ultimately, success in this field requires that professionals recognize that the regulatory role is evolving and that this evolution must be matched by a new, broader focus in their education and career development. Fortunately, the resources exist to prepare for this evolved position and to build a career in this challenging, growing field — One might even say there has never been a more exciting time to be on the regulatory side of the medical device and diagnostics industry.

Acknowledgment

Contributions to this chapter have been made by Chris Nuesch, Bill Chiodetti, and Riddhi Roy, all from Deloitte Consulting LLP.

References

1. http://www.sidley.com/newsresources/newsandpress/Detail.aspx?news=5061.
2. http://www.pacificbridgemedical.com/newsletter/article.php?id=567.
3. http://www.rajpharma.com/productsector/medicaldevices/Malaysia-consults-on-four-draft-guidelines-for-IVD-sector-324052?autnID=/contentstore/rajpharma/codex/4072005d-15cc-11e1-bbe6-4d8e6a53eb99.xml.
4. http://www.emergogroup.com/blog/2011/11/ghtf-unveils-successor-organization.
5. "China Drug and Device Regulatory Update 2009", Pacific Bridge Medical Group, May 2009.
6. http://www.rajpharma.com/productsector/medicaldevices/Singapore-plans-to-introduce-new-framework-for-medtech-trials-in-2012-323092?autnID=/contentstore/rajpharma/codex/b5848548-046e-11e1-bbe6-4d8e6a53eb99.xml.
7. http://www.sidley.com/sidleyupdates/Detail.aspx?news=5019.
8. http://regulatorycareers.raps.org/jobs/4660783/regulatory-affairs-specialist.
9. http://regulatorycareers.raps.org/jobs/4699968/sr-manager-regulatory-affairs-cmc-biologics.

Chapter 3

Ensuring Smooth Product Launch: Regulatory Interfaces with Marketing and Supply Chain

Alok Mishra
Asia Pacific, Strategic Business Systems,
Johnson & Johnson Medical Singapore
amishra@its.jnj.com

3.1 Introduction

The Regulatory step is perhaps the most critical step in the New Product Introduction process as it involves externalities — both within and outside the organization. In a large multinational device manufacturer, the product is often launched in geographies far from the originating company and involves a variety of regulatory and reimbursement authorities who can be quite different in their priorities, processes, requirements, and approach. This is key interfacial step in the launch and one that can create — or destroy — the significant value for the corporation.

A rough calculation can highlight the impact of achieving *speed to market*. Assume a product will achieve a forecast of $30 million

Handbook of Medical Device Regulatory Affairs in Asia
Edited by Jack Wong and Raymond K. Y. Tong

ISBN 978-981-4411-21-9 (Hardcover), 978-981-4411-22-6 (eBook)
www.panstanford.com

per year of peak sales. This translates to sales of over $82,000 per day. The company would lose a million dollars for each 12 days of delay! Alternatively, faster launch makes the company almost $2.5 million extra per month.

What does this have to do with Marketing and Supply Chain? To understand this, we need to look at *interfaces* and *delays*.

There are thus several areas where better communication processes can improve efficiency, reduce time to market, and thus have a positive impact on the bottom-line.

3.2 New Product Pipeline

In most cases, Marketing is exposed to new products in the pipeline much before anyone else. However, quite often they fail to convey this information to other parts of the organization — most importantly, Regulatory Affairs and Supply Chain — which creates suboptimal conditions later. Early information to regulatory affairs is critical for their being able to establish key connections for the documentation, providing heads up and getting feedback from regulators regarding possible requirements and overall being able to create appropriate Regulatory Strategy for the quickest path.

Information to Supply Chain is important as many new products, especially biologics and drug–device combinations, have unique storage requirements and its takes time to optimize vendors and locations to handle such products. In one case, the transportation cost of a biologic product was over 50% of the product's landed costs, and it took months of vendor negotiation to bring it down to a reasonable level.

3.3 Planned Launch Dates

It is important for Marketing to develop launch dates in early consultation with Regulatory Affairs as the latter are in the best position to assess Regulatory difficulty and provide guidelines for feasible dates. In addition, some products may have additional requirements, e.g., mandatory clinical trials, which need detailed budgeting and resource planning to be able to complete registration requirements.

3.4 New Product Forecasts

It is often said forecasting is difficult, especially of the future! The new product forecast of a medical device is a challenging task as it has several barriers that determine the growth rate. These are summarized as 4A's (Access, Adoption, Awareness, and Affordability) (Fig. 3.1).

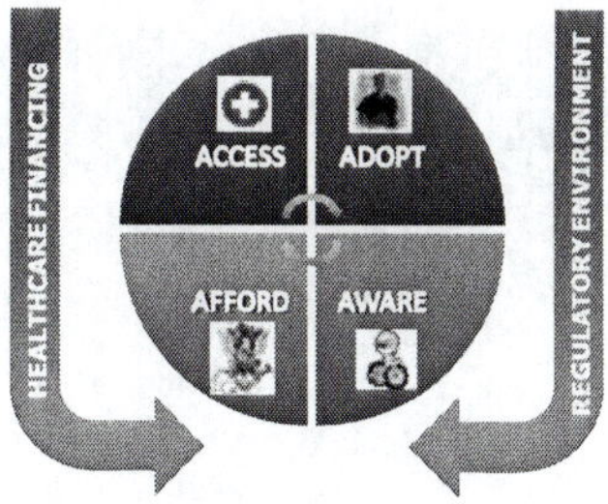

Figure 3.1 The four A's.

It is thus essential that the Marketing manager works with folks in Regulatory and Reimbursement to assess times and rates of approval and build good assumptions around rate of adoption and awareness to arrive at robust forecasts. The importance of this cannot be overemphasized as there is no bigger embarrassment than to have forecasted a wrong approval date and be sitting on valuable inventory when other parts of the world have shortages.

3.5 New Product Approval Dates

Finally, Regulatory Affairs also has an important responsibility to provide timely feedback to Marketing and Supply Chain so that they can plan the launch effectively and not waste resources by planning to early or miss revenue opportunity by not being prepared when the product approval comes through.

Working together of Regulatory Affairs, Marketing, and Supply Chain in a seamless fashion that identifies delays early and responds to problems proactively, thus minimizing the time to market, can be a key source of competitive advantage for a medical device company (Fig. 3.2). It is not easy but is worth all the time and money spent in making it happen.

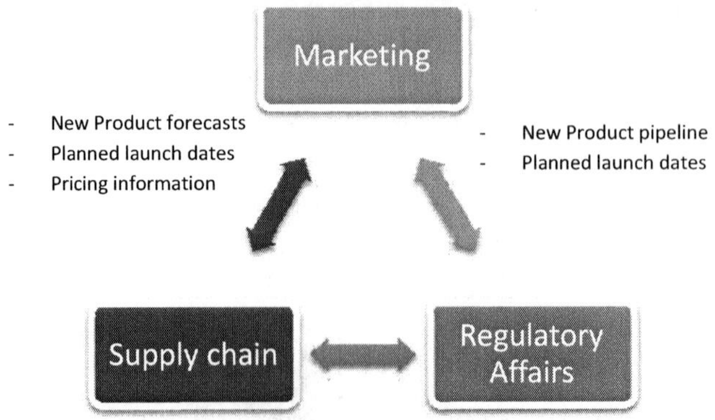

Figure 3.2 Team work for success.

Chapter 4

What Is the Right Thing to Do?

Jack Wong
Asia Regulatory Professional Association (ARPA)
speedxquality@yahoo.com

4.1 Right Job

I am a health care professional who graduated as a pharmacist and worked as a Regulatory Affairs officer in healthcare companies. I am very proud of working in the health care sector as my products or services are very important for people. My job as Regulatory Affairs officer is to make available new medical products to patients by utilizing scientific data from R&D, to ensure a good-quality system in manufacturers, to liaise with the health authority, and finally to obtain relevant certificates prior to supplying the products to patients who need it. To provide high-quality medical products to patients fast is my core job.

Handbook of Medical Device Regulatory Affairs in Asia
Edited by Jack Wong and Raymond K. Y. Tong

ISBN 978-981-4411-21-9 (Hardcover), 978-981-4411-22-6 (eBook)
www.panstanford.com

4.2 Two Key Challenges in Our Job

4.2.1 Quality

To ensure good quality, many international standard bodies (e.g., ISO and BSI) and local standard bodies in many countries such as the United States, Japan, and China actively develop better product standards for manufacturers so that products with better specifications are manufactured. After a product with good specifications has been developed, its production needs to be done within a good system, too (e.g., GMP and ISO 13485), and the process needs to be regularly audited by certification bodies and governments. As regulatory professionals, we need to understand this and explain this to relevant government bodies and finally obtain relevant approvals before supplying the product to patients.

4.2.2 Speed

Taking medical devices as an example, it usually takes 90 working days to get approval in the United States and Europe. Surprisingly, it can take up to 1–2 years to get approval in Asia. Health care sectors and governments in Asia are working hard to streamline the process.

4.3 Regulatory Affairs Job is a Combination of Science, Legal Affairs, and Moral

The following formula can explain our job aptly:

$$\text{RA} = (\text{Science} \times \text{Law})^{\text{Moral}}$$

The Science and Legal parts may be obvious to readers. I would like to explain the Moral part. To begin, I would like to start a story of moral situation.

4.4 Persons versus Things

To explain the moral part of the Regulatory Affairs job, I would like to start with a moral question/situation:

Suppose you were a trolley car driver driving at 60 miles an hour. Suddenly, you see five persons standing in your way. You try to stop, but the brakes do not work. You feel bad as the persons may die.
Then you notice a side track on your right hand side, but there is a person standing there. You can turn right hitting that one person but sparing the five.
What will you do? Sacrificing one life in order to save five seems the right thing to do.
Now consider another version of the trolley car situation:
You are not the driver but an onlooker standing on a bridge overlooking the track, and there is no side track this time. Along the track, there are five persons. The trolley car cannot stop as the brakes do not work, and it is about to crash into the five persons. You feel desperate to help them. Suddenly, you notice a heavy man standing next to you. You can push him off the bridge into the path of the trolley car. He could die, but the five persons would be saved. (Assume that this approach will work and the option of you jumping onto the track will not help as you are too small to stop the trolley).
Will you push the heavy man?

I studied some literature on human rights and philosophy to look for an answer to this question and came up with the following statement:

It is wrong to use people for the sake of the general welfare. Pushing the heavy man onto the track to block the trolley uses him as a means and, hence, fails to respect him and his dignity.

We value things not just "more" or "less," but in qualitatively higher and lower ways.

The Right Thing to Do

A human being is not an object but a person with dignity. As health care professionals, our sole aim is to help them receive good medical services/products fast. **By respecting human dignity, we should put human dignity first and minimize all administrative, bureaucratic, and political issues**. This drives our work in Regulatory Affairs.

Chapter 5

Affordable Access to Medical Devices in Developing Countries

Rosanna W. Peeling[a] **and Tikki Pang**[b]

[a]*London School of Hygiene and Tropical Medicine, London, UK*
[b]*World Health Organization, Geneva, Switzerland*
rosanna.peeling@lshtm.ac.uk, pangtikki@gmail.com

5.1 Introduction

National regulatory approval for drugs provides safeguards for the safety and effectiveness of drugs used in a country. Most countries have established a process for reviewing the evidence from drug trials to support the introduction of new drugs. Over time, this has improved the quality of drugs used in developing countries. Unfortunately, in the developing world, apart from tests used for blood banking, more than 50% of countries do not regulate *in vitro* diagnostics (IVD) for infectious diseases [1, 2]. More broadly, medical devices are often sold and used in most of the developing world without any formal evaluation of their performance and effectiveness. Access to good-quality medical devices is problematic in these countries as companies with good-quality products are often unable or reluctant to compete in a market that is flooded with cheap, poor-quality products.

Handbook of Medical Device Regulatory Affairs in Asia
Edited by Jack Wong and Raymond K. Y. Tong

ISBN 978-981-4411-21-9 (Hardcover), 978-981-4411-22-6 (eBook)
www.panstanford.com

In countries that do regulate medical devices, the regulatory landscape is highly variable and continuously changing, resulting in greater challenges associated with transparency, language barriers, and costs. Regulatory reviews consist of technical and administrative components which can vary significantly between countries, even in the same region. Time frames for approval and the complexity of the approval process vary widely. Because of the onerous process and costs, companies tend to target countries with markets that allow for a substantial return for investment. Smaller countries in the developing world are currently paying significantly higher prices for medical devices than countries with sizeable markets, largely because of the many distribution channels that health program and providers need to go through to access the products that they need. Another important outcome of this scenario is that these complex, lengthy and variable regulatory approval processes have driven up the cost of goods making products unaffordable and become a major disincentive to innovation.

Recent investments in the development of tools to improve global health will soon lead to the commercialization of novel classes of medical devices. However, regulatory directives have not kept pace with technological development [3].

In recent years, the global economic crisis has led to drastic cutback in health programs. Companies have less resources for the research and development of medical devices. International aid programs for HIV have declined from US$ 8.7 billion in 2009 to US$ 7.6 billion in 2010. The Global Fund, one of the major sources of support for global health, recently announced that no new projects will be funded until 2014. But now more than ever, affordable medical devices, in particular IVDs, are urgently needed in the developing world and these products need to be accessible and affordable to patients in the developing world.

5.2 Why Is Affordable Access to Medical Devices Important for Developing Countries?

In times of the global financial crisis, limited resources and competing priorities, affordable and sustainable access to medical devices in developing countries represents a critical first step in ensuring the optimal delivery of health care. In particular, access to rapid, point-of-care (POC) diagnostic tests is fundamental in emergency preparedness, in ensuring health system efficiency and, ultimately, for achieving health equity.

5.2.1 Emergency Preparedness

A rapid and accurate identification of a new or a re-emerging pathogen is the critical first step in the investigation of a potential epidemic or pandemic emergency. Together with standard public health measures to contain an outbreak, surveillance activities are dependent on the availability of rapid, accurate, sensitive, and specific diagnostics which can provide critical information relating to the most appropriate treatment (which drugs?), preventive strategies (are there any vaccines available?), and appropriate public health measures (border controls?). Coupled with standard microbiological procedures and molecular biology techniques in reference laboratories, rapid tests can quickly help to pin down the identity of a new (or re-emerging, or mutant) infectious agent. For example, a suspected dengue fever outbreak in Nicaragua several years ago proved, after rapid diagnosis, to be leptospirosis instead with important repercussions and implications for the needed public health measures, i.e. there are differences in strategies for dealing with a mosquito-borne virus as compared to a water-borne bacterial infection. Early identification of outbreaks leading to appropriate control interventions will also reduce the socioeconomic burden often associated with epidemics.

5.2.2 Efficiency and Effectiveness of Health Systems

Beyond emergency response and preparedness, diagnostics can have very significant impact on the efficiency and effectiveness of the health system as a whole. In the context of both infectious and non-infectious diseases, an accurate diagnostic test can clearly lead to more rational therapy decisions, e.g., deciding the use of an antibiotic or an anti-viral drug. Because of limited access to rapid point of care (POC) diagnostic tests, many treatment decisions in the developing world are made based on clinical/syndromic manifestations, which, arguably, is the cause of wrong, under-, or over-treatment thus resulting in wastage, inefficiency, and the potential selection for resistant strains of microbes. At the population level, a rapid and accurate diagnostic can also guide public health measures needed to contain a potential outbreak as mentioned previously. Finally, the recent trend towards generic, common platforms for multiple rapid diagnostic tests, potentially also including tests for chronic diseases, also promises standardization, increased efficiency and cost savings to the health system. As an example, a generic open platform (see below) will obviate the need to specially train laboratory staff to perform a variety of different diagnostic tests.

5.2.3 Health Equity

Ultimately, however, access to medical devices which improve efficiency of health care delivery in the developing world can help achieve the higher objective and mission of the World Health Organization of "the attainment by all peoples of the highest possible level of health" and the more recent goal of achieving universal health care. Gross inequities in health standards continue to exist between the developed and developing countries, and ensuring access to affordable diagnostics can bridge the equity gap. However, and despite enormous progress in the prevention, diagnosis, and treatment of diseases, developing countries often remain excluded from the benefits of innovations. High-quality diagnostic tests are often not affordable or accessible to patients in the developing world because of health infrastructure constraints. In other words, the inequity extends to the practical aspect of access to diagnostics.

In order to address this inequity, the Bill & Melinda Gates Foundation and Grand Challenges Canada, for example, have created a joint initiative, Grand Challenges in Global Health — Point of Care (POC) Diagnostics. The goal of this initiative is to create a sustainable market for high-performance, low-cost, POC tests for the developing world. Currently, POC diagnostic components are not inter-operable, leading to higher costs of goods and customised training for each test. The vision of this initiative is to develop open platforms that can support an extended menu of tests from different manufacturers, including those based in developing countries. Ideally, a future user will be able to purchase one of these open technology platforms on which a menu of tests can be run according to local needs and capacities. An analogous example would be USB memory sticks which are made by many companies but can work with any computer for data storage and transfer. To make progress towards this vision of a more equitable and "level playing field", it is critical that a diagnostic technology framework be developed with four related sets of standards: Product Standards, Interface Standards, Regulatory Standards and Business Standards.

Finally, it should be emphasized that all three aspects of emergency preparedness, efficiency and equity must be considered in the context of health systems as a holistic, integrated entity. A fundamental commitment to correct inequities is the foundation for the development of stronger, more robust and more efficient health systems which are well-prepared to deal with emergency situations.

5.3 Case Studies

5.3.1 Delay in Eligibility to Treatment for HIV

- Not only access to HIV treatment has been shown to be beneficial for HIV-infected patients, but also it plays a major role in the prevention of onward transmission.
- Eligibility to HIV treatment depends on a white blood cell count (CD4 assay), which is an indicator of the immune status of the patient.
- These assays require sophisticated equipment and are neither affordable nor accessible, especially to patients living outside of urban centres in the developing world.
- The first POC test for CD4 count has been developed, but the company has had to conduct 29 trials in Africa and 49 trials worldwide to obtain regulatory approval.
- The WHO estimates that currently 11 million HIV patients are waiting for CD4 testing to determine eligibility to treatment. The cost of these trials will inevitably be passed onto the cost of goods making the product unaffordable.
- The lengthy approval processes will lead to delays in getting patients on treatment and, in some cases, death.

5.3.2 Delay in Access to Early Diagnosis of Tuberculosis

- The WHO estimates that 1.8 million people die of tuberculosis (TB) every year.

- TB diagnostic trials are lengthy and expensive.
- A new POC TB test has been developed and is commercially available.
- The introduction of this novel life-saving technology will is likely to take 2–5 years for regulatory approval.
- Without expedited approval and harmonization, 4–9 million TB patients will die before this new technology can be widely used to save lives.

5.3.3 Misleading Claims of Test Performance for Dengue Rapid Tests

- One-third of the world is at risk of dengue.
- Countries need accurate diagnostics to rapidly identify the cause of outbreaks so that appropriate public health interventions can be put in place to control the outbreak without delay.
- However, many dengue tests are sold and used with misleading claims of test performance (see Table 5.1).
- New and improved dengue tests are being developed, but approvals may delay their deployment to identify and control outbreaks.

Table 5.1 Misleading claims of test performance for dengue IgM tests

	Manufacturers' claims accuracy (%)		WHO evaluation accuracy (%)	
Test	**Sens**	**Spec**	**Sens**	**Spec**
Test A	100	100	23	99
Test B	NS	NS	18	98
Test C	80	>99	63	69
Test D	NS	NS	9	100
Test E	70	100	65	98
Test F	93	100	22	99
Test G	100	100	6	99

Note: NS, not stated.

Adapted from Blacksell *et al., Clin Infect Dis* 2006; 42:1127.

5.3.4 Case Study — Access versus Performance: Basis for FDA Approval of the First Over-the-Counter Rapid HIV Test in the United States

5.3.4.1 Background

An HIV-infected person does not show any remarkable symptoms in the early stages of infection but is capable of transmitting the virus to others. A key component of the prevention and control of HIV is the early detection of infection through a blood test and counseling or treatment to interrupt the chain of transmission within the population. Laboratory methods to detect HIV infection have been used for more than two decades, but individuals need to take the initiative to present at a clinic for testing. Simple rapid HIV tests, available since the 1990s, have made testing accessible beyond clinic settings, but at-risk individuals, who are typically drivers of the HIV epidemic, frequently remain stigmatized and marginalized from care. In the United States, it is estimated that 1.2 million people are infected with HIV, of whom 18% do not know their HIV status and are continuing to transmit their infection to their sexual partners (http://www.cdc.gov/hiv/resources/factsheets/us.htm). In recent years, a simple rapid HIV test that can be used with oral fluids instead of blood has become available for purchase by consumers over-the-counter. This first-of-a-kind test offers the opportunity for testing in the privacy of one's home. The US FDA examined the personal and public health risks and benefits of approving the OraQuick® In-Home HIV Test to support its decision-making. http://www.fda.gov/AdvisoryCommittees/CommitteesMeetingMaterials/BloodVaccinesandOtherBiologics/BloodProductsAdvisoryCommittee/ucm298652.htm

5.3.4.2 Performance expectations

A US FDA Advisory Committee recommended that the OraQuick test should have sensitivity and specificity that are >95%, as the lower bound of the 95% confidence interval (CI) around the point estimates for the over-the-counter test (vs. 98% for professional use rapid HIV tests). Performance studies showed that, for professional use, the sensitivity and specificity the HIV test exceeded the recommended threshold of >98% as the lower bound of the 95% confidence interval. Likewise, the specificity of the over-the-counter

OraQuick test exceeded the minimum recommended performance. However, the OraQuick test sensitivity failed to reach the threshold of the minimum recommended lower 95% CI bound of 95% as shown follows:

Performance measure	Professional Use OraQuick Test performance (2-sided 95% CI*)	Minimum recommended performance	Over-the-counter OraQuick Test performance (2-sided 95% CI*)	Minimum recommended performance
Sensitivity	99.3% (**98.4**–99.7%)	**98%** (lower bound of the 2-sided 95% CI)	92.98% (**86.64**–96.92%)	**95%** (lower bound of the 2-sided 95% CI)
Specificity	99.8% (**99.6**–99.9%)	**98%** (lower bound of the 2-sided 95% CI)	99.98% (**99.90**–100%)	**95%** (lower bound of the 2-sided 95% CI)

*95% CI = 95% Confidence Interval.

5.3.4.3 Risk benefit analysis

The FDA performed a risk analysis to understand the public and individual health implications of approving a test with these performance characteristics. Potential outcomes evaluated included the following:

- Estimated test results for numbers of individuals projected to be tested annually who would not otherwise be tested, including number of true positives and negatives and false positives and negatives
- Estimated the net transmissions averted through the use of this test (assuming a change in behavior following a positive test result)
- The impact of switching from professional testing to self-testing
- The impact of who will use the test
- Do the benefits outweigh the risks?

A risk assessment model was developed, and the projected outcome in the first year of use was that there would be a projected net public health benefit from use of the OraQuick® In-Home HIV Test resulting from the net increase in the number of HIV infections newly identified among HIV-infected individuals who were unaware of their HIV status (approximately 4,500 individuals) and 2,700,000 who would test negative. The FDA concluded that the public health benefit of averting 4,000 transmissions would outweigh the individual risk of increased numbers of false negative results (approximately 1,100).

The fact that individual risk remained prompted FDA to address this risk through messages in the test kit labeling:

- A positive result with this test does not mean that you are definitely infected with HIV, but rather that additional testing should be done in a medical setting.
- A negative result with this test does not mean that you are definitely not infected with HIV, particularly when exposure may have been within the previous three months.
- Testing is recommended if you test negative and continue to engage in behavior that puts you at risk for HIV infection.
- A negative result does not imply it is safe to engage in risk behavior for HIV infection.

5.4 The Way Forward

The regulation of medical devices is critical in assuring their safety and effectiveness. However, regulatory oversight in much of the developing world is limited, leading to products being sold and used without evidence of effectiveness. In countries with regulatory authorities, the approval process often lacks transparency and can be costly and lengthy. This is a major barrier to innovation and access. What is needed is the development of a clearly defined set of standards and a critical pathway for preclinical and clinical testing of medical devices within a transparent framework that takes into account benefit for patients while ensuring safety and effectiveness [4]. While there are strong political and financial incentives for national regulatory authorities to insist on their own approval processes, there is a compelling need for harmonization or convergence of regulatory approval standards so that companies would not be required to conduct clinical trials in every country, thus reducing the cost of goods and decreasing lengthy delays. As the Global Harmonization Task Force (GHTF) transitioned to the International Medical Devices Regulatory Federation (IMDRF), there is hope that progress will continue to be made in harmonization of regulatory standards for medical devices and in particular, for

IVDs. The Asian Harmonization Working Party has made good progress with the result that countries from other regions have joined this initiative. Regional initiatives such as the formation of the Latin America IVD Association and the Pan-African Harmonization Working Party illustrate the need to ensure affordable access of medical devices in these regions. Similar harmonization efforts are being considered to expedite the approval of badly needed vaccines [5]. Regulatory authorities and the regional harmonization working parties need to work with the medical devices industry, departments of health, and standards setters to develop models for rapid assessment and efficient approval of novel classes of medical devices, and for the harmonization of regulatory processes in the developing world to ensure that patient needs are met in all resource settings.

References

1. Peeling RW, Smith PJ, Bossuyt PMM (2006) A guide for diagnostic evaluations. *Nat Rev Microbiol Suppl*: S2–S6. January 10, 2012. From http://www.nature.com/nrmicro/supplements.
2. World Health Organization. Regulation of *in vitro* diagnostics: a global perspective. Annex in: *Diagnostics for Tuberculosis: Global Demand and Market Potential.* Geneva: WHO 2006; pp. 194–203.
3. Gibbs JN (2011). Regulating molecular diagnostic assays: developing a new regulatory structure for a new technology. *Expert Rev Mol Diag*; 11:367–381. United Kingdom.
4. Woosley RL (2007). The FDA's Critical Path Initiative. *Pharmaco Vigilance Rev*; 1:16–18. Euromed Communications Ltd, United Kingdom.
5. Mahoney R, Chocarro L, Southern J, Francis DP, Vose J, Margolis H (2011). Dengue vaccines regulatory pathways: A report on two meetings with regulators of developing countries. *PLoS Med*; 8(2): e1000418. doi:10.1371/journal.pmed.1000418. United Kingdom and USA.
6. Mabey D, Sollis K, Kelly H, Benzaken A, Bitarakwate E, Changalucha J, Chen XS, Yin YP, Garcia P, Strasser S, Chintu N, Pang T, Peeling RW. Point-of-care tests to strengthen health systems and save newborn lives: The case of syphilis. *PLoS Med.* 2012 Jun; 9(6):e1001233. Epub 2012 Jun 12. PMID: 22719229.

Chapter 6

A Story of Attention to Detail

Richard Liu
MCI Shanghai
richard.liu@mci-group.com

MCI is a globally integrated company that helps companies, governments, and associations bring people together to create meaningful connections and provide professional event service to various conferences, seminars or board meetings. Beginning my job as a team lead for Johnson & Johnson two years ago, I mainly focused on providing professional conference/meeting services to our customer.

Today I would like to tell you a story about a drop of water. It might be something that you are indifferent to, or something you may ignore even if you are aware of it. From my point of view, it is something crucial that might determine the final success. Once I served for Johnson & Johnson regulatory meeting in China in March 2012. When a waitress served water for the Johnson & Johnson staff, a drop of water fell on the table. My first response would be to

Handbook of Medical Device Regulatory Affairs in Asia
Edited by Jack Wong and Raymond K. Y. Tong

ISBN 978-981-4411-21-9 (Hardcover), 978-981-4411-22-6 (eBook)
www.panstanford.com

quickly and gently wipe it away. In my opinion, it is not something related to hygiene only, but it is something that may cause problem; for instance, it may spoil the customer's important documents or it may lead to the breakdown of the customer's e-products. To provide professional and best service, it is required that people always pay attention to detail.

Do you think it is a very minor issue? You may remember an interesting instance in the movie *Mission Impossible.* When Tom Cruise hangs down to take his mission target, a disc with top secret data, a drop of sweat trickles down. In that essential moment, Tom stops what he was doing and makes an attempt to trap the drop of sweat. If the drop of sweat touches the desk, it will raise an alarm and the mission would become impossible to achieve. To me, a drop of water is, to some extent, what a drop of sweat is to Tom in the movie.

As explained by Johnson & Johnson, in regulatory work, we need to pay attention to detail. The above story may explain what the right attitude to provide service to the customer should be. Sometimes, a tidier dossier will make product registration quicker!

Part 2

Medical Device Safety and Related ISO Standards

Chapter 7

Biomedical Devices: Overview

Piu Wong

The Whitehead Institute for Biomedical Research, Cambridge, USA

pwong0610@gmail.com

7.1 Historic Aspect of Medical Devices

Medical devices are part of our daily life. They could range from simple equipment such as a thermometer to a highly sophisticated machine such as a pacemaker for a person with heart problem. They all serve to meet the medical needs. In contrast to pharmaceutical products, their modes of action are not pharmacological, metabolic, or immunological. Some of the landmarks in medical device development are illustrated in Table 7.1 [1–2].

Handbook of Medical Device Regulatory Affairs in Asia
Edited by Jack Wong and Raymond K. Y. Tong

ISBN 978-981-4411-21-9 (Hardcover), 978-981-4411-22-6 (eBook)
www.panstanford.com

Table 7.1 Landmarks in medical devices

Year	Device	Inventor
1943	Dialyzer	Dutch physician, Willem Kolff
1950	Artificial hip replacement	Performed by English surgeon Sir John Charnley
1951	Artificial heart valve	US team led by electrical engineer Miles Edwards
1952	External cardiac pacemaker	US cardiologist Paul Zoll
1960	Internal pacemaker	US electrical engineer Wilson Greatbatch
1970	Computerized axial tomography (CT) scanner	Nobel Prize winners Godfrey Hounsfield and Allon Cormack
1977	Magnetic resonance imaging	US team led by physician Raymond Damadian
1982	Artificial heart	Willem Kolff
1985	Implantable cardioverter defibrillator	Polish cardiologist Michel Mirowski
2000–2010	Robotic medical devices, such as NeuroArm and CyberKnife	Various inventors (http://www.mritechnicianschools.org/twelve-amazing-robots-that-are-revolutionizing-medicine/)

Between 1980 and 2000, high-resolution imaging devices, in particular, radiographic and fluoroscopic units, became more commonly used in hospitals and clinics. Devices designed for the real-time monitoring of cardiovascular parameters such as heart rate and blood pressure were part of the standard equipment. Moreover, there was no effective treatment for some of the diseases such as chronic kidney failure until dialysis machines were used to greatly improve their quality of life. Computerized axial scanners (CT) and magnetic resonance imaging (MRI) have become crucial tools in medical imaging to supplement X-rays and ultrasound for screening disease such as patients with a high risk of colon cancer.

It is estimated that approximately 50,000 people died because of the human error [3]. From 2000 onward, robotics became a reality and began to be used in clinical procedures where extreme precision is critical. For example, a minor error in neurosurgery will lead to paralysis. NeuroArm combines MRI and a surgical robot to perform microsurgery and biopsy-stereotaxy with high precision [4].

Another advantage is that remote-controlled surgery is possible if the doctor is not next to the patient. Da Vinci Surgical System has developed over 100 devices so that surgeons can remotely access the machine and perform surgery such as double vessel bypass surgery in the human heart [5].

7.2 Biomedical Market Environment

Aging population, enhanced awareness of the patients, and improved quality of the medical system are the driving forces for the continued demand and growth of the medical device industry in Asia. HSBC's "The Future of Retirement" report estimates that the number of people aged 65 or older will reach 1.4 billion by 2050. The United Nations also predicts that the number of people aged 60 or older will reach 2 billion by 2050, representing 32% of the world's population. For example, in China, 25% of the population will be over 65 by 2050. In Japan, 35.6% of the population will be over 65 by 2050. Standard & Poor's (S&P) reported that 80% of the older individuals suffer from at least one of the chronic health conditions, such as arthritis and cataracts [6, 7]. Therefore, there is a strong need and market to develop technologies to better diagnose disease and improve the treatment for the aging population.

The global medical devices industry has generated revenues in excess of $300 billion in 2011 worldwide [8]. Despite the fact that Asia has more than 60% of the world's population, the healthcare expenses constitute about 15% of the global healthcare expenditure. This suggests that there is an enormous upside potential in the Asian market to improve the healthcare system possibly by better diagnosis and treatment using advanced medical devices. For example, China's import of US medical devices has increased steadily, and it is the second largest market for US medical devices after Japan, with 1.5 billion US medical devices imported in 2008 [9].

The United States is the largest producer of medical devices worldwide. S&P reports that US medical device manufacturers receive 40–50% of their revenues from the foreign markets. The largest US-based medical device companies based on S&P Healthcare products and supplies survey, 2010, are Johnson & Johnson, GE Healthcare, Medtronic, Boston Scientific, Abbott Labs, Becton Dickinson, Stryker, Zimmer, and St. Jude Medical. Companies based outside the United States, such as Siemens (Germany), Hitachi Medical Corporation, and Toshiba (Japan), are major players in the biomedical device industry [10]. US firms are building manufacturing and marketing centers in Asia to streamline manufacturing and distribution efficiencies. High-technology medical products that address the prevalent health issues, especially for the aging population, have a very positive outlook in the future. Here I will illustrate the importance of medical devices by focusing on only diagnosis and treatment of age-related diseases such as arthritis and vision degeneration.

7.3 Orthopedics

7.3.1 Market

Approximately 1 million patients worldwide are treated annually for total replacement of arthritic hips and knees joints. One in forty persons requires orthopedic surgery because of the common joint disorder, osteoarthritis. The number is increasing because of the aging population and enhanced awareness among patients. Stryker Corporation reported that the 2009 worldwide market for reconstructive devices was in the order of $12 billion in size [11]. Knee reconstruction is the most common surgery, constituting 50% of the total joint replacement market. For example, DePuy Rotating Platform Knee mimics the human knee's natural range of motion (Fig. 7.1). Spinal surgery such as thoracolumbar (relating to thoracic and lumbar region of the vertebral cord) implant generates about $5.5 billion worldwide revenue. The United States contributes about 60% of the global orthopedic device market. Major players include Johnson & Johnson (DePuy), Stryker, Zimmer Inc, Medtronics, and Biomet [12].

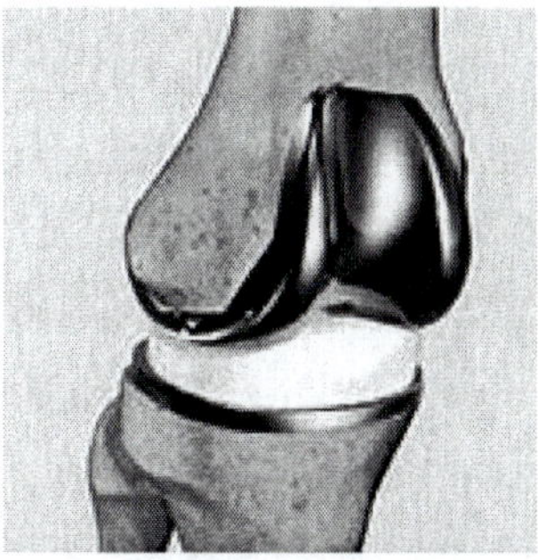

Figure 7.1 The DePuy Rotating Platform Knee mimics human knee's natural range of motion.

7.3.2 Materials

Lightweight, strength, and biocompatibility are the key requirements for the material to be chosen for medical implants. The most commonly used orthopedic implant materials are stainless steels, cobalt–chromium alloys, and titanium alloys (13). Stainless steel is often preferred for making bone plates, screws, pins, and rods because of its resistance to chemicals and environmental conditions found inside the human body. Cobalt–chromium alloys are used in joint replacement and fracture repair implants. Titanium alloys have a significantly higher strength-to-weight ratio than stainless steels. The higher flexibility offered by titanium alloys allows the design of shape-memory-based implants to aid in bone in-growth for better grip. Trabecular metal, which is made from tantalum over carbon, is also strong, flexible, and biocompatible and is porous enough to allow tissue in-growth. Ceramic materials are also used to make implant surfaces that rub each other but do not require flexibility, such as the surface of the hip joint [14].

7.3.3 Biocompatibility

The evaluation of medical device compatibility determines if the contacts of the device with the body produce any harmful local or systemic effect, e.g., degraded products are carcinogenic. The ISO 10993 guidelines have been developed to cover the testing of materials and devices that come into direct or indirect contact with the patient's body [15]. The very first consideration of the selection of materials shall be fitness for purpose with regard to characteristics of the materials such as chemical, toxicological, physical, electrical, morphological, and mechanical properties. The extent of the test depends on the existing pre-clinical and clinical safety data. More stringent tests will be carried out for a novel material. Some of the critical issues include characterizing the material for genotoxicity, carcinogenicity, and reproductive toxicity, irritation and skin sensitization *in vitro* cytotoxicity, and identification and quantification of degradation products from polymeric medical devices ceramics and metals. Importantly, testing should be done on the sterile final product, or representative samples processed in the same manner as the final products [16].

7.3.4 Fabrication

The characteristics of the metal or the biomaterial that I described earlier can be changed depending on the methods to shape the material into the implant, a process called fabrication. In other words, some fabrication methods can strengthen the material, while others can weaken them [17]. The most common fabrication methods used for metal implants are machining, investment casting, and hot and cold forging.

Machining of implant materials is usually performed with computer to allow high precision and reproducibility. For example, cobalt–chrome stem caps for hip transplant are often made using automated machining process. Investment casting is often employed for more complex shapes such as knee implants. Metal is melted and poured into a ceramic mold to create the desired shape of the implant. Forging process presses materials into shape between two molds. This often involves heat treating for molding (hot forging), or the metals are shaped at room temperature (cold forging) [18]. Implants made by forging are often stronger than similar parts made by casing.

7.3.5 Polyethylene Fabrication

Turning powdery polyethylene into a solid piece of polyethylene is called consolidation. Different ways of consolidation can influence the characteristics of the final implants. One of the consolidation processes is called ram extrusion. The polyethylene powder is heated and forced out through a tube. The combination of heat and pressure deposits the powder into the solid bar for further machining. Another way to fabricate polyethylene implants is called compression molding, where the raw powder is heated and then pressed into sheets that can be cut and shaped to create the implant. A slight variation of this process is called net-shape compression molding. The powder is directly deposited into the final implant shape, instead of some intermediate product. This method improves wear reduction of the finished material. After fabrication, heat-treating the metal implant and then slow cooling it reduces brittleness [19, 20]. Because of its durability and performance, metal-on-polyethylene has been the leading artificial hip component material chosen by surgeons since the approval by the US Food and Drug Administration (FDA) 30 years ago. The metal ball is cobalt chrome molybdenum alloy and the liner is polyethylene. This ability to adapt and customize during the surgical procedure is an important attribute of polyethylene (Fig. 7.2).

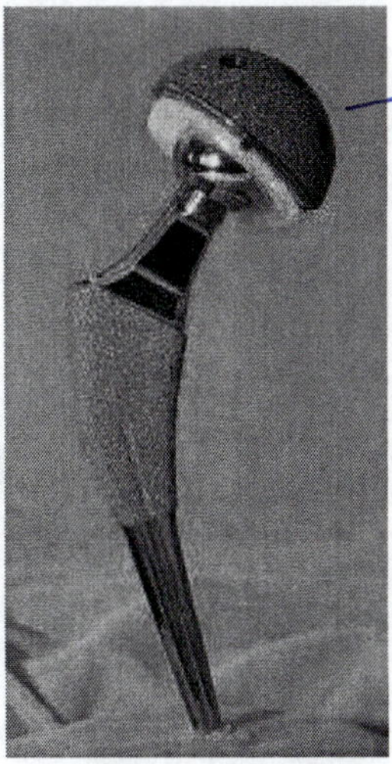

Figure 7.2 This artificial hip is composed of cobalt chromemolybdenum alloy made metal ball and polyethylene liner. Polyethylene liner provide flexibility during surgical procedure. (http://bonesmart.org/hip/hip-replacement-implant-materials/).

7.4 Vision Care

7.4.1 Market

Age-related vision disorders such as cataract, muscular degeneration, and glaucoma have boosted the growth of eye-care industry in the area of cosmetic surgery such as the implantation of refractive lens. BCC Research reported that the global market for ophthalmic devices, diagnostics, and surgical equipment was valued at $15.2 billion in 2009, excluding consumer eye-care products [21]. The market is estimated to reach $19 billion by 2014. Major manufacturers include Advanced Medical Optics, Bausch & Lomb, Canon, Nidek, Topcon, and Zeiss Meditec.

7.4.2 Diagnostic Devices

Diagnostic instruments are the key tools to identify diseases by high-resolution inspection of the cornea and the macula. One of the most commonly used equipment among ophthalmologist is slit lamp (Fig. 7.3). The most important field of application is the examination of the anterior segment of the eye, including the crystalline lens and the anterior vitreous body. The illumination system produces a slit image that is as bright as possible, at a pre-defined distance from

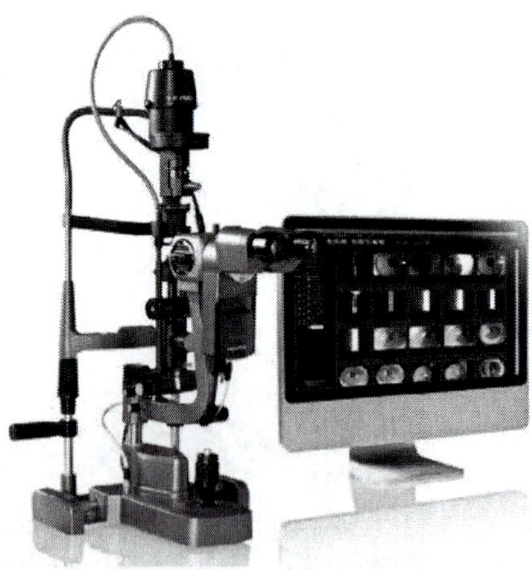

Figure 7.3 Digital slit imaging used for the detection of cataracts, corneal injury, and other eye diseases (http://www.in.all.biz/g182258/).

the instrument. The slit imaging system is used for detecting cataracts, corneal injury, muscular degeneration, and retinal detachment. Another commonly used procedure is tonometry, which is used to determine the intraocular pressure, the fluid pressure inside the eye. It is a critical test to evaluate the risk of glaucoma [22].

7.4.3 Treatment

Cataracts lead to blurred and cloudy vision. Cataracts grow very slowly and become denser over time. More than 90% people have a cataract and half of them will lose part of the vision by age 75 [23]. Cataract surgery is the most effective treatment. Further advancement of technology in intraocular lens implants such as multifocal refractive lens has significantly improved the vision of the cataracts patients [24], e.g., the implant of artificial lens such as ReZoom IOL, marketed by Abbott restore vision (Fig. 7.4), after the removal of patients' clouded native lens.

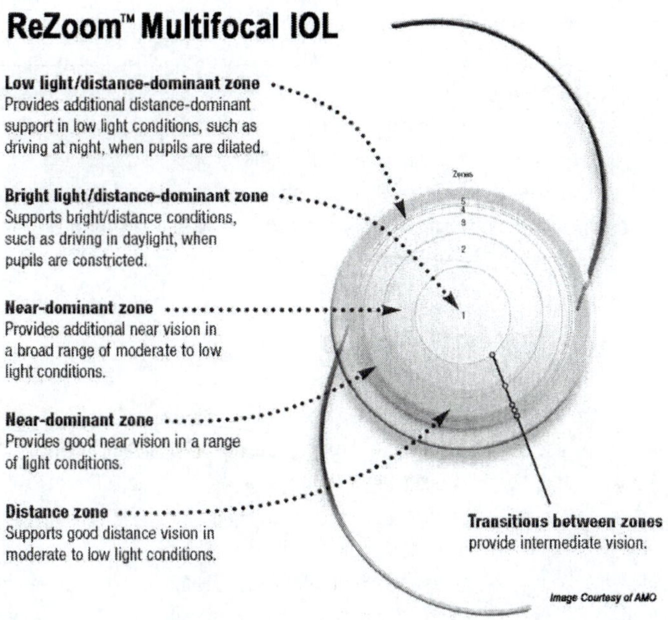

Figure 7.4 ReZoom is a multifocal refractive intraocular lens that scatters light over five optical zones, as indicated, to provide near, intermediate, and far vision.

7.5 Diabetics

Glucose monitoring is essential for diabetes management. LifeScan, J&J company One Touch Ultralink blood glucose monitoring system allows accurate estimation of blood glucose [25]. In combination of an insulin pump, proper dosing can be administered in response to blood glucose level before or after meals. To streamline these processes, an artificial pancreas system helps reduce the severity of a drop in glucose levels by automatically adjusting insulin flow. The system combines a continuous glucose monitor, an insulin infusion pump, and a glucose meter [26].

7.6 Obesity

Obesity is a major global problem affecting billions of people. Unfortunately, there is no single FDA-approved pill that can effectively stop this pandemic. In addition to the traditional obesity surgery to reduce the size of the stomach, there are a few less invasive devices that slow down digestion, making people feel fuller longer. EndoBarrier, is a flexible tube inserted into the small intestine, forming a barrier between food and intestinal walls. It has been approved in Europe and Australia and clinical trials are being run in the United States [27]. SatisSphere is a device that can be placed in the small intestine, mimicking the shape of duodenum. Therefore, the food journey is delayed and possibly gives the body wrong perception that plenty of food has been taken [28].

7.7 Vascular Disease

One of the major vascular diseases, abdominal aortic aneurysms (AAA) is a localized swelling (ballooning) of the abdominal aorta, caused by the weakness of the aortic wall. Untreated condition is likely to cause rupture and associated death in one-third of patients. Although there are about 27 million people worldwide suffering from AAA, only 20% are detected [29]. Ultrasound screening for AAA can be adopted to improve the accuracy of the detection. Endovascular aneurysm repair (EVAR) is a minimally invasive procedure that is also used in the treatment of AAA. In an EVAR, a manufactured device known as a stent-graft is deployed under x-ray guidance inside the aneurysm to exclude it from the circulation (30). The principle is illustrated in Fig. 7.5.

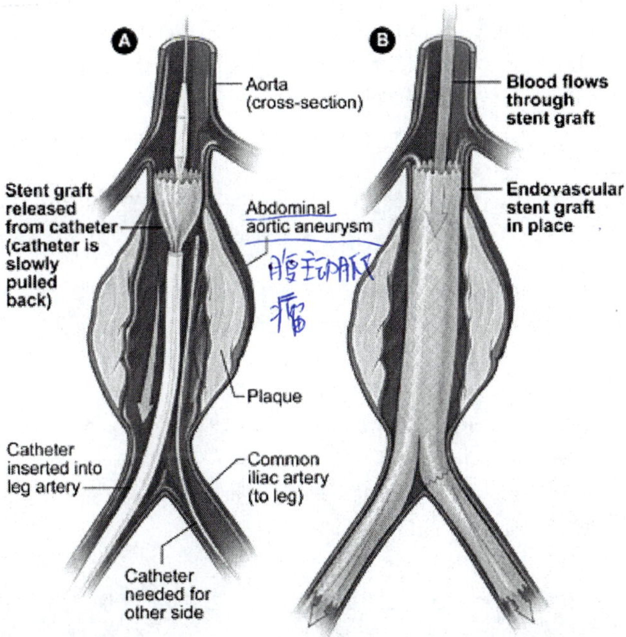

Figure 7.5 Reconstruction of a stent graft in AAA. (A) A catheter is inserted into the weakened artery. The stent graft is then released. (B) The stent supports the artery walls and divert the blood to pass through the aneurysm, therefore preventing it from rupture (http://www.hearthealthywomen.org/treatment-and-recovery/pvd-treatment-and-recovery/aortic-aneurysm-repair/page-3.html).

7.8 Concluding Remarks

Biomedical devices are diverse and rapidly evolving. This brief introduction aims to highlight representative examples, and we hope the readers will gain an appreciation of medical devices in everyday life. Recent trends have indicated that various health care-related disciplines such as biological sciences, nanotechnology, cognitive sciences, information technology, and material sciences converge into the development of medical devices. This will ultimately improve the quality of medical devices.

References

1. Health Technologies Timeline. Retrieved October 10, 2011, from http://www.greatachievements.org/?id=3824.
2. Reiser SJ. (1978). *Medicine and the Reign of Technology*, Cambridge University Press, New York.
3. Kohn LT, Corrigan JM, Donaldson MS (1999). *To Err Is Human: Building a Safer Health System,* National Academy Press, Washington, D.C.
4. Neuroarm. Retrieved October 11, 2011, from: http://www.neuroarm.org/.
5. The *da Vinci*® Surgical System. Retrieved October 11, 2011, from http://www.davincisurgery.com/davinci-surgery/davinci-surgical-system/.
6. *World Health Statistics 2009.* (2009). Geneva, World Health Organization. Retrieved October 20, 2011, from *www.who.int/entity/.../**world_health_statistics**/EN_WHS09_Full.pdf.*
7. Department of Economic and Social Affairs, Population Division (2002). *World Population Ageing, 1950–2050.* United Nations, New York.
8. Medical Device Revenue to Top $300 Billion This Year: Kalorama. Retrieved February 25, 2012, from http://www.kaloramainformation.com/about/release.asp?id=1826.
9. U.S. Department of Commerce and the U.S. International Trade Commission (2009). *Medical Devices Industry Assessment.* US Trade Department, USA.
10. Industry Surveys Healthcare Product and Supplies. Retrieved October 19, 2011, from http://issuu.com/alanahealthcare/docs/s-p-healthcare-product-and-supplie_20110819_142411.
11. Handout on Health: Osteoarthritis. Retrieved October 30, 2011, from http://www.niams.nih.gov/health_info/osteoarthritis/default.asp.
12. Tanna S (2004). *Osteoarthritis — Opportunities to Address Pharmaceutical Gaps.* Geneva, World Health Organization, Switerland.
13. Breme HJ, Helsen JA (1998). *Metals as Biomaterials*, Chichester, John Wiley & Sons, United Kingdom.
14. Alireza N, Peter DH, Cui'e W (2007). Biomimetic Porous Titanium Scaffolds for Orthopedic and Dental Applications, Institute for Technology Research and Innovation, Deakin University, Australia.

15. Practical Guide to ISO 10993. Retrieved October 30, 2011, from www.distrupol.com/images/ISO_10993.pdf.

16. Use of International Standard ISO-10993, "Biological Evaluation of Medical Devices Part 1: Evaluation and Testing" Retrieved October 28, 2011, from http://www.fda.gov/MedicalDevices/DeviceRegulationandGuidance/GuidanceDocuments/ucm080735.htm.

17. Nakajima H (2007). Fabrication, properties and application of porous metals with directional pores. *Progress in Materials Science*, **52**, 1091–1173.

18. Ryan G, Pandit A, Apatsidis DP (2006). Fabrication methods of porous metals for use in orthopaedic applications. *Biomaterials*, **27**, 2651–2670.

19. Avitzur B (1987). Metal forming, *Encyclopedia of Physical Science & Technology*, **8**, 80–109.

20. Drozda T; Wick C, Bakerjian, Ramon V, Raymond F, Petro L (1984). *Tool and Manufacturing Engineers Handbook: Forming, SME.*

21. Global Markets for Ophthalmic Devices, Diagnostics and Surgical Equipment. Retrieved October 30, 2011, from http://www.bccresearch.com/report/ophthalmic-devices-markets-hlc083a.html.

22. Amm M, Hedderich J (2005). Transpalpebral tonometry with a digital tonometer in healthy eyes and after penetrating keratoplasty. *Ophthalmologe*, **102**(1), 70–76.

23. Cataract. Retrieved October 27, 2011, from: http://www.who.int/topics/cataract/en/.

24. ReZoom multifocal lens. Retrieved 25 October 2011 from http://www.rezoomiol.com/rezoom_multifocal_lens.html.

25. One touch. Retrieved October 25, 2011, from http://www.onetouch.com/our_products.

26. Artificial pancreas system. Retrieved October 25, 2011, from http://www.fda.gov/MedicalDevices/ProductsandMedicalProcedures/HomeHealthandConsumer/ConsumerProducts/ArtificialPancreas/default.htm.

27. Endobarrier. Retrieved October 24, 2011, from: http://www.endobarrier.com/.

28. Columbus may be the home to the next big craze in weight loss. Retrieved October 22, 2011, from http://www.examiner.com/extreme-weight-loss-in-columbus/columbus-may-be-the-home-to-the-next-big-craze-weight-loss.

29. First patients enrolled in Cordis Trial of New Stent Graft System to Treat Abdominal Aortic Aneurysm. Retrieved October 23, 2011, from http://www.investor.jnj.com/textonly/releasedetail.cfm?ReleaseID=457755.

30. Greenhalgh RM, Powell JT (2008). Endovascular repair of abdominal aortic aneurysm. *N. Engl. J. Med.*, **358**(5): 494–501.

Chapter 8

Labeling, Label, and Language: A Truly Global Matter

Evangeline D. Loh and Jaap L. Laufer
Emergo Group
evangeline@emergogroup.com, Jaap.Laufer@dekra.com

8.1 Introduction

For most medical devices, the label on the product is the primary interface between the user and the product. As an integral part of the product proper, it provides a visual way to verify that the product in the packaging is what the user intends to use and ensures the packaging is used as intended (e.g., for a sterile, double packed product). But labeling is a lot more — it encompasses the whole interface between the user and the manufacturer. Labeling tells the reader what the product may be used for and when not, what benefits and risks it is expected to have, and which precautions the user should take or consider when used as intended. Some legal labeling definitions include any and all promotional utterances, while others restrict its remit to the printed materials that accompany the

Handbook of Medical Device Regulatory Affairs in Asia
Edited by Jack Wong and Raymond K. Y. Tong

ISBN 978-981-4411-21-9 (Hardcover), 978-981-4411-22-6 (eBook)
www.panstanford.com

product. Labeling also establishes the use intended by the manufacturer and depending on the classification of the product, may have been reviewed in the regulatory submission.

But all labeling must be based on the risk management performed by the manufacturer during design and development, no exceptions. This pivotal document dictates not only in essence the labeling content but also the fundamentals upon which the clinical evaluation of the product should be based. So, as the product is on the market, the experience gained in the "post-market" phase will dictate through its feedback on the risk management an evolution of the labeling content commensurate with the stage in the life cycle of the device.

Labeling and languages are often mentioned in one breath. However, languages required by the respective countries or economies are just a subsection of the need to adapt the language of the instruction for use to the intended user or users. Complicated use of even absence of the native language of a user may defy the purpose of communicating the essential elements of the information required to use the device safely and for its intended use. So, labeling language should be interpreted in those two distinct ways. It constitutes a critical aspect of Human Factors in Design and other core considerations when creating a new product or adapting an existing one.

An aspect not always appreciated is that "world" languages such as English, French, Spanish, and increasingly, Mandarin Chinese, have an (often unintended) impact beyond the national borders of the jurisdiction for which they were intended. This may lead to conflicting versions of label content in different countries and, thus, cause confusion among the readers. This calls for a global harmonization of labeling content — a lofty but often elusive goal. Note that label content is distinguished from the indications for use, which is also conveyed by the labeling. There can often be different indications for use based on what the manufacturer was able to substantiate in their regulatory submission in a particular market. (Or stated another way, what the regulatory authorities in a particular market were comfortable to accept as indications for use based on the clinical data.)

Finally, the revolution in information has impacted the requirements put forward by notably hospitals and other electronically advanced users. While we included the information available at this time, this is most certainly the aspect that will need to be updated in the next five years.

8.2 Definition of Labeling

Labeling means different things in different countries. The European Medical Devices Directive 93/42/EEC as amended by Directive 2007/47/EC (the MDD) does not define labeling per se or its constituent components. Apart from the ubiquitously present stipulations in the MDD when and where the CE-marking must be affixed, par. 13 of Annex I (Essential Requirements) spells out in great detail which information must be supplied by the manufacturer. The elements of labeling mentioned there are limited to the information accompanying the device (i.e., package insert or instruction for use, which includes a manual for large or complex devices) and the label(s) proper for individual units either on the product itself or on the unit packaging, on the "sales packaging." Terms such as "shipping carton," labeling for double packaging, and other commonly used designations have not been codified in the law.

One of the key elements of labeling in the near future will be the use of a UDI, a unique device identifier. While the idea itself makes eminent sense, it must be feared that in absence of a well-defined electronic structure allowing for the proper handling and management of the huge quantity of data influx, the objective of the electronic tracing of individual products from the manufacturer to the user will stay an illusion for many years to come. To this end, the Global Harmonization Task Force (GHTF) has issued guidance on UDI [1] (UDI System, September 16, 2011) which implores countries to consider the GHTF guidance in promulgating regulations on UDI. It would appear the USA FDA will be the first in line to publish a draft rule (expected in the fall of 2011) [2]. The FDA has published this draft UDI as a proposed rule (Federal Register, Vol. 77, No. 132, 10 July 2012). http://www.gpo.gov/fdsys/pkg/FR-2012-07-10/html/2012-16621.htm; however, the EU, with their revision of the medical devices directives, will similarly seem to require UDI [3]. The draft Medical Device Regulation introduces the use of UDI. http://www.gpo.gov/fdsys/pkg/FR-2012-07-10/html/2012-16621.htm.

As the concept of "labeling" in Europe means different things in the respective EU Member States, vastly different regulatory regimens exist. France, Germany, the United Kingdom, and even Italy and Spain show an increasingly strong enforcement of their respective laws concerning promotion, including the Internet. The enforcement of a harmonized label content (especially concerning intended uses, indications, and claims as well as contra-indications) is just beginning, enhanced by the COEN (Committee of Enforcement), and lately by the CMC (Central Management Committee), two Member State-only committees that promotes a coordinated approach toward interpretation and implementation of laws and regulations for devices.

Based on Title 21, Section 820.1 of the Code of Federal Regulations (CFR), the United States has had a long and historically driven tradition of strong and sometimes even heavy-handed enforcement of labeling compliance. Labeling in the United States means any written or verbal expression of information accompanying or concerning the device and controlled in any way by the manufacturer, including but not limited to labels in the strict sense, promotional materials, any verbal statement by company representatives, the Internet, and even information about products not yet approved but shown to the public at trade fairs. The FDA is strictly monitoring the compliance of labeling content with the claims approved. Any proof that a manufacturer is intentionally or commercially exploiting the often gray area of "off-label" use can lead to draconian fines and/or criminal prosecution.

In Korea, a medical device label is one attached onto the outer most packaging though there does not appear to be an official reference to the definition of labeling. In China, SFDA Order No. 10 regulates the labeling (Instructions, Labels, and Packaging of Medical Devices). There are 23 Articles in the Order. Countries such as Singapore and Hong Kong, which use more GHTF (or AHWP)-like regulatory systems, have similarly defined labeling as in the EU.

8.3 Elements of Labeling

Labeling may consist of

- The label proper (see above) increasingly including the UDI code.
- A manual, instruction for use, package insert, etc., intended for the intended user(s).

- Where applicable or demanded by laws or regulations, promotional materials where they relate to the "approved" claims or intended uses. For instance, where an insulin pump must not be used when the user is swimming, the manufacturer or distributor cannot show a lady on the beach wearing that pump. (Historic example! The case was whistle-blown by a competitor and the manufacturer cancelled the ad.)
- Materials placed by a manufacturer or a distributor of the product on the Internet or spread by e-mail, social media, involuntary pop-ups, etc. This is such a growing and complicated subject that we will treat it separately further in this chapter. Suffice it to say here that electronic utterances that are in perfect compliance with the laws in one country may be offensive in another, even when the national language of the latter country is not used. A historic example springs to mind: When a representative of a UK-based company showed a training video to illustrate the use of a new invasive surgical device (hardly glamorous) to physicians, he was arrested in Libya for "pornography." The video had used a female patient.

A good source for labeling content guidance is the GHTF document "SG1-N70:2011 Label and Instructions for Use for Medical Devices," issued on September 22, 2011. It is a bit general but gives a solid basis for which aspects of labeling should absolutely be considered before placing a device on the market. Also, while there are country differences and deviations, there is generally a core set of elements in labeling, which is captured in the GHTF guidance.

In many countries in Asia, South America, and even North America (Mexico specifically), there is a requirement that the medical device registration number be included on the labeling.

In Korea, labeling is generally a sticker that is attached onto every product intended for the Korean market, which must include the information about the following: KFDA registered model number, manufacturer information, Korean license holder information, KFDA registration number, manufacturing date/lot number, etc. In China in particular, the SFDA Order No. 10, Article 8, stipulates the number of the Import Medical Device Registration Certificate (IMDRC) number as well as the reference to the relevant technical standards.

The Australian system leverages the EU system, and generally labeling developed for the EU can be used in Australia with the addition of the Australian Sponsor. In New Zealand, the Medicines Regulations 1984, Regulation 12(4) [4], establishes the requirements for the labeling of medical devices. The regulation states, "No person shall sell any medical device that does not bear the name of the manufacturer of the medical device or the name of the manufacturer's distributor in New Zealand."

In Hong Kong, the Medical Device Administrative Control System (MDACS) is modeled on the recommendations of the GHTF, and, thus, compliance should not be particularly burdensome for products that have already met the criteria in the EU. The labeling requirements are delineated in Appendix 3, Additional Medical Device Labelling Requirements of the guidance, GN 01. Again, the device's Listing Number ("HKMD No. ####") needs to be on the label. There is guidance on labeling in the form of the Singapore Health Sciences Authority (HSA) GN-23 Guidance on Labelling for Medical Devices, August 2009; and, again, the medical device regulatory system in Singapore is largely based on the GHTF guidance documents.

The applicable Brazilian labeling requirements are described in Resolution RDC No. 185, Annex III.B, information on the labeling and IFU for medical devices. The name and address of the Brazilian importer should be included if appropriate (2.1), but more specifically, the Brazilian Registration Holder, technical expert certified by ANVISA, technical expert's name must be delineated on the label (2.11). Also, once ANVISA has accepted the application, the ANVISA registration number must be included on the product label preceded by "ANVISA" (2.12). For the most part, Resolution RDC No. 185, Annex III.B, resembles the MDD, Annex I, ER, Section 13. Information supplied by the manufacturer.

In Chile, at the writing of this section, only a limited number of products are subject to mandatory control by the ISP: examination gloves, surgical gloves, condoms, and sterile hypodermic needles and syringes for single use. The regulatory framework for medical devices is based on Law 19,497 and Products Control Regulations and Medical Use Elements (DS No. 825/98), and Article 26 discusses the labels. Again, as observed in many countries, the Chilean device registration number issued by the ISP must be included as well as all the standard elements.

8.4 Risk Management, Clinical Evaluation and Labeling: The Core Triangle for Safe and Effective Use of the Device

Few risk analyses are concluded without specific inclusion of risk mitigating statements in the labeling, mostly in the instructions for use. These statements are commonly divided into contra-indications, warnings when used as intended, precautions to be taken before or after device use, and which side effects may be expected, as well as other considerations. Most countries do not define under which header a particular statement must be placed; however, this aspect is usually emphasized by a regulatory authority whenever a risk mitigating statement is insufficiently complied with by the user, sometimes replete with the instruction to print bold or similar.

Clinical evaluation and investigation are the tool to validate critical labeling content, e.g., under what conditions the device should be used, what performance specifications may be expected, what precautions need to be taken, etc. Very important, the specific nature, relevance and incidence of adverse events or incidents must be critically evaluated, as it directly relates to the expectations expressed in the initial risk assessment. The final conclusion about the risk/benefit ratio is frequently determined by the capability to address the residual risks adequately by explicitly stated warnings in the instruction for use or the manual. Any risk that turns out to have been underestimated in any way will have to be reassessed, especially whether it can be mitigated by improved design and/or labeling content, or poses an insurmountable block to further use.

So, even though the labeling content is drafted in the course of the design development, the adequacy of the instruction for use can only be verified when it is applied in practice, i.e., in a clinical investigation or in the post-market phase. (Note also, the regulatory authority review of the regulatory submission can lead to changes in the labeling content as well.) Consequently, the post-market surveillance (PMS) is the single most important feedback phase in the life cycle of a label. This is where refinements of the actual handling, expanded indications (if they do not require further corroboration), more detailed warnings, precautions, etc., as well as government-dictated insertions occur. For instance, in a case not too long ago, the United Kingdom demanded that for a relatively low-risk device, a cautionary statement be included about the lack of data for pediatric use, and consequently, the restricted use in patients under 16. In another case, the French agency determined that the package insert of mammary implants must display a warning that such products may interfere with the effectiveness of classic mammography.

This leads to one more consideration: In this global age, any intervention at the government level of one country will lead to inquiries by other regulatory authorities, especially if the initial intervention originated in one of the GHTF founding countries, but increasingly also in emerging economies. This puts a big stake in the proper formulation of label content.

In conclusion, any significant deviations between the risk assessment, the results of clinical evaluation, and the labeling will likely lead to problems for the manufacturer. Both competitors and regulatory authorities are watching this matter closely!

8.5 Labeling and Promotion

A general rule is that promotion must be consistent with labeling. A medical device cannot be promoted beyond the comments delineated in the labeling for which the manufacturer obtained the regulatory approval, clearance, or registration. It is not common for manufacturers of medical devices to be marketing professional-use medical devices to consumers.

Widely different regulatory regimens exist for promotional materials for devices. For example, in the EU, promotion and advertising are not explicitly discussed in the MDD, nor in the proposed Draft Revision of the Directives.

Promotion directed to patients or lay users may also be regulated differently [5]. This is specifically the case in Australia, where a code exists: the Therapeutic Goods Advertising Code 2007 [6]. Advertisements related to medical devices directed to consumers must comply with this code.

Many lesser developed economies do not have specific regulations for promotional materials, or they may be regulated by pharmaceutical laws.

8.6 e-Labelling, Web Sites, Internet, and Social Media: A Brave New World for Labeling

While the term e-labeling has been widely accepted to mean electronic labeling, the official reference to the source was not readily apparent, of course, an adoption from the moniker electronic mail, "email." For the purposes of this discussion, electronic should mean non-paper though this is a moniker that each regulatory environment will need to define.

At the time of this writing, Europe appeared to have made the greatest accomplishment with e-labeling. A European guidance, MEDDEV, was published in 2007 on e-labeling of IVDs [7]. The guidance established the use of the other-than-paper format IFUs (different media) by different means of supply for certain categories of *in vitro* diagnostic devices. There were, of course, very stringent provisions that needed to have been addressed in order to supply IFUs by different media and through different means of supply, not withstanding a toll-free telephone number. A toll-free number within the 27 EU member states as well as Norway, Iceland, Lichtenstein, and Switzerland is quite a feat! In the summer of 2011, the European Commission issued draft regulations on electronic labeling (e-labeling) and shared these publically as part of their WTO Technical Barriers Trade activities [8]. At that time, the publication date was December 14, 2011. While this date has passed, this legislation is expected in Q1 2012. There is now published an EU Commission Regulation (Regulation (EU) No 207/2012) on electronic instructions for use of medical devices. http://eur-lex.europa.eu/LexUriServ/LexUriServ.do?uri=OJ:L:2012:072:0028:0031:EN:PDF.

While recitals are in essence background comment without legal merit, Recital (3), of the draft indicates: "In order to reduce potential risks as far as possible, the appropriateness of the provision of instructions for use in electronic form should be subject to a specific risk assessment by the manufacturer." Ultimately, provided the medical device meets the provisions of the legislation, this still needs to be considered. This, of course, is similar to the recommendation for labeling, provided the device in the EU is a category that qualifies for e-labeling; ultimately, the decision is risk management related.

> *"The draft Regulation sets out conditions according to which instructions for use in paper form may be replaced by electronic instructions for use. It limits the possibility of providing instructions for use in electronic form to defined medical devices and accessories intended to be used in specific conditions. Furthermore, it contains a range of procedural safeguards. Thus instructions for use have to be provided in paper form on request, and a specific risk assessment by the manufacturer and information on how to access to the instructions for use is needed."*

The draft Regulation also sets up a few basic safety requirements for the following:

- *instructions for use in electronic form which are provided in addition to complete instructions for use in paper form*
- *Web sites containing such instructions for use*

Article 1 of the draft legislation states the premise that information supplied by the manufacturer may be in "electronic form instead of in paper form." Article 2(2) describes electronic IFUs: electronic form by the device, electronic storage medical with the device, and on a Web site. Only manufacturers of explicit categories of medical devices can consider e-labeling (Article 3(1)): fixed installation, implanted medical devices, devices built-in system visually displaying the IFUs, software, and professional use.

As it stands, many of the AHWP members do not accept e-labeling. In Korea, the package insert including intended use, instructions for use, etc., can be provided in an electronic format such as a CD ROM [9]. In China, e-labeling is not permitted, *per se*, but can certainly be provided in addition to the paper version.

At this time, one can comfortably assert that there is nothing to preclude provision of hard copy labeling with e-labeling. Whether e-labeling alone is accepted is an entirely different matter and will likely be increasingly permitted over time.

Early 2012, social media have yet to make a visible impact on the sale or promotion of medical devices. It is to be expected that we will see an increased use of sale channels especially for "OTC" devices. This is addressed cursorily in the proposed European Draft Regulation to become enforceable later in this decade.

8.7 Language, Language Level and Intended User

One of the more critical aspects of the labeling content is the language. The famous non-verbal IKEA® "manuals" and labels do not use any language predicated on the assumption that every individual will recognize certain pictures and symbols. The same is true for the universally recognized symbol for "exit." So, the problem posed by the limited space (as well the high cost) on most devices relative to the need for translation in national languages has been partially resolved by the use of symbols. Insofar these have been included in the "Harmonized Standard" European standard EN 980, there is a "presumption of compliance" with the respective subsections of the ER 13 of Annex I of the MDD. Any other symbols, including but not limited to those in ISO 15223, must be explained in the instruction for use in all applicable languages. That said, EN 980:2008 at the time of publication of this text will have been withdrawn, and the EN harmonized standard EN ISO 15223-1:2012.

In the United States, the use of symbols is much less appreciated. There, as well as in many other mainly Anglosaxon jurisdictions, culture dictates a graphic description of details in the instruction for use, which in the United States is also driven by the fear of liability for anything not explicitly expressed in the labeling. Health Canada does not explicitly state that symbols are accepted and Health Canada does not recognize EN 980 or ISO 15223 though Health Canada appears to accept symbols. While this attitude is most outspoken in the Anglosaxon cultures, it tends to become also increasingly prominent in other ones. The ultimate result is an instruction for use or manual that is for most intended readers, at best difficult to access or comprehend.

Brazilian RDC No. 185, Annex III.B, Section 1.4, permits the use of symbols; however, symbols must comply with regulations and technical standards. If there are no regulations or technical standards applicable, symbols used must be described in the IFU. The standards that are published by Associação Brasileira de Normas Técnicas (ABNT) include ABNT NBR ISO 15223-1:2010 titled *Productos para a saúde — Símbolos a serem utilizados em rótulos, rotulagem e informações a serem fornecidas de produtos para saúde.*

This dilemma between readability and completeness has been partially resolved by demanding that manufacturers develop and enclose instruction for use that represents a language comprehension of a 12-year-old individual, taking into account that the language used is native. The use of a language other than the native language(s) is in most countries of the world restricted to higher professional users or specialists. For instance, an insulin pump might be used by an array of users from a highly educated physician diabetologist to a semi-literate elderly person. An implantable left ventricular assist device (LVAD) may have up to four different manuals for the respective users of the device and its accessories.

The EU requires that the knowledge and experience of the user be considered (MDD Annex I, Section 1). In the United States, there has been greater emphasis on human use factors [10]. One should not dismiss the standard of IEC 62366:2007, Medical Devices — Application of Usability Engineering to Medical Devices. Human use factors have implications on the labeling, which should also be considered.

Then there is the language proper. Especially in multi-country or -language areas (most of the world, actually....), it is very difficult for a manufacturer to develop an instruction for use with sufficient coverage of languages to satisfy the users' needs. Oddly enough, it is here that e-labeling (see elsewhere in this article) accessible by smartphones could provide a very legitimate solution. This appears to be a very cost-effective, environmentally friendly, and practical solution for many sparsely populated or developing regions of the world, with the only limitation being expressed by the saying "you can lead the horse to the well, but you cannot make it drink": The user — even an educated one — should at least a few times, read the instructions for use and not discard them unread when opening the package.

8.8 Conclusion

Labels and labeling are among the most important parts of a medical device. While cultures, educational levels, reading proficiency, and familiarity with a product do vary, manufacturers must pay utmost attention to the formulation of content for the respective components of labeling to ensure the safe use of the device when used as intended. The use of language commensurate with the various intended users is critical, as is the effort by the manufacturer to keep the labeling contents current to the knowledge gained by the use of the product in practice.

References

1. GHTF Guidance on UDI. Retrieved December 2011 from http://www.ghtf.org/documents/ahwg/AHWG-UDI-N2R3.pdf.
2. US FDA Draft Rule on UDI. Retrieved December 2011 from http://www.fda.gov/MedicalDevices/DeviceRegulationandGuidance/UniqueDeviceIdentification/default.htm. http://www.gpo.gov/fdsys/pkg/FR-2012-07-10/html/2012-16621.htm.
3. EU UDI. Retrieved December 2011 from http://ec.europa.eu/health/medical-devices/specific-areas-development/udi/index_en.htm.
4. New Zealand Regulations. Retrieved December 2011 from http://www.legislation.govt.nz/regulation/public/1984/0143/latest/DLM96155.html.
5. TGA Online. Retrieved December 2011 from http://www.tga.gov.au/industry/legislation-tgac.htm.
6. Australia Regulation. Retrieved December 2011 from http://www.comlaw.gov.au/Details/F2007L00576.
7. E-labelling of IVD. Retrieved December 2011 from http://ec.europa.eu/health/medical-devices/files/meddev/2_14_3_rev1_ifu_final_en.pdf.
8. EU Draft regulation on e-labelling. Retrieved December 2011 from http://ec.europa.eu/enterprise/tbt/index.cfm?fuseaction=Search.viewDetail&Country_ID=EEC&num=381&dspLang=en&nextpage=1&basdatedeb=&basdatefin=&baspays=&baspays2=&basnotifnum=&basnotifnum2=&bastypepays=ANY&baskeywords=electronic%20instructions&fromform=viewKeyword".
9. Korean Ministry of Health and Welfare (2011) *Korea Medical Device Act No. 0564, Amended as of April 7, 2011 effective from October 08, 2011.*
10. US FDA. Retrieved December 2011 from http://www.fda.gov/downloads/MedicalDevices/DeviceRegulationandGuidance/GuidanceDocuments/UCM095300.pdf.

11. Council of the European Parliament (July 12, 1993), Council Directive of 14 June 1993 concerning Medical Devices (MDD 93/42/EEC), as amended by Directive 2007/47/EC of the European Parliament and of the Council of 5 September 2007, *Official Journal of the European Communities (OJ)* L169, p1.

12. CEN/CENELEC EUROPEAN STANDARD (May 2008), *Symbols for use in the labelling of medical devices*, EN 980, ICS 01.080.20; 11.120.01.

13. CEN/CENELEC EUROPEAN STANDARD (October 2008), *Information supplied by the manufacturer of medical devices*, EN 1041.

14. Code of Federal Regulations, Title 21, Volume 8 (Revised as of April 1, 2011), Title 21-Food and Drugs, Chapter I-Food And Drug Administration, Department of Health and Human Services, Subchapter H — Medical Devices, *Part 820 — Quality System Regulation*, CITE: 21CFR820.1.

Chapter 9

Clinical Trials: Legal and Ethical Considerations of Increasing Globalization

Paula Celine Trepman
Massachusetts Institute of Technology,
4316 Forest Avenue SE, Mercer Island, WA 98040, USA
ptrepman@mit.edu

9.1 Introduction

Clinical trials constitute a critical aspect of regulatory affairs in the biomedical device industry. Class III devices, which are defined as highly regulated, high-risk instruments that may pose significant risk or injury, must go through pre-marketing approval.[1] These include central life-saving devices such as pacemakers, joint implants, and cardiac catheters. Before a device becomes approved by health authorities and merchandisable for use in humans, it must be proven to be harmless to patients and be able to deliver its expected benefits.[2] Clinical trials are the primary means of obtaining this assurance. Within the growing biomedical device industry in

Handbook of Medical Device Regulatory Affairs in Asia
Edited by Jack Wong and Raymond K. Y. Tong

ISBN 978-981-4411-21-9 (Hardcover), 978-981-4411-22-6 (eBook)
www.panstanford.com

Asia, running proper clinical trials will guarantee the safety and efficacy of newly developed medical devices.

9.2 The Increasing Trend of Offshore Clinical Trials

Offshore clinical trials are becoming increasingly more common in testing biomedical devices. Outsourcing can reduce costs by 10–30%, due to less expensive recruitment and labor costs, site fees, and compensatory payments; they can also be completed up to seven months sooner in low-cost countries compared with the United States and Western Europe.[3] In 2011, total clinical trials registered on Clinicaltrials.gov,[4] a service of the National Institutes of Health in the United States, were distributed as shown in Fig. 9.1.

Table 9.1 Total clinical trials in 2011 arranged by region and quantity performed

Region	Number of trials
North America	63,591
Europe	30,509
East Asia	9183
Middle East	4637
South America	3834
Pacifica	3320
Africa	2549
Southeast Asia	2222
North Asia	2084
South Asia	2034
Central America	1641

Note: As of 2008, 40% of trials conducted by US-owned companies were performed outside of the United States. By the end of 2011, this figure is expected to rise to 65% among these FDA-approved studies.[5] The general trend is toward an increase in offshore trials as a means of bringing devices to the market more quickly and inexpensively.

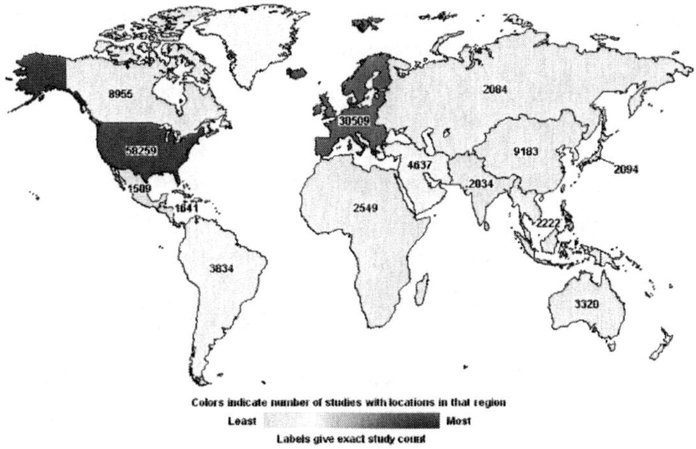

Figure 9.1 Geographic distribution of clinical trials registered by the United States National Institutes of Health.

9.3 International Standards to Protect Patients

The *Guidelines for Good Clinical Practice* determined by the International Conference on Harmonization of Technical Requirements for Patient Use (ICH-GCP) contain specific recommendations to protect the rights, safety, and well-being of trial subjects in clinical trials globally.[6] The ICH-GCP also serves to minimize human exposure to untested devices, increase the quality of scientific data, speed up marketing of new devices, and aid in lowering costs to both producers and consumers. Following inspection, devices are approved for sale on the market. To ensure safety of devices and study design, all clinical trial protocols should be approved prior to the start of the study.[7]

In addition, regulatory institutions play a key role in the integrity of clinical trials.[8] Health authorities are responsible for verifying compliance to ICH-GCP and approved protocols, accuracy of record-keeping, and proper informed consent of patients. Infrastructure at the testing site is also closely examined. Prior to inspection, health authorities may require documentation, such as curriculum vitae of trial investigators and monitoring reports. With a month of inspection, a Corrective and Preventative Action Plan (CAPA) is issued, with classification of No Action Indicated (NAI),

Voluntary Action Indicated (VAI), and Official Action Indicated (OAI). In the case of OAI classification, remedial measures may be required within the following month. Currently, the number of warning letters issued has increased, from 3 in 2005 to 23 in 2009; rejection of CAPA plans by the FDA has also increased.[8] These realities emphasize the importance of following ICH-GCP guidelines in trial design.

9.4 Breaches of Clinical Trial Legality

Failure to follow standard ICH-GCP protocols can result in infringement of patient rights and sometimes illness or death. Legal action may be raised against the device companies. For example, in the United States court case Friter v. Iolab Corp., the hospital had contracted with the FDA to test intra-ocular lenses.[7] The FDA had required the hospital to receive signed patient consent forms since the devices had not yet been tested, but the hospital failed to do so. Friter, who had just undergone cataract surgery, had not been notified that an experimental lens was being tested in his eye, but as a result of the experimental lens, he endured hemorrhage, corneal damage, and other complications. The trial ruling was found to be in favor of Friter, and the hospital was liable for $1.75 million in damages. The Council of Europe's Convention on Human Rights and Biomedicine also entitles injured parties to fair compensation. Following ICH-GCP and receiving pre-approval of experimental devices by health authorities can minimize legal actions and reduce amount of damages paid.

In transnational biomedical trials, the case falls under national protocols of private international law. This can raise issues for consumers in court systems that lack proper infrastructure or are corrupt. For instance, in 1996, an experimental antibiotic called Trovan was tested that caused paralysis, deafness, and blindness in a number of child subjects.[9] In the Trovan Trial Litigation of 2001, the ethics of the trial protocol were examined. However, the case was dismissed 14 times in the country in which the trial occurred; similarly, the case against the US-based pharmaceutical company was dismissed on grounds that the case should be raised in the country of the clinical trial. Current debate exists on the role of courts in transnational lawsuits and the hurdle of *forum non conviens*, when courts refuse to take jurisdiction over trials run by companies in their districts but executed in another region.

9.5 Issues of Informed Consent

Receiving patient consent is a complicated but important aspect of conducting ethical clinical trials; this is especially true in the case of offshore trials. Several factors may influence an individual's decision to take part in clinical trials, including the patient's culture and education level, subject vulnerability within the healthcare system, and economic background.

9.6 Cultural and Social Factors

Cultural and language barriers, as well as differences in education level, can make proper patient consent difficult to obtain. First, patients may be unclear about the risks associated with the trial; they may think that they are receiving approved, established treatment rather than a device that is still being developed and evaluated. Additionally, there may not be a clear understanding of placebo groups in the study among poorly educated individuals or those unfamiliar with standard scientific methods.[10] There may also be deviation from approved protocols due to miscommunications in the amount or frequency of dosage; greater confusion may exist in regions where units of time may differ from standard days or weeks or where the concept of time differs from the United States and Europe.

Individuals frequently are recruited to participate in trials via advertisements. To ensure ethical recruiting practices, the health authorities should review advertisements to ensure that they do not promise specific results or coerce the patients into participating. Additionally, these advertisements should not state the product's safety, efficacy, or superiority over existing devices. It is also important that subjects are aware that research is not the only option available for them. Whenever possible, viable alternatives should be discussed with patients. Potential subjects should be provided with specific data including the risks, benefits, and alternative courses of treatment before deciding to participate in the trial and signing consent forms.[7] In the case of a cultural or language barrier, it is ideal if an interpreter with a similar cultural background can be made available. This is important for overcoming cultural barriers in explaining scientific theories and methods. To aid in translation and the crossing cultural barriers, it is suggested that the language of the consent document be as clear and short as possible. Through conservative advertising and comprehensive patient education, patient consent can be obtained in an ethical manner.

9.7 Vulnerable Patient Populations

Vulnerability of the population may also affect enrollment in trials. Extra precautions must also be taken in the consent of individuals who may not be in the position to give consent themselves, such as children, the elderly, and the mentally ill.[11] These populations may not have the capacity to make value judgments, so a court-appointed official often aids these subjects in decision-making. An unequal patient–doctor relationship may also persuade patients to take part in trials. Doctors are often viewed as prominent and trustworthy individuals in society; due to hierarchical class structures, patients are more likely to listen to doctors' encouragements to participate without fully understanding the associated risks. Therefore, it is critical that the entire consent document is reviewed with each patient. In vulnerable or underprivileged populations, the presence of proper court-appointed officials or supportive family members may aid in assessing trial participation.

9.8 Economic Considerations

When financial disparities are a major constraint, patients may not have other treatment options available or may be drawn by money. In individuals lacking medical coverage, patients may not be able to afford treatments that are already on the market. They may also be compensated heavily for participation, strengthening the incentive to participate in low-income or unemployed populations. In fact, in offshore settings, companies often take advantage of the ready-to-recruit strategy because patient pool consists primarily of individuals with intractable health conditions, no health insurance, and economic need. From a financial standpoint, it is suggested that the device being tested not be commercialized by charging investigators or subjects a higher price than is required to cover device and study costs. Conversely, participants should not be overcompensated to participate in clinical trials as this may lead to patient oversight of potential risks of involvement. Over compensation can affect the integrity of the results as well as overall enrollment in the trials. Through fair reimbursement, financial factors will be eliminated from the decision-making process, ensuring careful consideration of the risks of the trial.

9.9 Comparison of Trial Population to Target Population

Another problem arises when studies are conducted in areas not representative of the final target population. Clinical research should be responsive to the needs of the communities where it is conducted; yet in the case of offshore trials, the most prevalent illnesses in high-income countries may be vastly different from those in the developing world. This discrepancy can result from genetic mutations or environmental factors that may affect treatment efficacy.[12] For example, although cardiovascular disease and cancer are prevalent problems in the developed world, infectious diseases such as malaria and tuberculosis are much more rampant in low-income areas. Even when similar diseases are present in both settings, populations with geographically distinct populations can have genetic profiles that markedly affect the efficacy and safety of biomedical devices.

The treatment setting can also cause differences in device efficacy. Organization of hospitals and clinics, preferred treatments, and available quality of care may differ markedly between state-of-the-art facilities with expert physicians and clinics with minimal resources and doctors with less experience. Therefore, even if the same biomedical devices existed in both resource-poor and wealthier settings, if doctors in underprivileged areas are not as well trained, devices may be less effective. In large-scale clinical trials, however, information on physician training and existing medical infrastructure is generally not provided.

Also, treatment naïve patients are more difficult to find in the developed world; in fact, some patients may be enduring several existing therapies. This differs from low-income and rural settings, where patients are less likely to have previous exposure to medications due to cost and geographical barriers. So for this target population of developed-world individuals, it would remain unclear if combining novel treatments with established regimens would improve, reduce, or have no effect on patient outcomes.

Even among different nations in the developing world, biomedical theories and priorities may diverge, in part due to the role of the government in providing health care. For instance, in the United States, with its privatized system of medicine, individuals are more likely to have undergone invasive heart procedures than Canadians, who are an otherwise fairly comparable patient population.[13]

There are several means of addressing disparities between clinical trial and target populations. One method is to include standard treatments as controls in place of a placebo. In 1994, a clinical trial for the antiretroviral AIDS drug azidothymidine (AZT) was run using a placebo control. This led to a controversy regarding placebo use, since a proven AIDS treatment existed at the time and the control group was knowingly not given this treatment.[14] Following this incident, the Helsinki Declaration, which provides guidelines for human biomedical research, was modified to state that when known treatments exist, they should be utilized in place of a placebo. This eliminated the ethical concerns of withholding treatment when effective treatments are available. From a scientific perspective, comparison against standard treatments may be more useful as well, allowing results to be more accurately assessed for populations of the first world and of the upper-class of the developing world. The environmental variables for which offshore trials are often criticized can be accounted for by comparing efficacy data of standard treatments in offshore populations (to be used as the clinical control) to existing data in developed regions. Statistical analyses should also be used to draw comparisons between testing and targeted populations such that environmental and genetic differences are accounted for.

Another way to minimize such discrepancies is to collect data on physician training in addition to patient data during the trial. It may then be determined if the caliber of the facility or past experience of the doctors influence outcome. This, in turn, would increase the scientific quality of the trial by allowing for adjustment in efficacy based on available healthcare facilities. Using standard treatment controls in place of placebo controls while accounting for variation in facilities and training will aid in determining treatment efficacy in the target population.

9.10 Conclusion

Clinical trials serve to ensure effectiveness and safety of biomedical advices prior to sale on the market. Offshoring of clinical trials is a growing trend to reduce costs and shorten time to completion. To prevent ethical and legal misconduct, the ICH-GCP should be followed and proper approval should be received from the health authorities prior to the implementation of the trial. One key aspect of the ICH-GCP is obtaining informed consent from trial subjects. This is oftentimes complicated by cultural, social, and financial factors. Difficulties also exist in relating the results from trial population to the targeted population for the device. To eliminate ethical concerns and improve scientific legitimacy of clinical trials, potential trial subjects should be informed accurately and completely prior to the start of the trial. Other involved parties should be included in the decision-making process if appropriate, and patients should not be over- or undercompensated for trial participation. Last, standard treatment controls may be used in place of placebo controls and statistical analyses should be performed to account for differences among clinical trial and target populations. These measures will ensure trials are performed ethically and that results accurately represent the efficacy of the device in the targeted population.

References

1. Bailey W, Cruickshank C, and Sharma N. *Make Your Move: Taking Clinical Trials to the Best Location,* Vertical View, A.T. Kearney, **2**:56–62 (online), available (2012): http://graphics.eiu.com/upload/gtf/1571871942.PDF.
2. Barnes K. China "Most Attractive" Offshore Clinical Trial Location, *Outsourcing-Pharma.com* (online), available (January 4, 2007) http://www.outsourcing-pharma.com/Clinical-Development/China-most-attractive-offshore-clinical-trial-location.

3. ClinicalTrials.gov. *Map of All Studies in Clinical Trial.gov* (online), available (2011): *http://clinicaltrials*.gov/ct2/search/map.
4. Dunne G (2011). Medical Device Clinical Trials: The Changing Scene, *Regulatory Affairs Medtech* January/February, 18–19 (Clinica/United Kingdom).
5. Ford J, and Tomossy G (2004). Clinical Trials in Developing Countries: The Plaintiff's Challenge, (1) *Law, Social Justice & Global Development Journal (LGD)*. http://elj.warwick.ac.uk/global/issue/2004-1/fordtomossy.html (Australia).
5. Glickman SW, *et al.* (2009). Ethical and Scientific Implications of the Globalization of Scientific Research, *New England Journal of Medicine*, **360**: 816–823 (United States).
6. Goldenberg M (2004). Recent Controversies in Consumer Lawsuits: When Biomedical Devices Fail, *Pharmacy and Therapeutics*, **29**(9): 581–583 (United States).
7. International Conference on Harmonisation of Technical Requirements for Registration of Pharmaceuticals for Human Use (2002). *ICH Harmonised Tripartite Guideline, Guidelines for Good Clinical Practice*, 6th edition, revision 1.
8. London AJ (2011). *Offshoring Science: The Promise and Perils of the Globalization of Clinical Trials*, IRB: Ethics and Human Research (The Hastings Center/United States).
9. Solovay K. Medical Device Firms Do Many Trials Offshore. Here's Why, Healing Innovation, *Medcity News* (online), available (April 4, 2011): http://www.medcitynews.com/2011/04/medical-device-firms-do-many-clinical-studies-offshore-heres-why.
10. Manthei J, Thoelke KR, and Haas JB (2008). *Global Clinical Trials: Potential Pitfalls of Offshore Trials*, BAYBIO2008 (online), available (2008): http://www.baybio.org/files/AC08_T4S3_Global_Clinical_Trials.pdf.
11. Marwah R, Van de Voorde K, and Parchman J (2010). Good Clinical Practice Regulatory Inspections: Lessons for Indian Investigator Sites, *Perspectives in Clinical Research*, **1**(4): 151–155 (Bristol-Myers Squibb/United States).
12. Schipper I and Weyzig F (2008). *Ethics for Drug Testing in Low and Middle Income Countries: Considerations for European Market Approval*, Center for Research on Multinational Corporations (Stichting Onderzoek Multinationale Ondernemingen/the Netherlands).

13. Singer N (February 18, 2009). Outsourcing of Drug Trials Is Faulted, *The New York Times* (United States).
14. Stiffler H (2003). Guidelines for Obtaining Informed Consent for Clinical Research, *Applied Clinical Trials.*
15. Sunita, Service Outsourcing Opportunities in Medical Device Market Worth US$26.77 Billion by 2014, *PR Newswire* (online), available (November 12, 2009) http://www.prnewswire.com/news-releases/service-outsourcing-opportunities-in-medical-device-market-worth-us2677-billion-by-2014-69837522.html.
16. Pozgar G. (2012). *Legal Aspects of Health Care Administration* (Jones and Bartlett Publishers/ United States).
17. Yuling F, *et al.* (2000). Canadian-American Differences in the Management of Acute Coronary Syndromes in the GUSTO IIb Trial, *Circulation,* **102**(12): 1375–1381 (Canada).
18. Wenland CL (2008). Research, Therapy, and Bioethical Hegemony: The Controversy Over Perinatal AZT Trials in Africa, *African Studies Review,* **51**(3): 1–23 (African Studies Association/ United States).

Chapter 10

Regulatory Affairs for Medical Device Clinical Trials in Asia Pacific

Seow Li-Ping Geraldine

Johnson & Johnson Medical Asia Pacific,
No. 2 International Business Park,
#07-01, Tower One, The Strategy, 609930 Singapore
lseow@its.jnj.com

10.1 Introduction

Over the past decade, the Asia-Pacific region has grown to become an important player in global clinical research development and has contributed to the provision of quality clinical data to gain market access for new products. Even though the most remarkable growth has been observed mainly in pharmaceutical clinical trials, industry stakeholders have recognised the high potential of medical device clinical trials which have hitherto been unregulated in most Asia-Pacific countries. In recent years, more regional regulators have too been turning their focus on the regulation controls required for medical device clinical trials. As both regulators and industry stakeholders seek for direction in this changing landscape, there is a generated demand for regulatory affairs professionals

Handbook of Medical Device Regulatory Affairs in Asia
Edited by Jack Wong and Raymond K. Y. Tong

ISBN 978-981-4411-21-9 (Hardcover), 978-981-4411-22-6 (eBook)
www.panstanford.com

to participate actively in this quest, and work synergistically with their clinical research colleagues, to ensure that any additional regulatory controls would be better managed without impeding the path to market access for new medical devices. It is therefore pertinent for regulatory affairs professionals to gain a good understanding of medical device clinical trials and develop expertise in related regulatory requirements.

10.2 Medical Device Clinical Trials versus Pharmaceutical Clinical Trials

For those who are new to the world of medical device clinical trials, it would be fair to assume that there are differences between medical device clinical trials and pharmaceutical clinical trials, whereas they share a similar overall clinical trial process (Fig. 10.1).

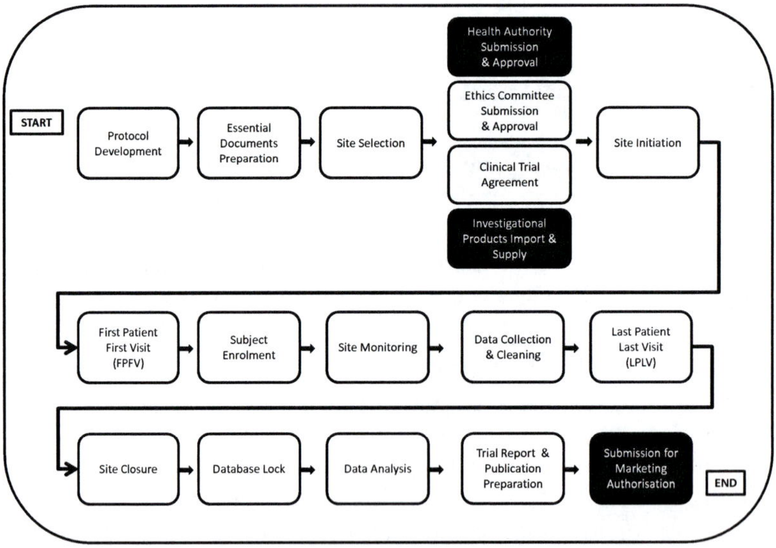

Figure 10.1 The clinical trial process (simplified).

The most obvious difference would be the product types involved in the trial. Medical devices vary in complexity and would include a wide range of health or medical instruments used in the treatment, mitigation, diagnosis or prevention of disease or abnormal physical condition. Medical devices with pharmaceutical components may be categorised as a combination product or a medical device or a pharmaceutical product. Interestingly, some medical devices are classified and regulated as drugs in a few countries. The classification of the investigational medical device should be clarified upfront by the sponsor with the relevant regulatory bodies as this would influence the requirements for conducting the clinical trial.

Trials are designed to answer medical questions. The purpose of a trial is to test out a hypothesis about the effect of a particular intervention upon a disease or condition. This effect could be tested using a single-arm (uncontrolled) design or a comparative (controlled) design (Fig. 10.2). The comparator could be (1) no intervention, (2) a sham device/procedure (placebo in pharmaceutical studies), or (3) existing therapies. The use of placebo or a blinded product may not always be ethical or possible in medical device trials. A comparator could be an existing product which has either been first in the market or has proven efficacy and safety, or an existing procedure which uses different products and instrumentation but has similarities to the investigational procedure, or existing standard of care which may not be linked to a product or a procedure. The added clinical value compared to an existing medical device is of interest to healthcare providers, patients and payers. Due to the innovative nature of medical devices, this "gold standard" may not always exist. For first in class medical devices, it is also a challenge to identify the comparator to be used for the study. Alternatively some trials are conducted with a single arm design, only to compare the results with those from a historical trial involving a predecessor.

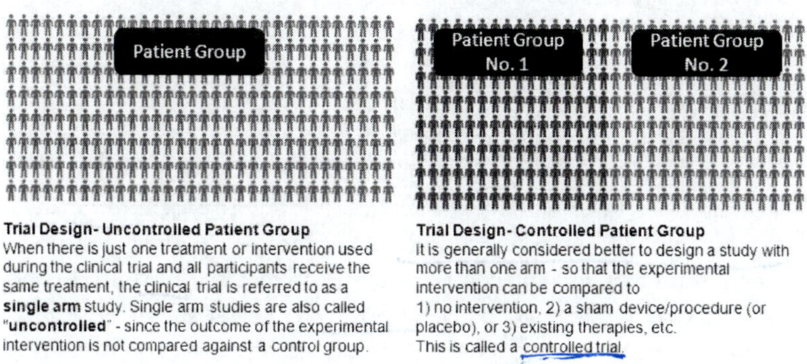

Figure 10.2 Uncontrolled versus controlled trial design.

The focus in a pharmaceutical clinical trial is solely on the investigational drug. In the medical device context, the investigational device is but part of a complex system comprising the device, the instrumentation or accessory devices and the procedure for using the device. Sometimes all components are unregistered products and the indicated procedure has an investigational status. The clinical trial protocol needs to address how the device is the only investigational component without being influenced by the variability from the other components of this system, for example, through standardised certified surgical technique training before using the device in the trial. Another relevant consequence would be the scope of safety and complaints reporting which should cover all components and the expectedness of events, unless otherwise specified in the protocol.

The pharmaceutical phasing of trials from phase 1 to 4 does not apply to medical device clinical trials. Instead the 4Ps are commonly used: Preclinical trials including *in vitro*/bench-top testing and animal studies, Pilot trials, Pivotal trials and Post-marketing studies (Table 10.1). Generally, the clinical development of a medical device tends to move at a faster pace in order to attain the innovative leader position for the technology involved and to ensure that the customers can access to the latest device. Some devices, depending on their classification and the selected regulatory path, do not even require clinical data for registration which is based on literature evaluation of data from predicate or previously approved devices, thus some regulatory bodies warrant the need for post-marketing studies to monitor long-term effects and to gain additional safety and effectiveness clinical data for the new device.

Many similarities exist between medical device clinical trials and pharmaceutical clinical trials. Those with experience in pharmaceutical clinical trials could leverage on this experience and apply their knowledge with an open mindset and adaptability to the different scenarios in medical device clinical trials. The principles of the Good Clinical Practice Guideline by the International Conference on Harmonisation of Technical Requirements for Registration of Pharmaceuticals for Human Use (ICH) Guideline, or commonly referred to as ICH GCP [1], that form the ethical foundation for pharmaceutical clinical trials, do apply to medical device clinical trials.

Table 10.1 Phases of clinical trials involving medical devices

	Phase	Description
Preclinical trials	***In vitro* (benchtop) testing**	*In vitro* research takes place in the laboratory. Laboratory researchers attempt to simulate conditions of the human body, conducting multiple tests to establish whether the device is effective, safe, and functioning properly.
	Animal studies	Initial tests to *establish safety* of the product or materials in question will be conducted *on animals*.
Clinical trials	**Feasibility (pilot) studies**	A feasibility, or pilot, study will be conducted to *test safety and performance* of the product in question, usually a multi-centre study, involving 30 to about 200 subjects and lasts for 30 days to 6 months.
	Pivotal trials	Pivotal trials are conducted to *gain evidence of safety and effectiveness*, also usually multi-centre studies, with 100 to over 1,000 subjects and lasts for 30 days to several years. Used to obtain regulatory approval from the relevant approval body.
	Post-marketing studies	After the launch of a product, post-marketing studies will be conducted to *monitor long-term effects and to gain additional safety and effectiveness data*.

10.3 Regulation of Clinical Trials

Basically, regulation of clinical trials is necessary to ensure

(i) The safety, well-being and rights of the clinical trial subjects
(ii) The scientific conduct of the clinical trial
(iii) The credibility of the clinical trial data

This is in coherence with a Regulatory Authority's role in the governance of public health and safety. When a clinical trial application is submitted to the regulatory authorities for approval, the reviewers would typically evaluate the protocol, the informed consent form as well as product-related essential documents like the Investigator's Brochure to establish an expert opinion on whether the trial should be conducted from a scientific perspective and whether there are measures in place to ensure the safety, well-being and rights of the subjects. Credibility of clinical trial data, which would be analysed and collated into a clinical trial report, is reviewed as part of the evaluation of a product registration dossier. In some countries, these aspects are further verified through inspections performed by the health authority either during or after the trial. Other basic aspects of regulation would also cover standards for the conduct of the clinical trial, reporting of safety-related events, product defects and regular trial status updates, and labelling, import, accountability and traceability of investigational medical devices which should be manufactured according to relevant standards. A risk-based approach to the scope of control is adopted by most regulatory authorities. Observations of latest regional trends also reveal that Regulatory Authorities are going beyond merely enforcing regulation by playing a more contributing role, to enhance the local clinical research infrastructure and competency of clinical trial personnel, through organising training programmes in medical device clinical trials for clinical trial personnel, provisioning for the registration of trials in a public clinical trial registry, and even revising their local version of GCP to keep up with the changing clinical trial environment (Table 10.2).

Table 10.2 Possible areas of regulation

New clinical trial application	Local GCP
Protocol & amendment review	Reporting of trial status & deviations
Informed consent form review	Reporting of safety-related events
Investigator's brochure review	Reporting of product defects
Surgical technique review	Clinical trial report review
Label & packaging review	Inspection-sponsor, site, CRO, warehouse
Instructions for use review	Clinical personnel qualification & training
Product import into country	Public clinical trial registry
Product accountability	Certification of competent sites

Apart from the Regulatory Authority, the responsibility of upholding the above-mentioned three ethical pillars of a clinical trial is also shared by the other major stakeholders in a clinical trial albeit from different perspectives: the Investigator, the Sponsor and the Institutional Review Board (IRB), which is sometimes also referred to as the Ethics Committee (EC) (Fig. 10.3). In fact, although ICH GCP, being a guideline to be followed when generating clinical trial data that are intended to be submitted to regulatory authorities, is commonly used as a basis to regulate clinical trials, it does not have a section specifically for "Regulatory Authority". The Declaration of Helsinki, which describes the ethical principles for medical research involving human subjects, is addressed primarily to physicians, i.e. the Investigator [2]. The other common reference for medical device clinical trials, ISO14155:2011 (E) [3], does not describe the role and responsibilities of the regulatory authority. Hence, while regulatory affairs professionals from the Sponsor organisations have guidance on the scope of their responsibility, those from the regulatory authorities need to establish their specific role and responsibilities within their own clinical research environment.

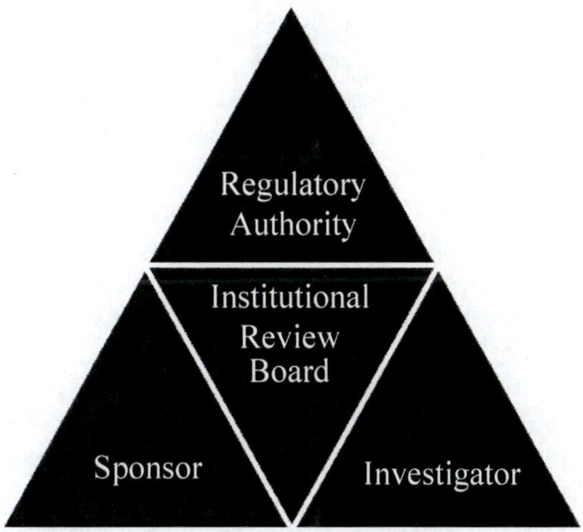

Figure 10.3 Major stakeholders in a clinical trial.

The harmonisation of regulation within the region and the opportunity to learn about the implementation of regulation in other countries including outside the Asia-Pacific region will definitely help local regulators and regulatory affairs professionals to formulate regulation that would effectively meet the needs of their country as well as to increase acceptance of local clinical trial data in overseas submissions. The US Food and Drug Administration (US FDA) would be a forerunner in medical device clinical trial regulations since implementing medical device amendments to the Federal Food, Drug & Cosmetic Act on 28 May 1976. The European Medical Directives, which were implemented in the last decade, adopt a different regulatory approach through a combination of regional and local laws, ISO standards and notified bodies. Within the region, within the last decade, the regulatory authorities in

Japan, South Korea and Taiwan have implemented changes to their organisations and clinical trial regulations to address the needs of the growing number of local medical device clinical trials.

From an operational perspective, using the same clinical trial reviewer team who has been evaluating pharmaceutical clinical trials may seem like an easily adaptable and convenient approach to undertake the task of evaluating medical device clinical trials. However, a copy and paste success should not be expected without investing in equipping and/or building up the team with knowledge and experience in medical device clinical development process, investigational methodology and the greater emphasis on technology expertise, diagnostic approach and surgical techniques. A similar consideration should be made for the team who traditionally reviews safety reports and product complaints for pharmaceutical products. This scaling up of clinical trial and safety vigilance resources should be part of the medical device regulation development strategy. Due to the rapidness and specificity of the technology and innovation involved in medical device clinical development, the engagement of independent experts to perform the evaluation could help to augment the required resources to support this effort.

Industry stakeholders who often take on the role of the Sponsor or clinical research organisations are watching these developments closely. Changes to clinical trial regulations have an impact on clinical trial operations and more crucially affect the clinical development pathway in terms of speed and complexity. Proper change management coupled with effective organisational strategy for regulatory affairs and clinical research will help to cushion the impact of these changes and prepare the industry to take on the challenges of a changing regulatory landscape.

Interestingly, there is a heavy reliance on the IRB to be the only ethical and scientific "third party" gatekeeper to evaluate and approve medical device clinical trials when the regulatory authority's approval is not required. Inadvertently, most of these regulatory authorities would have guidelines regarding IRB's organisation and procedures. In 2001, the Association for the Accreditation of Human Research Protection Programs, Inc. (AAHRPP), an independent human research protection accreditation program, was established in the United States and has defined domains of responsibility: Organization, Institutional Review Board (IRB) or Ethics Committee (EC), and Researchers and Research Staff. AAHRPP has even accredited eight organisations outside the United States among which there are three each from India and South Korea and one each from China and Singapore.

In the United States, clinical evaluation of devices that have not been cleared for marketing requires an Investigational Device Exemption (IDE); if the clinical trial involves a significant risk device, the IDE must also be approved by the US FDA. The scope and strategy for regulation of medical device clinical trials varies within the Asia-Pacific region. This could be influenced by the maturity of medical device regulation, the adoption of medical device clinical trial regulation from other countries, the available infrastructure, regulation and resources for pharmaceutical clinical trials, the role and responsibilities of the IRBs, and the local demand for regulation of medical device clinical trials, among others. Most countries require compliance to ICH GCP or a localised version of GCP in their regulations, noting that localised GCP or local regulation will generally prevail over ICH GCP requirements where there is a conflict between the local and international references. Some implement more stringent controls on clinical trials involving unapproved products than those involving approved registered products. Countries with well established regulatory organisations for evaluation of pharmaceutical clinical trials, for example Australia, Japan, South Korea and Taiwan, have leveraged on their experience and allocated dedicated teams for evaluation and consultation for medical device clinical trials. In Southeast Asia, Singapore is taking the lead in the implementation of medical device clinical trial regulation from 2013. In a few countries where the specific regulations are not implemented, certain regulations for pharmaceutical clinical trials could sometimes apply to medical device clinical trials on a case-by-case basis; for these countries, prior consultation with the relevant authorities would be advised. As of the end of 2011, Hong Kong and Malaysia currently do not have any regulation on medical device clinical trials and import of investigational medical device for clinical trial use.

10.4 Country Regulations

Figure 10.4 describes the typical regulatory activities that are relevant to the clinical trial process.

Table 10.3 Overview of the current regulation of medical device clinical trials in some Asia-Pacific countries

Country	Regulatory authority	Submission	Notification	Approval	Import licence	Safety reporting	Inspection
Australia	Therapeutic Goods Administration (TGA)	Sequential	Within 10 business days (CTN scheme)	Within 50 days (CTX scheme for review of safety of device)	Part of CTN/CTX	Local SUADEs/SUSARs within 7–15 days	NA
China	Center of Medical Device Evaluation, State Food and Drug Administration (CMDE, SFDA)	Sequential (Before IRB submission)	Yes (protocol only)	NA	NA	SAE within 24 hours	Site-specific
Hong Kong	Medical Device Control Office, Department of Health	NA	NA	NA	NA	Voluntary	NA
India	Medical Device Division, Central Drugs Standard Control Organization, Drugs Controller General (India) (DCGI)	Parallel	NA	About 12–16 weeks. Prior IRB approval required	Yes	Local SUADEs/SUSARs within 14 days	NA
Malaysia	Medical Device Control Division, Ministry of Health (MOH)	NA	NA	NA	NA	Yes	NA
New Zealand	New Zealand Medicines and Medical Devices Safety Authority (Medsafe)	Sequential	Within 45 business days.	NA	NA	Local SUADEs/SUSARs within 7–30 days	NA
Singapore	Clinical Trials Branch & Medical Device Branch, Health Sciences Authority (HSA)	NA	NA	NA	Yes	Local SUADEs/SUSARs within 48 hours or 10–30 days	NA
South Korea	Medical Device Safety Bureau, Korean Food & Drug Administration (KFDA)	Parallel	NA	Officially 30 days	Per import	Local SUADEs/SUSARs within 7–15 days	NA
Taiwan	Division of Medical Device and Cosmetics, Taiwan Food and Drug Administration (TFDA)	Parallel	NA	1–3 months	Yes	Local SUADEs/SUSARs within 7–14 days	GCP inspection by TFDA
Thailand	Thailand Food and Drug Administration	NA	NA	NA	Yes	NA	NA

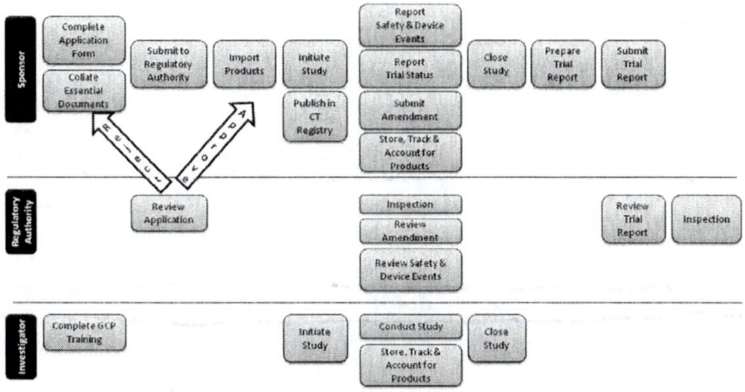

Figure 10.4 Typical regulatory activities in the clinical trial process.

Table 10.3 shows an overview of the current regulation of medical device clinical trials in some of the Asia-Pacific countries.

10.4.1 Australia

Medical devices that are not in the Australian Register of Therapeutic Goods (ARTG) can be legally supplied in a clinical trial through the Clinical Trial exemptions mechanism (Clinical Trial Notification (CTN) Scheme or the Clinical Trial Exemption (CTX) Scheme), which is managed by the Therapeutic Goods Administration or TGA. In addition, prior quarantine clearance must be obtained to import any material of biological origin (human, animal, plant or bacterial) and questions about requirements for an import permit should be directed to the Australian Quarantine & Inspection Service (AQIS). The responsibility for monitoring a clinical trial rests with the Sponsor, Institution in which the trial is being conducted, the Ethics Committee and the Investigator. Clinical trials must be approved by a Human Research Ethics Committee (HREC) which must be constituted and operating in accordance with the NHRMC's National Statement on Ethical Conduct in Human Research. The HREC is responsible for considering the scientific and ethical issues of the proposed clinical trial protocol. Approval of a trial is required from a HREC with jurisdiction over the specific site where the trial is conducted. The Sponsor decides whether to use the CTN CTX Scheme when the trial involves any device which is not included in the ARTG or used beyond the conditions of its marketing approval. The Sponsor in this scenario must be an Australian clinical trial Sponsor. Clinical trials in which the medical devices are used within the conditions of their marketing approval are not subject to CTN or CTX requirements but still require approval by a HREC before the start of the trial.

The CTN process involves a notification only to the TGA with a nominal notification fee, thus no approval or decision is made by the TGA. CTN trials cannot commence until the appropriately completed CTN scheme form and the notification fee is submitted to the TGA who will send the clinical trial sponsor an acknowledgement letter. The notification of the CTN form and the associated fee automatically creates the exemption necessary to allow lawful supply of the unapproved medical devices for the clinical trial.

In the CTX approval process, TGA reviews the safety of the device by assessing the summary data and usage guidelines for a proposed clinical development programme within 50 working days, and if approval if granted, subsequent trials must be carried out under the terms of the approval and be notified to the TGA. The CTX application does not require the submission of the clinical trial protocol which should be reviewed by the HREC. A CTX trial cannot commence until TGA has provided written advice that the application has been approved, and a HREC and the institution at which the trial will be conducted have provided approval for the conduct of the trial.

The clinical trial Sponsor needs to notify TGA of the data of trial completion and the reason for completion. TGA does not require notification of protocol amendments which clarify the use of, and/or monitoring of treatment but may require if there is a major change to the protocol and the HREC requires a change to the conditions of their approval.

In terms of adverse event reporting, the clinical trial Sponsor is required to report to TGA about serious and unexpected adverse device events. Fatal or life-threatening adverse device events must be reported initially within 7 calendar days of knowledge, followed by a full report within 8 additional calendar days. Other serious unanticipated device events must be reported within 15 calendar days of knowledge. The Investigator is responsible for adverse event reporting to the HREC as required by the HREC and to the Sponsor as required by the protocol [4–7].

10.4.2 China

Submission of a clinical trial application in China is currently limited to Class III medical devices implanted into human body that are not yet available in the market, or those medical devices that are based on the theory of traditional Chinese medicines only [8]. The clinical trial protocol should be filed with the Center of Medical Device Evaluation (CMDE) of the State Food and Drug Administration (SFDA). Medical devices to be used in a clinical trial must fulfill certain conditions including measuring up to the registered product or industrial standard, possession of a testing report from the Sponsor and a qualified type testing report from a SFDA-recognised testing centre, as well as data from animal studies. Approval requirements are set on a case by case basis after consultation with SFDA since the need for a SFDA approval before commencing a clinical trial is not clearly stated in the regulations. Once the protocol has been filed with the CMDE, the Sponsor can proceed with the submission to the IRB for review and approval. All serious adverse effects must be reported to SFDA within 24 hours; however, there is no clear definition for "serious adverse effects" in the regulations. SFDA may conduct site inspections during or after the end of the trial. It is not mandatory to obtain local clinical data if global clinical data is available for imported medical devices. In addition, there is new regulation with regards to clinical data exemption for some class II medical devices [9]. As of the fourth quarter of 2012, China is in the process of revising its Medical Device GCP.

10.4.3 Hong Kong

Hong Kong has not implemented regulations for medical device clinical trials. Although reporting of serious adverse events in a medical device clinical trial is still done on a voluntary basis, the Medical Device Control Office would prefer to be notified of local reportable adverse events which have occurred at sites in Hong Kong.

10.4.4 India

Generally an approval from the Drugs Controller General (India) (DCGI) is required for first-in-man and pivotal clinical trials; this is also dependent on whether the investigational device is included in a list of notified devices which are classified by the DCGI as drugs. The medical device advisory committee (MDAC) reviews the submitted clinical trial application for completeness and, in the case of early phase of first-in-man trials, may refer the application to the Indian Council for Medical Research for scientific review. The application dossier is rather comprehensive and consists of many sections requesting for most essential documents including the insurance certificate and indemnity agreement but excluding the clinical trial agreement with each site. Both DCGI approval and IRB approval for the institution(s) where the trial will be conducted are required before the trial can commence. An import licence is required for importing investigational medical devices into India.

The application for an import licence for the investigational medical devices is submitted together with the clinical trial application. Any unexpected serious adverse event (SAE), as defined in the Indian GCP Guidelines, occurring during a clinical trial should be communicated promptly (within 14 calendar days) by the Sponsor to the Licensing Authority and to the other Investigator(s) participating in the study [10–12].

10.4.5 Malaysia

As of end of 2011, regulation of medical device clinical trials has not officially implemented in Malaysia. Future guidelines based on the recently passed Medical Device Bill will provide more information on the regulation of medical device clinical trials in Malaysia.

10.4.6 New Zealand

Clinical trials of medical devices do not require approval under New Zealand legislation, but the New Zealand Medicines and Medical Devices Safety Authority or Medsafe would like to be informed by email of such trials. However, Health and Disability Ethics Committee approval should be obtained for medical device clinical trials. If the medical device used in a clinical trial contains a hazardous substance or a new organism, an approval under the requirements of the Hazardous Substances and New Organisms Act 1986 (HSNO Act) is required. Any medical device imported for use in a clinical trial is exempted from mandatory notification to the Web Assisted Notification of Devices (WAND) database [13].

All clinical trials conducted in New Zealand are expected to be conducted in accordance with the CPMP Note for Guidance on Good Clinical Practice, regardless whether an approval under the Medicines Act is required for the trial. The Sponsor, who must be a person in New Zealand, assumes responsibility, including legal liability, for the trial in New Zealand in terms of preservation of records, reporting adverse events, submit 6 monthly progress reports, notifying protocol changes and ensuring that the trial is conducted in accordance with both New Zealand law and Good Research Practice standards. Expedited reports of all fatal or life-threatening suspected unexpected serious adverse reactions (SUSARs) occurring in New Zealand trial participants must be sent to Medsafe by the Sponsor within 7 days of knowledge. The Sponsor is required to hold reports of all worldwide SUSARs which may be requested by Medsafe. Adverse events that cause injury and that are associated with medical devices should also be reported to Medsafe, initial reports within 7 calendar days for actual or potential death or serious injury and within 30 calendar days for those with or without actual or potential injury [14].

Medsafe also administers a self-certification scheme for clinical trial sites that have patients in residence, and maintains a list of sites for which it has received evidence of compliance with GCP requirements.

10.4.7 Singapore

Import of unregistered medical devices into Singapore for use in clinical trials requires the approval of the Health Sciences Authority (HSA). An application form for Clinical Trial Test Materials (CTM for Medical Devices) must be submitted by the the Sponsor [15, 16]. Upon importation of the investigational medical devices into Singapore, the Sponsor is responsible for complying with safety and defects reporting, notification of device recalls, and device labelling, accountability and traceability requirements. Although currently medical device trials do not require regulatory approval, all adverse events or defects in medical device trials must be reported. Adverse events that represent a serious threat to public health must be reported within 48 hours while those that have led to the death, or a serious deterioration in the state of health, of a patient, a user of the medical device or any other person must be reported within 10 days. Events where a recurrence of which might lead to the death or a serious deterioration in the state of health, of a patient, a user of the medical device or any other person must be reported within 30 days. Initial reports should be followed by a final report within 30 days of the initial report, detailing the investigation into the adverse event.

During the final phase of implementation of the medical device regulatory framework in Singapore in the fourth quarter of 2012, the new Health Products (Clinical Trials) Regulations will introduce regulations for medical device clinical trials in Singapore using a risk-based approach. Proposed changes, which affects clinical trials to determine safety and performance of all Class C and D registered and unregistered medical devices, will include a new Clinical Trial Notification route for listed investigational devices versus a Clinical Trial Approval route for unregistered investigational devices. Clinical trials involving Class A and B medical devices, non-invasive and non-confirmatory *in vitro* diagnostic products as well as observational trials are excluded from this scope of regulation. Changes to current safety reporting requirements are also expected. Another proposed change of interest is the allowance of a trial to have more than one Sponsor in order to address various industry business and outsourcing models where the Sponsors may have joint or allocated responsibilities. All unregistered medical devices which are imported for non-investigational purpose in the conduct of a clinical trial, regardless of product risk class, will be regulated under the Health Products (Medical Device) Regulations instead.

10.4.8 South Korea

From 2007 to 2011, the Korean Food and Drug Administration (KFDA) has approved 120 medical device clinical trials. Applications for clinical trial protocol and amendment approval and reporting for adverse events, product defects, trial status updates and import quantities are submitted online via the KiFDA Electronic Filing System. For trials where the essential documents are prepared in English, a Korean translation of the protocol and participant-facing written material must be prepared and submitted in addition to the English versions. Otherwise all remaining essential documentation can be submitted in English. Submission to KFDA can be done in parallel with the submission to the IRB, however KFDA requires an IRB approval for the site where the trial is conducted before KFDA issues the approval. Although the official review time for a clinical trial application is 30 days, this timeline could be delayed by, for example, IRB-required changes to the informed consent form.

Device-related death or life threatening adverse events must be reported within 7 days for the initial report and a follow-up detailed report within the next 8 days; all other types of SAEs must be reported within 15 days of knowledge of the event [17–19].

KFDA has even taken one step further by creating a new system requiring hospitals and medical doctors to be qualified specifically as medical device clinical centres. To be qualified, hospitals must have standard operating procedures according to GCP and medical doctors must have training in medical device clinical development and GCP. By the end of September 2011, a total of 94 university hospitals were registered by KFDA as medical clinical device centres nationwide.

10.4.9 Taiwan (TFDA)

The regulatory system for investigational medical devices in clinical trials consists of regulation for GMP (Good Manufacturing Practice) or QSD (Quality System Design), determination of device classification and regulation for import of these devices. The documents required for the import of investigational medical devices used in a clinical trial and the clinical trial approval include the Certificate of Free Sale in marketed countries, the protocol and the informed consent form as well as most other clinical trial essential documents including the clinical trial agreement, insurance certificate and indemnity agreement. If the Certificate of Free Sale in marketed countries is not available, technical data including preclinical safety and functional tests plus the IRB approval letter must be provided. The clinical trial application can be submitted in parallel both to the IRB and the Division of Medical Device and Cosmetics, Taiwan Food and Drug Administration (TFDA) for review. After the clinical trial results are submitted as reference for product registration, a TFDA review team will perform a GCP inspection at the site before approving the use of these results as reference for product registration. To shorten the review time for medical device clinical trials, the review process has recently been simplified for clinical trials which have obtained US FDA approval and for those with minor changes to the protocol (excluding safety and design changes).

In addition, TFDA has implemented a local version of GCP as well as established a list of good clinical research centres, mandated attendance of compulsory GCP training programme for clinical trial personnel and organised training on clinical trials involving medical devices and technology for regulators, industry and site personnel.

Reporting of adverse medical device reactions (ADR) and product defects can be done online, using the National Reporting System of Adverse Medical Device Reactions and the Medical Product Defect Reporting System respectively, by consumers, medical personnel and manufacturers. For SAEs, manufacturers are expected to provide an oral or initial report is expected within 7 days of knowledge of the event, followed by a full report within 14 days [20].

10.4.10 Thailand

To date, the Thailand Food and Drug Administration (Thai FDA) does not have any regulation on the conduct of medical device clinical trials in Thailand. Only the import of unapproved medical devices used in clinical trial must be pre-approved by Thai FDA who will issue an import licence that specifies the approved quantity before the products can be shipped into Thailand.

10.5 Moving Ahead as Regulatory Affairs Professionals

Existing regulations will change as the learning curve progresses. The clinical research environment and the regulations for medical device clinical trials will evolve to meet the demands and challenges in the conduct of medical device clinical trials in the Asia-Pacific region. A careful effort to streamline regulations governing clinical trials could reduce redundancy in the system while ensuring ethical conduct [21]. In order for Asia Pacific to contribute even more significantly to the globalisation of evidence based medicine, the crucial role of regulatory affairs professionals in this evolution could be enhanced by exploring various possibilities of continuous personal development of regulatory affairs and clinical research knowledge and trends, and through collaborations with their clinical research colleagues in the same quest using a synergistic goal approach. Implementation of new or revised regulations should be coupled with motivated considerations for appropriate change management measures within the organisations. Resources could be dedicated to extend the organisation's knowledge database, outside their area of jurisdiction or countries, about sites, investigators, participants, other key stakeholders, clinical research practices and the quality of trial data. The continuation of using a risk-based approach may not be disadvantageous, though more long-term benefits could be derived from a proactive strategy than a reactive one. Meanwhile, where regulations are not yet available, the principles of globally recognised good clinical practice guidelines, like ICH GCP, should be used as foundation beacons to guide the management and conduct of medical device clinical trials.

References

1. International Conference On Harmonisation Of Technical Requirements For Registration Of Pharmaceuticals For Human Use (10 June 1996). International Conference on Harmonisation (ICH) Tripartite Guideline, Guideline for Good Clinical Practice E6 (R1). Retrieved 10 January 2011, from http://www.ich.org/fileadmin/Public_Web_Site/ICH_Products/Guidelines/Efficacy/E6_R1/Step4/E6_R1__Guideline.pdf.
2. World Medical Association (2008). Declaration of Helsinki: Ethical Principles for Medical Research Involving Human Subjects. Retrieved 10 January 2011, from http://www.wma.net/en/30publications/10policies/b3/17c.pdf.
3. International Organisation for Standardisation (2011). ISO 14155:2011: Clinical Investigation of Medical Devices for Human Subjects- Good Clinical Practice.
4. Therapeutic Goods Administration, Australia *Government* (March 2006). The Australian Clinical Trial Handbook. Retrieved 10 January 2011, from http://www.tga.gov.au/industry/clinical-trials.htm.
5. Therapeutic Goods Administration, Australia *Government* (May 2011). Australian Regulatory Guidelines for Medical Devices version 1.1.

Retrieved 10 January 2011, from http://www.tga.gov.au/industry/devices-argmd.htm.

6. Therapeutic Goods Administration, Australia Government (October 2004). Access to Unapproved Therapeutic Goods: Clinical Trials in Australia. Retrieved 10 January 2011, from http://www.tga.gov.au/industry/clinical-trials.htm.
7. National Health and Medical Research Council. Australian Government (October 2007). National Statement on Ethical Conduct in Human Research. Retrieved 10 January 2011, from http://www.nhmrc.gov.au/health-ethics/human-research-ethics-committees-hrecs/human-research-ethics-committees-hrecs/national.
8. State Food and Drug Administration, P.R. China (17 January 2004). Provisions of Clinical Trials for Medical Devices, SFDA Order No.5. Retrieved 10 January 2011, from http://eng.sfda.gov.cn/WS03/CL0768/61644.html.
9. State Food and Drug Administration, P.R. China (24 November 2011). Notification about Clinical Data Exemption for Certain Class II Medical Devices (In Chinese). Retrieved 10 January 2011, from http://www.sda.gov.cn/WS01/CL0845/67233.html.
10. Central Drugs Standard Control Organisation, Ministry of Health, India (December 2008). Guidance for Industry on Submission of Clinical Trial Application for Evaluating Safety and Efficacy, CT/71108, Version 1.1. Retrieved 10 January 2011, from http://cdsco.nic.in/CDSCO-GuidanceForIndustry.pdf.
11. Central Drugs Standard Control Organisation, Ministry of Health, India (04 August 2010). Requirements for Conducting Clinical Trial(s) of Medical Devices in India - Draft. Retrieved 10 January 2011, from http://cdsco.nic.in/Requirements%20for%20Conducting%20Clinical%20Trial(s)%20of%20Medical%20Devices%20in%20India.PDF.
12. Ministry of Health and Family Welfare, Government of India (20 April 2010). List of Notified Medical Devices. Retrieved 10 January 2011, from http://cdsco.nic.in/Medical_div/medical_device_division.htm.
13. New Zealand Medicines and Medical Devices Safety Authority (May 2011). Guideline on the Regulation of Therapeutic Products in New Zealand Part 11: Clinical Trials- Regulatory Approval and Good Clinical Practice Requirements, Edition 1.1. Retrieved 10 January 2011, from http://www.medsafe.govt.nz/regulatory/clinicaltrials.asp.
14. New Zealand Medicines and Medical Devices Safety Authority (10 May 2011). Information for Medical Device Suppliers: Medical Device Adverse Event Reporting. In *MedSafe Regulatory Information.*

Retrieved 10 January 2011, from http://www.medsafe.govt.nz/regulatory/devicesnew/9adverse-event.asp.

15. Health Sciences Authority, Singapore (01 September 2010). Health Products Act (Chapter 122D): Health Products (Medical Devices) Regulations 2010. Retrieved 10 January 2011, from http://www.hsa.gov.sg/publish/etc/medialib/hsa_library/health_products_regulation/legislation/health_products_act.Par.69129.File.dat/HEALTH%20PRODUCTS%20(MEDICAL%20DEVICES)%20REGULATIONS%202010.pdf

16. Health Sciences Authority, Singapore (01 September 2010). Health Products Act (Chapter 122D): Health Products (Medical Devices) (Exemption) Order 2010. Retrieved 10 January 2011, from http://www.hsa.gov.sg/publish/etc/medialib/hsa_library/health_products_regulation/legislation/health_products_act.Par.94239.File.dat/HEALTH%20PRODUCTS%20(MEDICAL%20DEVICES)(EXEMPTION)%20ORDER%202010.pdf.

17. Korean Food and Drug Administration, South Korea (25 November 2011). Guideline for Medical Device Korean Good Clinical Practice (In Korean). Retrieved 10 January 2011, from http://www.kfda.go.kr/index.kfda?mid=90.

18. Korean Food and Drug Administration, South Korea (28 November 2010). Enforcement Regulations of the Medical Device Act. Retrieved 10 January 2011, from http://www.kfda.go.kr/eng/eng/index.do;jsessionid=VAnDsf9zaa5M8jZvOtuhIQi8TiICe6RPiZA5PK1o3UtxBONueQ7AEtlQxPaNsgTE?nMenuCode=46&searchKeyCode=125&page=1&mode=view&boardSeq=66026.

19. Korean Food and Drug Administration, South Korea (01 September 2010). Enforcement Decree of the Medical Device Act. Retrieved 10 January 2011, from http://www.kfda.go.kr/eng/eng/index.do;jsessionid=VAnDsf9zaa5M8jZvOtuhIQi8TiICe6RPiZA5PK1o3UtxBONueQ7AEtlQxPaNsgTE?nMenuCode=46&searchKeyCode=125&page=1&mode=view&boardSeq=66026.

20. Taiwan Food and Drug Administration, Taiwan (12 April 2006). Guidelines for the Registration of Medical Devices. Retrieved 10 January 2011, from http://www.fda.gov.tw/eng/people_laws_list.aspx.

21. Seth W. Glickman, *et al* (2009). *Ethical and Scientific Implications of the Globalization of Clinical Research.* N Engl J Med 360:816–823.

Chapter 11

Medical Device Classification Guide

Patricia Teysseyre

Johnson & Johnson Medical Asia Pacific,
No. 2, International Business Park,
#07-01, Tower One, The Strategy, 609930 Singapore

pteyssey@its.jnj.com

11.1 How to Carry Out Medical Device Classification

11.1.1 Scope

It is the responsibility of the manufacturer to determine the classification of its medical device as early as possible in the device development. Its determination should be based on rules derived from the potential of a medical device to cause harm to a patient or user and thereby on its intended use and the technology it utilizes.

The manufacturer should first clearly define the intended use of the device [1]. The next step is to consider the applicable classification regulations in force in the country where the product is going to be registered before being marketed. Most countries have their own classification scheme, such as Japan, People's Republic of China [5], and India. The classification schemes of Canada and

Handbook of Medical Device Regulatory Affairs in Asia
Edited by Jack Wong and Raymond K. Y. Tong

ISBN 978-981-4411-21-9 (Hardcover), 978-981-4411-22-6 (eBook)
www.panstanford.com

Australia/New Zealand resemble the European one, whereas the one in the United States is different. Efforts are under way to effect a global harmonization of classification. For instance, Study Group 1 of the Global Harmonization Task Force (GHTF/SG1/N15:2006) [8] has made progress and has been taken as a reference in some Asian countries such as Singapore, but it can still be noticed that systems differ and it is the up to the manufacturer to check and adapt its medical device class to the appropriate local classification scheme. Although different in many jurisdictions, they carry remarkable resemblance in most cases, having 4 categories of risks identified and treating *in vitro* diagnostics in their own right [3]. A large percentage of the products would be in the same class across the globe, but care should be taken to examine individual product classifications carefully. GHTF consolidates the classes as A to D, with A being the lowest risk, and D the highest.

In accordance with the classification rules, the manufacturer should document and justify the class of the device.

The class determination can be influenced by several factors, including the duration of device contact with the body, the degree of invasiveness, whether the device delivers medicinal products or energy to the patient.

In general, when two or more classification rules may apply to the device, the device is allocated to the highest level of classification. In case of doubts, the appropriate Notified Body or Regulator should be consulted.

11.1.2 Definitions

Central circulatory system: the major internal blood vessels including the following: arteriae pulmonales, aorta ascendens, arcus aorta, aorta descendens to the bifurcatio aortae, arteriae coronariae, arteria carotis communis, arteria carotis externa, arteria carotis interna, arteriae cerebrales, truncus brachiocephalicus, venae cordis, venae pulmonales, vena cava superior, vena cava inferior.

Central nervous system: means brain, meninges, and spinal cord.

Duration

Transient: Normally intended for continuous use for less than 60 minutes.

Short term: Normally intended for continuous use for not more than 30 days.

Long term: Normally intended for continuous use for more than 30 days.

Intended use/intended purpose: means the use for which the device is intended according to the data supplied by the manufacturer on the labelling, in the instructions and/or in promotional materials.

Invasiveness

Invasive devices: A device which, in whole or in part, penetrates the body, either through a body orifice or through the surface of the body.

Body orifice: Any natural opening in the body, as well as the external surface of the eyeball, or any permanent artificial opening, such as a stoma.

Surgically invasive device: An invasive device which penetrates inside the body through the surface of the body, with the aid of or in the context of a surgical operation.

Implantable device

Any device which is intended

(i) to be totally introduced into the human body or

(ii) to replace an epithelial surface or the surface of the eye by surgical intervention which is intended to remain in place after the procedure.

Any device intended to be partially introduced into the human body through surgical intervention and intended to remain in place after the procedure for at least 30 days is also considered an implantable device.

11.2 Main Classifications

11.2.1 Medical Devices

The flow chart in Fig. 11.1 shows the main steps to be taken and questions to be addressed when carrying out a medical device classification. This decision tree is based on the GHTF (GHTF/SG1/N15:2006) [8] and MEDDEV 2.4/1 Rev. 9 Guidance [6].

11.2.2 Active Devices

The classification of rules for active medical devices in some jurisdictions differ from the medical devices ones and are shown in Fig. 11.2, as they are defined in the European Medical Devices Directive 93/42/EEC [2]. Figure 11.2 is an extract from the MEDDEV 2.4/1 Rev. 9 Guidance [6]. It should be noted that these are additional classification rules for active devices. The general rules 1–8, and the higher-numbered special rules may be applicable as well.

11.2.3 IVD Devices

Regarding *in vitro* diagnostic devices, their classification is well defined in each local regulation, which usually provides the class corresponding to the assay or reagent (and the associated equipment).

For instance, GHTF has a separate risk based classification. Europe uses risk assessment from 10 years ago. Health Canada has a separate classification for IVD but bringing them individually into the generic 4 risk classes.

In vitro Diagnostic (IVD) product means any reagent product, calibrator, control material kit, instrument, apparatus, equipment or

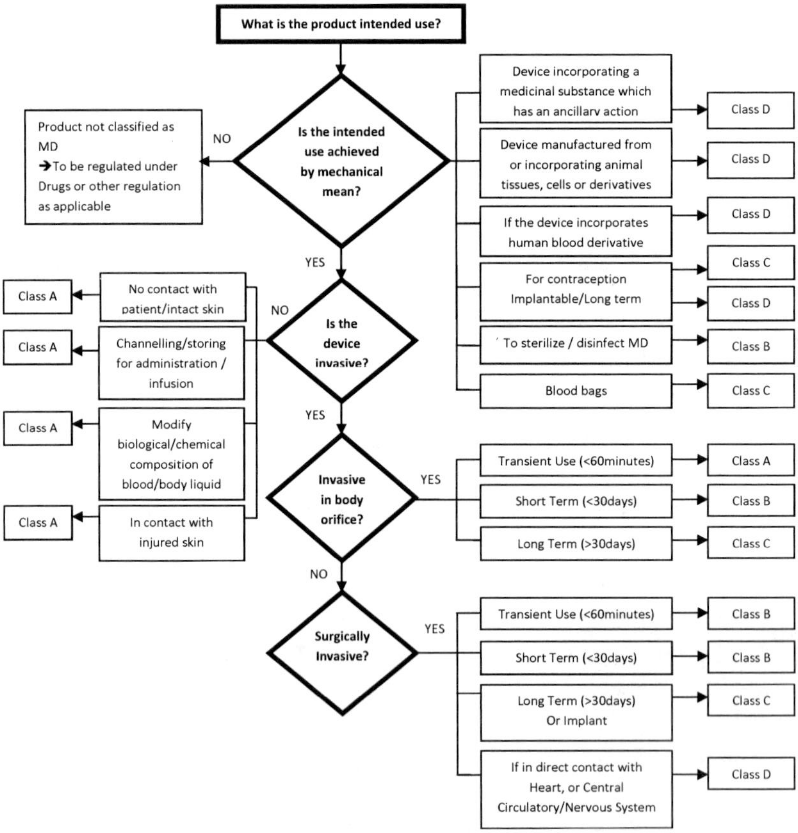

Figure 11.1 Steps to be considered while carrying out medical device classification.

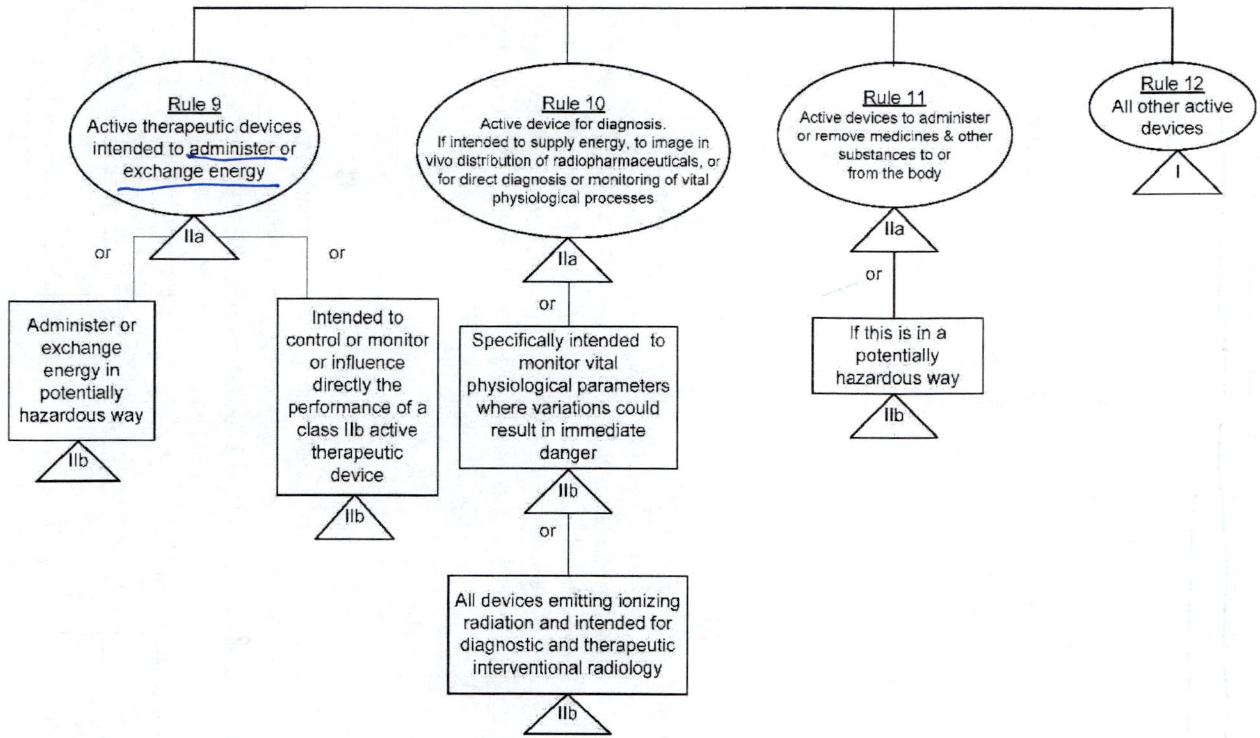

Figure 11.2 Classification of rules for active medical devices.

system, whether used alone or in combination, that is intended by its product owner to be used *in vitro* for the examination of specimens, including blood and tissue donations, derived from the human body, solely or principally for

(i) providing information concerning a physiological or pathological state,
(ii) providing information concerning a congenital abnormality,
(iii) determining the safety and compatibility of donations, including blood and tissue donations, with potential recipients, or
(iv) monitoring therapeutic measures

and includes a specimen receptacle but not a product for general laboratory use, unless that product, in view of its characteristics, is specifically intended by its product owner to be used for *in vitro* diagnostic examination

According to GHTF standards [7], IVD medical devices are classified into four classes, based on the individual risk and public health risk level (Table 11.1).

Table 11.1 Classification system for IVD Medical Devices

Class	Risk level	Device examples
A	Low individual risk and low public health risk	Clinical chemistry analyser, prepared selective culture media
B	Moderate individual risk and/or low public health risk	Vitamin B_{12}, pregnancy self-testing, anti-nuclear antibody. urine test strip
C	High individual risk and/or moderate public health risk	Blood glucose self testing, HLA typing, PSA screening. Rubella
D	High individual and high public health risk	HIV blood donor screening, HIV blood diagnostic

11.2.4 IVD Case Study

IVDs are medical devices intended to perform diagnoses from assays in hematology, immunology, microbiology, etc. Table 11.2

Table 11.2 Classification overview of Chlamydia serological reagents in different legislations

Country/ region	US	Canada	EU	Singapore
Class	Class I	Class III	List B	Class C
Rule	21CFR866.3120	Rule 2(b) (ii) of SOR/ 98-282) SCHEDULE 1 (Section 6)	Directive 98/79/EC — Annex. II	GN-14 Guidance on the Risk Classification of *in vitro* Diagnostic Medical Devices

illustrates the Chlamydia serological reagents. The exercise conducted around it aimed to determine its classification within different regulations; the rules which served as a reference to determine the class are highlighted.

11.2.4.1 US FDA

- **Rule: 21CFR866.3120 [10]:**

Title 21 — Food And Drugs: Chapter I — Food And Drug Administration Department Of Health and Human Services Subchapter H — Medical Devices Part 866 — Immunology and Microbiology Devices

Subpart D — Serological Reagents

Sec. 866.3120 Chlamydia serological reagents.

(a) *Identification.* Chlamydia serological reagents are devices that consist of antigens and antisera used in serological tests to identify antibodies to chlamydia in serum. Additionally, some of these reagents consist of chlamydia antisera conjugated with a fluorescent dye used to identify chlamydia directly from clinical specimens or cultured isolates derived from clinical specimens. The identification aids in the diagnosis of disease caused by bacteria belonging to the genus Chlamydia and provides epidemiological information on these diseases. Chlamydia are the causative agents of psittacosis (a form of pneumonia), lymphogranuloma venereum (a venereal disease), and trachoma (a chronic disease of the eye and eyelid).

(b) *Classification.* Class I (general controls).

11.2.4.2 Canada

- Medical Devices Regulations (SOR/98-282) [9] SCHEDULE 1 (Section 6) Classification Rules for Medical Devices Part 2, *in vitro* Diagnostic Devices Use With Respect to Transmissible Agents
- **Rule 2(b) (ii):**

An IVDD that is intended to be used to detect the presence of, or exposure to, a transmissible agent is classified as Class II, unless

(a) it is intended to be used to detect the presence of, or exposure to, a transmissible agent that causes a life-threatening disease if there is a risk of propagation in the Canadian population, in which case it is classified as Class IV; or

(b) it falls into one of the following categories, in which case it is classified as Class III:

(i) it is intended to be used to detect the presence of, or exposure to, a transmissible agent that causes a serious disease where there is a risk of propagation in the Canadian population,

(ii) **it is intended to be used to detect the presence of, or exposure to, a sexually transmitted agent,**

(iii) it is intended to be used to detect the presence of an infectious agent in cerebrospinal fluid or blood,

or

(iv) there is a risk that an erroneous result would cause death or severe disability to the individual being tested, or to the individual's offspring.

11.2.4.3 EU

Directive 98/79/EC [3] — Annex II — List of Devices Referred to in Article 9(2) and (3)

- **Rule: List B**
  - — Reagents and reagent products, including related calibrators and control materials, for determining the following blood groups: anti-Duffy and anti-Kidd,
  - — reagents and reagent products, including related calibrators and control materials, for determining irregular anti-erythrocytic antibodies,
  - — reagents and reagent products, including related calibrators and control materials, for the detection and quantification in human samples of the following congenital infections: rubella, toxoplasmosis,
  - — reagents and reagent products, including related calibrators and control materials, for diagnosing the following hereditary disease: phenylketonuria,
  - ⇒ **reagents and reagent products, including related calibrators and control materials, for determining the following human infections: cytomegalovirus, chlamydia,**
  - — reagents and reagent products, including related calibrators and control materials, for determining the following HLA tissue groups: DR, A, B,
  - — reagents and reagent products, including related calibrators and control materials, for determining the following tumoral marker: PSA,
  - — reagents and reagent products, including related calibrators, control materials and software, designed specifically for evaluating the risk of trisomy 21,

— the following device for self-diagnosis, including its related calibrators and control materials: device for the measurement of blood sugar.

11.2.4.4 Singapore

Health Sciences Authority GN-14 Guidance [4] on the risk classification of *in vitro* Diagnostic Medical Devices

- **Rule: 2**

Tests to detect infection by HIV, HCV, HBV, HTLV. This Rule applies to first-line assays, confirmatory assays and supplemental assays.
Rule 2: IVD medical devices intended to be used for blood grouping, or tissue typing to ensure the immunological compatibility of blood, blood components, cells, tissue or organs that are intended for transfusion or transplantation , are classified as **Class C,** except for ABO system [A (ABO1), B (ABO2), AB (ABO3)], rhesus system [RH1 (D), RH2 (C), RH3 (E), RH4 (C), RH5 (e)], Kell system [Kel 1 (K)], Kidd system [JK 1 (Jka), JK2 (Jkb0)] and Duffy system [FY1 (Fya), FY2 (Fyb)] determination which are classified as Class D.

Rationale: The application of this rule as defined above should be in accordance with the following rationale: A high individual risk, where an erroneous result would put the patient in imminent life-threatening situation places the device into Class D. The rule divides blood-grouping IVD medical devices into two subsets, Class C or Class D, depending on the nature of the blood group antigens the IVD medical device, is designed to detect, and its importance in a transfusion setting.

11.3 Medical Device Classification: Practical Examples

Figures 11.3–11.8 provide examples of the way to use the classification decision trees provided in the various guidelines when classifying a medical device. These examples focus on one type of medical device (i.e. a syringe). Depending on its intended use, a simple syringe can be classified in each of the categories, from the lowest one (lower risk) to the highest one (higher risk). The rules taken as reference for this case study are the ones from the European regulation as laid down in Appendix IX of the Medical Devices Directive 93/42/EEC with the supporting charts from the MEDDEV 2.4/1 Rev. 9 Guidance [6].

Syringe without needle

↳ Intended use: **channel or store substances which will eventually be administered to the body; typically, it can be used in transfusion, infusion, extracorporeal circulation**

Invasive?

↳ NO

↳ Rule 2: Channelling or storing for eventual administration

↳ **Class I**

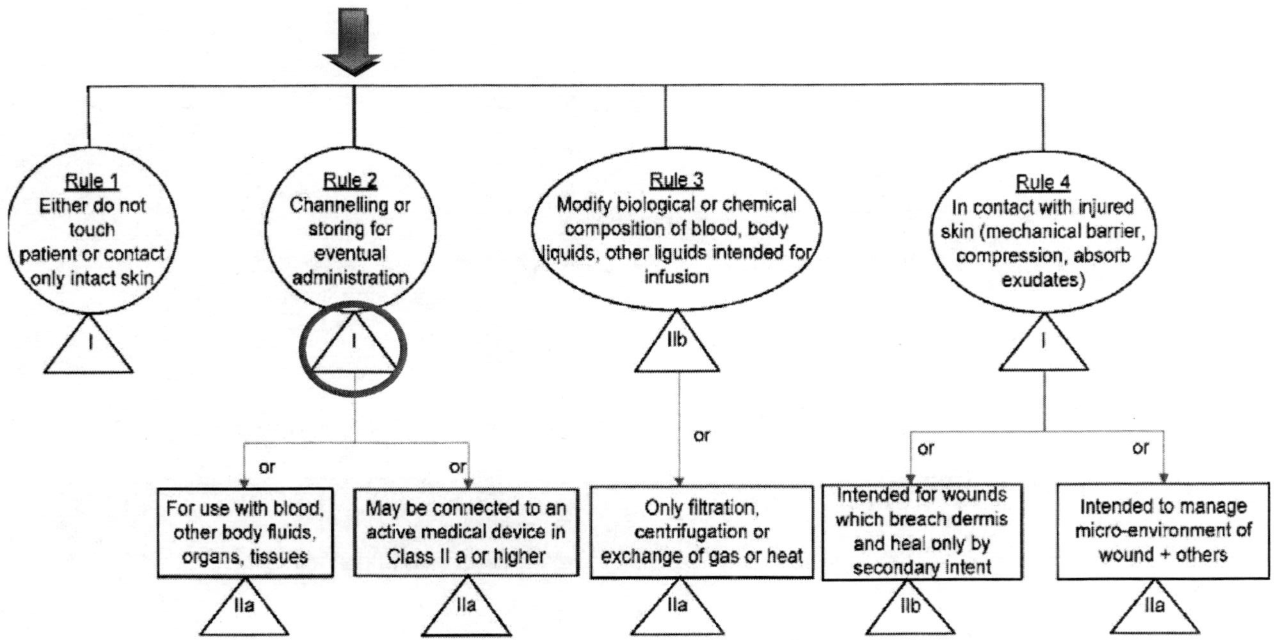

Figure 11.3 MEDDEV 2.4/1 Rev. 9 — Non-Invasive Devices.

Syringe without needle

↳ Intended use: **channel or store substances which will eventually be administered to the body; to be used on infusion pumps**

Invasive?

↳ NO

↳ Rule 2: Channelling or storing for eventual administration

It may be connected to an active medical device (infusion pump)

↳ **Class IIa**

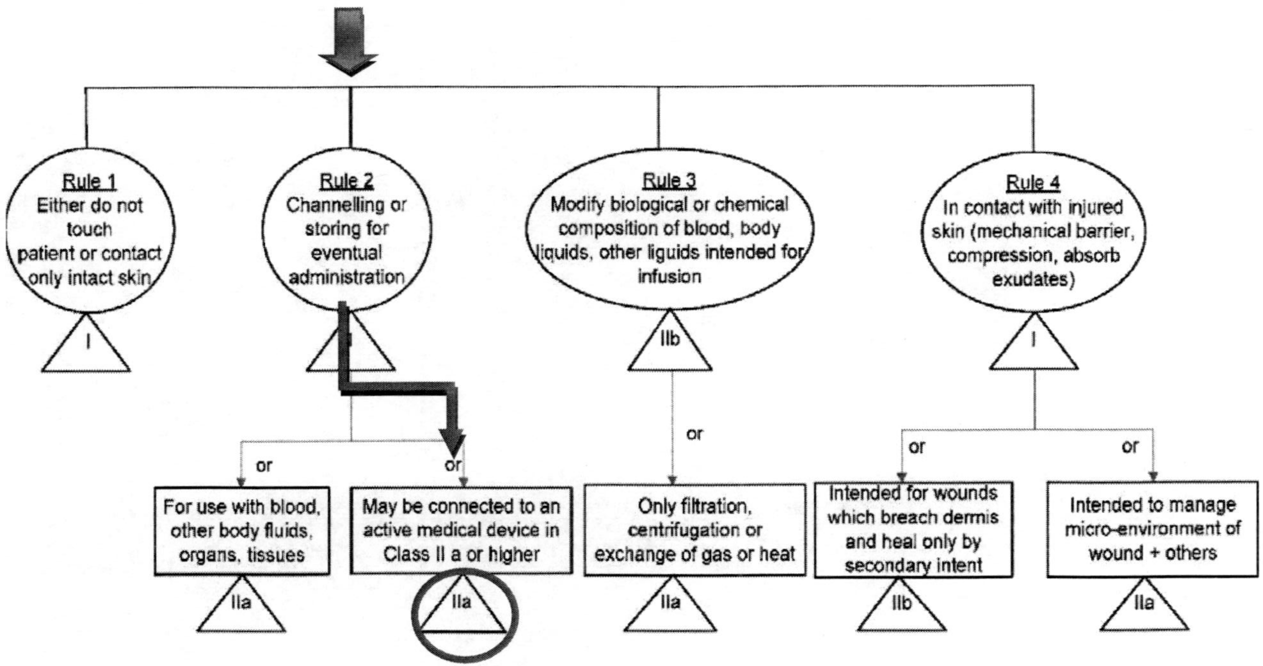

Figure 11.4 MEDDEV 2.4/1 Rev. 9 — Non-Invasive Devices

Syringe without needle

↳ Intended use: **deliver oral medication**

Invasive?

↳ YES

Invasive in body orifice?

↳ YES

Transient Use?

↳ YES (the the syringe is aimed to be used for less than 60 minutes)

Class I

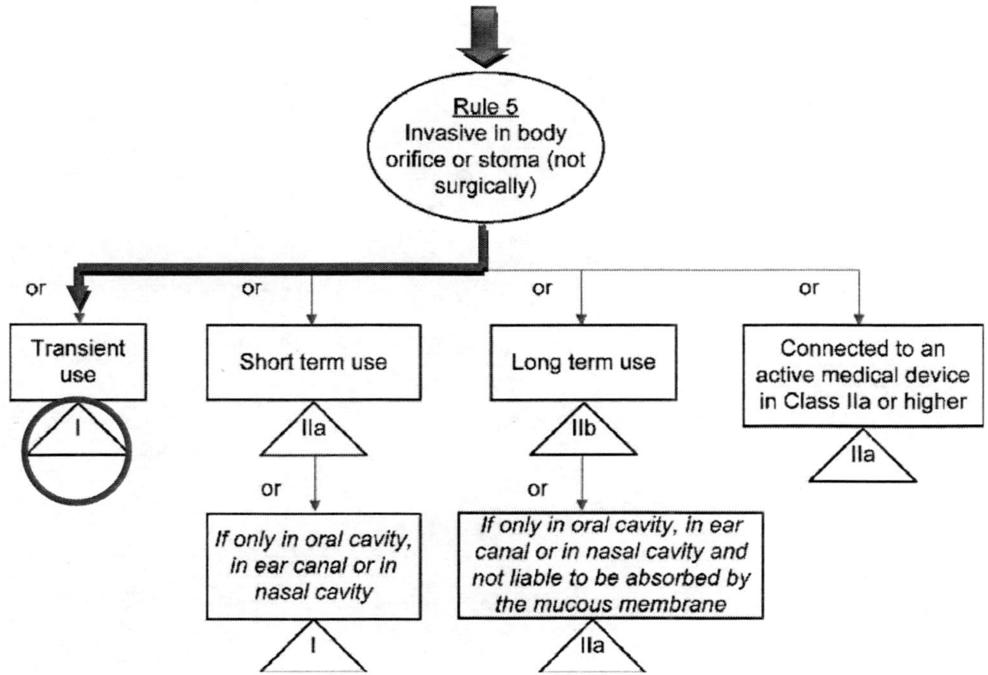

Figure 11.5 MEDDEV 2.4/1 Rev. 9 — Invasive Devices.

Syringe with needle

↳ Intended use: **to administer substances to the body**

Invasive?

↳ YES

↳ Invasive in body orifice?

↳ NO

Surgically invasive?

↳ YES

Transient Use?

↳ YES (the syringe is aimed to inject medicine for less than 60 minutes)

↳ Class IIa

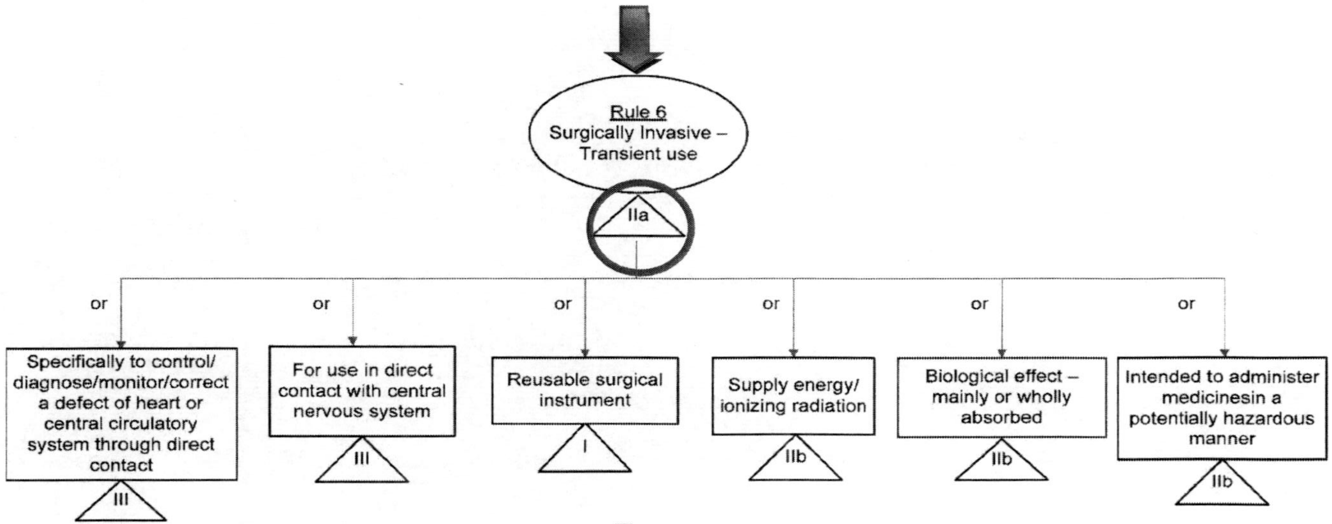

Figure 11.6 MEDDEV 2.4/1 Rev. 9 — Surgically Invasive Devices.

Syringe with needle

↳ Intended use: **to administer or withdraw substances in the spine**

Invasive?

↳ YES

↳ Invasive in body orifice?

↳ NO

Surgically invasive?

↳ YES

Transient Use?

↳ YES (the syringe is aimed to be in contact with the body in less than 60 minutes)

For use in direct contact with the Central Nervous System

↳ **Class III**

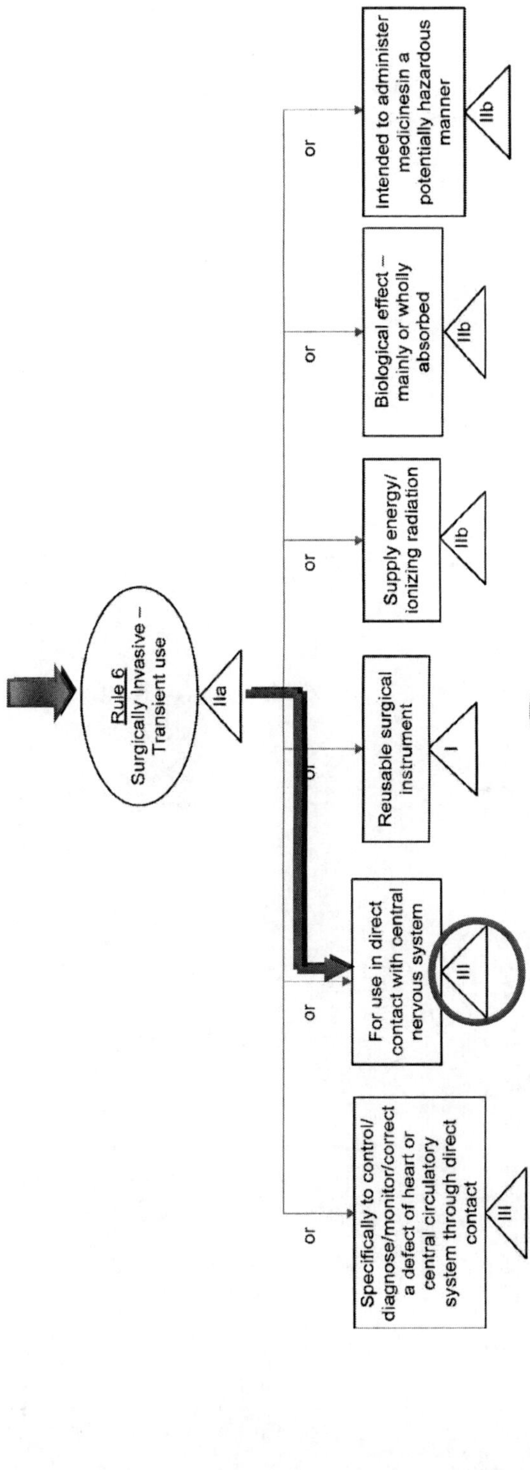

Figure 11.7 MEDDEV 2.4/1 Rev. 9 – Surgically Invasive Devices.

Syringe without needle, pre-filled with Sodium Chloride Solution

⮡ Intended use: **to rinse vascular access devices**

Mechanical?

⮡ YES (rinsing, flushing catheters)

⮡ Device incorporating a substance, which, if used separately, can be considered to be a medicinal product, and which acts on the human body with an ancillary action

Class III

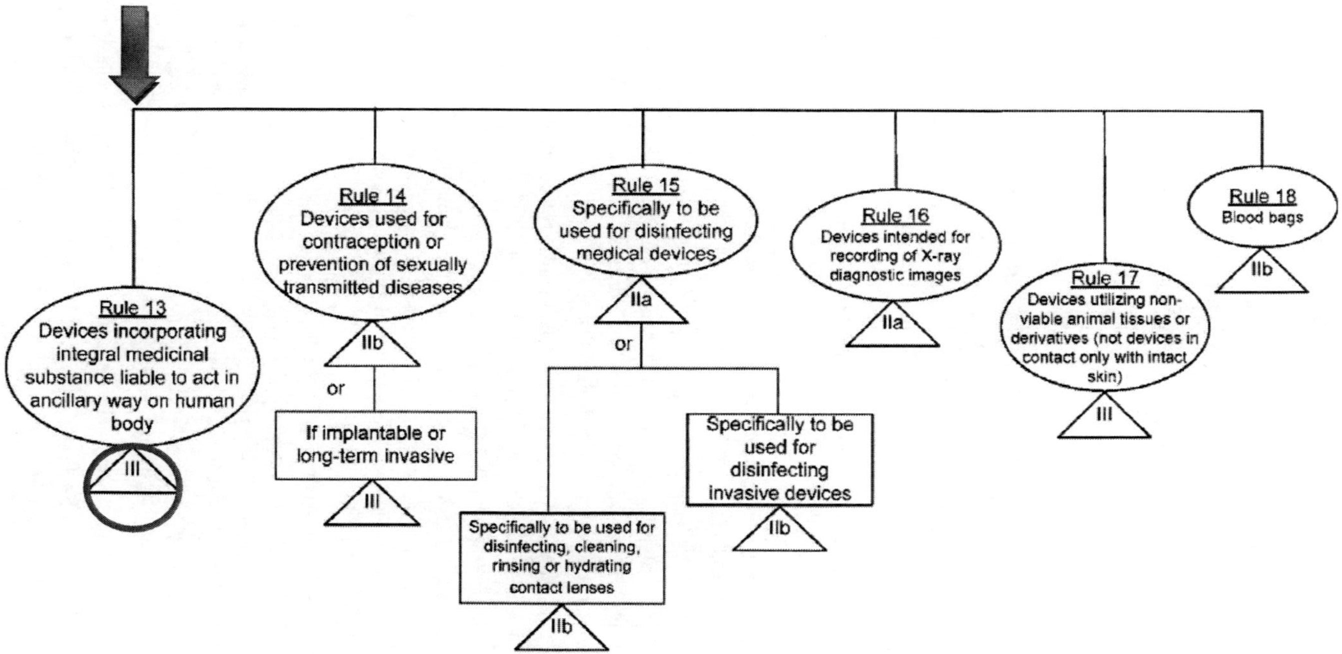

Figure 11.8 MEDDEV 2.4/1 Rev. 9 — Special Rules.

Note: If the syringe is prefilled with a drug, the entire combination is reviewed under the pharmaceutical legislation in Europe. If it would be filled with degradable hyaluronic acid for injections in knees as lubricant, they would be class III, based on rule 8; filled with bovine collagen they would be class III under rule 17 and animal tissue directive would be applicable as well.

References

1. Classification of Medical Devices in Europe — An Overview Dr Jaap Laufer, President, European Medical Device Consultants (EMDC).
2. Council of the European Parliament (5 September 2007) Directive 2007/47/EC of the European Parliament and of the Council of 5 September 2007 amending Council Directive 90/385/EEC on the approximation of the laws of the Member States relating to active implantable medical devices, Council Directive 93/42/EEC concerning medical devices and Directive 98/8/EC concerning the placing of biocidal products on the market, *Official Journal of the European Communities* OJ L247 p. 21.
3. Council of the European Parliament (27 October 1998), Directive 98/79/EC of The European Parliament and of The Council of 27 October 1998 on *in vitro* diagnostic medical devices, *Official Journal of the European Communities* OJ L331 p. 1.
4. GN-14 Guidance on the Risk Classification of *In Vitro* Diagnostic Medical Devices Revision 1 (2008). Medical Device Guidance, Health Sciences Authority, Singapore.
5. Guidance Notes: GN-01 Overview of the Medical Device Administrative Control System Government of the Hong Kong Special Administrative Region, The People's Republic of China Date of Issue: 1 September 2005, Department of Health.
6. European Commission — DG Health and Consumer — Directorate B, Unit B2 "Cosmetics and medical devices" — June 2010 MEDDEV 2. 4/1 Rev. 9 — Guidelines Relating to the Application of the Council Directive 93/42/EEC on Medical Devices, OJ L 169, 12.7.1993, p. 1.
7. Principles of IVD Medical Devices Classification SG1 Final Document GHTF/SG1/N045:2008, Global Harmonization Task Force.
8. SG1(PD)/N77R4 Global Harmonization Task Force — (Revision of GHTF/SG1/N15:2006) Title: Principles of Medical Devices Classification — Authoring Group: Study Group 1 of the Global Harmonization Task Force — Date: October 3, 2011.

9. Medical Devices Regulations (SOR/98-282) Schedule 1 (Section 6) Classification Rules for Medical Devices Part 2, *in vitro* Diagnostic Devices Use With Respect To Transmissible Agents. Retrieved 06 April 2012, from: http://laws.justice.gc.ca/eng/regulations/SOR-98-282/page-23.html#h-68.
10. Title 21 — Food And Drugs: Chapter I —Food And Drug Administration Department Of Health And Human Services Subchapter H—Medical Devices Part 866 — Immunology And Microbiology Devices Subpart D — Serological Reagents Sec. 866.3120 Chlamydia Serological Reagents. Code of Federal Regulations, Revised as of April 1, 2011, CITE: 21CFR866.3120. Retrieved 06 April 2012, from: http://www.accessdata.fda.gov/scripts/cdrh/cfdocs/cfcfr/CFRSearch.cfm?fr=866.3120.

Chapter 12

ISO 13485:2003 Medical Devices — Quality Management Systems — Requirements for Regulatory Purposes

Ann Goodall and Gert Bos

British Standards Institution (BSI) — Healthcare,
Kitemark Court, Davy Avenue, Knowlhill, Milton Keynes, MK5 8PP, UK

ann.goodall@bsigroup.com, gert.bos@bsigroup.com

This chapter describes the origin, implementation and use of the quality management system requirements in medical device globally based on a commonly used standard 13485 [1].

12.1 Introduction

A standard is, in essence, an agreed repeatable way of doing something. It is a document, published after collective work from one or more committees, which contains a technical specification or other precise criteria designed to be used consistently as a rule, guideline, or definition. Standards help make life simpler and to increase the reliability and the effectiveness of many goods and services we use. Standards are created by bringing together the experience and expertise of all interested parties such as the

Handbook of Medical Device Regulatory Affairs in Asia
Edited by Jack Wong and Raymond K. Y. Tong

ISBN 978-981-4411-21-9 (Hardcover), 978-981-4411-22-6 (eBook)
www.panstanford.com

producers, sellers, buyers, users and regulators of a particular material, product, process or service.

Standards are designed for voluntary use and do not impose any regulations. However, laws and regulations may refer to certain standards and make compliance with them compulsory.

The current basis for quality management systems is ISO 9000, which was first published in 1987. ISO 9001, which was based on the BS 5750 series of standards from the British Standards Institution (BSI), was proposed to ISO in 1979. However, Historically, ISO 9000 can be traced back some twenty years before that, to the publication of the UK Department of Defence MIL-Q-9858 standard in 1959 that through the NATO AQAP series of standards in 1969, the BS 5179 series of standards (1974), led to the development of BS 5750.

BSI has been certifying organizations for their quality management systems since 1978, and the first ever issued certification (FM 00001) still exists.

12.2 Background and Origins of ISO 13485:2003

ISO 13485:2003 is a Quality Management System (QMS) for medical devices specifically for regulatory purposes and whilst based upon the ISO9001:2000 quality management system standard is a standalone standard.

ISO13485:1996 was published by the International Standards Organisation Technical Committee 210 Working Group 1, following alignment with ISO9001:1994 — Quality Systems — Requirements. During December 2000, ISO 9001:2000 was published replacing the ISO9001:1994 series. There was a three-year transition period before the 1994 versions (ISO9001:1994 — complete MS-, EN ISO 9002:1994 — exclusion or design — and EN ISO 9003:1994 — exclusion for design and manufacturing) were withdrawn for those organisations that were already certified to the standards. The ISO 13485:1996 standard made reference to ISO9001 throughout and as such was not a standalone standard, but rather provided additional requirements for the medical device industry. There was also ISO 13488:1996, which was aligned to ISO 9002:1994, in essence focussing on all QMS aspects with the exception of design.

During April 2000, ISO 13485:1996 and ISO 13488:1996 were adopted as European standards and replaced the then existing sector specific European standards (i.e. EN 46001, EN46002, EN46003). Europe changed the harmonised reference to the European medical Devices Directives to the ISO series away from the European Norms.

ISO 13485:2003 is published by various organisations and when it is published by those organisations, this is recognised by letters being placed before the ISO 13485:2003. For example in the United Kingdom it is published by British Standards Institution (BSI) and this is denoted by the Standard being BS ISO 13485:2003 and as it is also a European Norm it is published as BS EN ISO 13485:2003.

Some of the changes that had been introduced with the publication of ISO9001:2000, including the reduction in the number of required documented procedures and the inclusion of concepts such as customer satisfaction and continual improvement, were not in alignment with the regulatory requirements for medical devices. The option of revising ISO 13485 and ISO 13488 in alignment with ISO 9001:2000 was considered but thought not to be appropriate and so the Technical committee decided that ISO 13485 should become a standalone standard (Fig. 12.1). This meant that in order to fulfil the regulatory requirements organization did not have to have certification to ISO 9001 as well as ISO 13485/8.

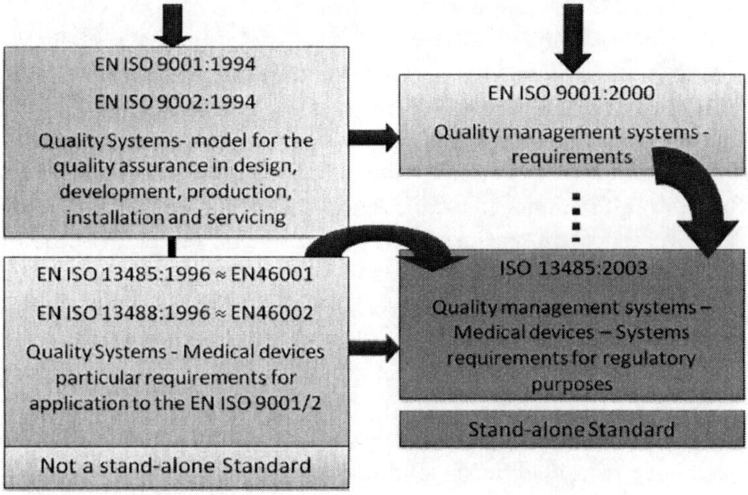

Figure 12.1 Initiation of a standalone healthcare QMS standard.

The standard ISO 13485:2003 Medical Devices — Quality Management Systems — Requirements for Regulatory Purposes is now becoming the certification standard of choice for medical device manufacturers. The requirements are specific to organisations that are providing medical devices or services to the medical device industry and this does not depend on the size or type of the organisation.

12.3 Management Systems Standard [2]

While ISO 13485:2003 is a standalone standard, it is based on ISO 9001:2000. Sub-Clause 3.1 of ISO 13485:2003 explains that those (sub-) clauses in ISO 13485:2003 quoted directly and unchanged from ISO 9001:2000 are in normal font. Where the text of ISO 13485:2003 differs from the text of ISO 9001:2000, the sentence or indent containing the text as a whole is shown in blue italics. The nature and reasons for the differences are noted in Annex B of the standard, providing further insight useful in implementing ISO 13485:2003.

The main difference between ISO 13485:2003 and ISO 9001:2000 is related to customer satisfaction and continuous improvement. These are not included in ISO 13485:2003. In ISO 13485:2003, processes are required for ensuring continuing effectiveness of the quality system to meet customer and regulatory requirements instead of continual improvement. The standard also promotes active systems for customer feedback related to if the organization is meeting customer and regulatory requirements.

In addition, the requirements of ISO 13485:2003 include many more requirements for documented procedures, documented requirements and records. This is due to the nature of the standard, i.e., it is there to support meeting regulatory requirements.

The relationship between ISO 9001:2008 and ISO 13485:2003 is evaluated in more detail in ISO/TC 210 N382 — Explanation of Differences Between ISO 13485:2003 and ISO 9001:2008. In moving ISO 9001 to the next level, there might well be more divergence between the two related standards in the future, as elements of added value auditing that might be introduced in ISO 9001 would not be directly related to the purpose of meeting regulatory requirements that forms the basis of ISO 13485.

12.4 Quality Management Systems

Quality management systems consist of common elements that are expressed as the organizational structure, processes, procedures, work instructions and resources needed to implement quality management (Fig. 12.2).

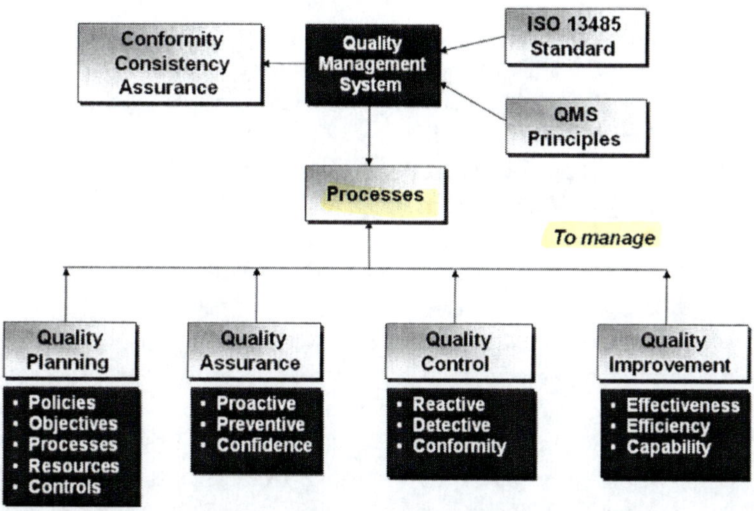

Figure 12.2 Essence of quality management system.

Shared elements of the organizational structure, authorities and responsibilities, methods and processes, data management, resources, training, maintenance, customer satisfaction/requirements, product quality and continuous improvement are based on eight principles of quality management:

(i) **Customer and regulatory focus**: By understanding current and future customer needs, organisations can meet their requirements whilst ensuring that all known applicable regulations are applied.

(ii) **Leadership on purpose and direction**: Leaders, by establishing unity of purpose and direction of the organization, should create and maintain the internal environment in which people can become fully involved in achieving the organizations objectives.

(iii) **Involvement of people at all levels**: People are the essence of an organization and their full involvement enables best performance in the organisation.

(iv) **Process approach to resources and activities**: This principle commonly leads to the PDCA approach of Plan–Do–Check–Act.

(v) **Systems approach to management**: The core in the system's smooth running is identifying, understanding and managing inter-related processes of a system as it contributes to the organizations effectiveness and efficiency in achieving its objectives and reducing overall process risks.

(vi) **Factual approach to decision making**: Decisions based on analysis of data and information are typically more effective. Monitoring and measuring will allow an organization to understand its ability to supply a safe and effective product and service.

(vii) **Mutually beneficial supplier relationships**: An organization is responsible for ensuring control of its outsourced processes, and with increasing regulatory pressure, supply chain management truly becomes one of the keys to success.

(viii) **Improvement as an ongoing objective**: Long withheld in medical device industry, legislation is now changing to stimulate product improvement in a continuous effort.

12.5 ISO 9000 and ISO 13485 Quality Management System Family of Standards

ISO 13485:2003 is commonly seen as part of the 9000 series of standards, despite it being a standalone standard. This means that effective implementation can best be achieved by combining the requirement of ISO 13485 with the content, views and guidance of a series of adjacent standards, representing further detail and in some cases national variations:

(i) BS EN ISO 9000:2000 describes the fundamentals and vocabulary.

(ii) BS EN ISO 9001:2000 provides the basic QMS requirements.

(iii) BS EN ISO 9004:2000 provides guidelines for performance improvement beyond general QMS requirements.

(iv) BS EN ISO 19011:2011 provides guidelines for quality and/or environmental management systems auditing, including internal audits.

(v) ISO/TR14969:2004 provides guidelines for application of ISO13485:2003.

In addition there is a standard used to supervise third party assessment bodies that audit against e.g. ISO13485:2003:

(i) ISO/IEC 17021:2006 provides requirements for bodies providing audit and certification of management systems.

12.6 ISO 13485:2003 and Regulatory Requirements Around the World

With the increasing use of ISO13485:2003 by regulatory authorities worldwide, the use of the standard by manufacturers and other organizations is increasing. ISO13485:2003 supports the regulatory compliance in several countries including the European Union for CE marking, Australia, Canada and Taiwan. Japanese Ministerial Ordinance (MO) No. 169 is similar to ISO 13485. In Europe it is a harmonised standard for the three medical devices directives, which means that adhering to it for the quality management systems aspects identified in these directives there is a presumption of conformity, details of which are specified in the so-called annexes Z found at the back of the European versions of the standards. For the USA ISO 13485:2003 is an option and may typically be the basis for the QMS that is used by many manufacturers, but it is not a distinct requirement. It can also be used for low risk devices manufacturers that are exempt from QSR's 21 CFR 820. The US FDA has been cooperating closely with the development of ISO 13485, in the attempt to further align ISO 13485 and QSR (Quality System Regulations) requirements.

With the growing interest in regulatory regimes in the Middle East, Asia, Africa, and Latin America, many more regulatory requirements are added to the equation. ISO 13485:2003 certification is a great tool to harmonise the various QMS requirements from all these existing and developing legislations, as it is very easy for national regulators to add some country specific requirements to the general framework provided in the global standard.

12.7 Good Reasons to Implement an ISO 13485:2003 Quality Management System

There are various reasons why an organisation implements a certified ISO13485:2003 quality management system, and this primarily includes meeting regulatory requirements when registering medical devices worldwide. In addition, it might help improve customer confidence and increase the organisation's competitive edge. As such it makes good business sense and forms an excellent basis for an efficient and effective business to be certified against ISO 13485:2003.

A well-implemented ISO13485-based QMS supports regulatory compliance and improves customer confidence. It improves the consistency and stability of the processes used by the organisation. It can reduce waste and defects and improve employee motivation and participation and is a basis for monitoring, managing or potentially improving the performance of suppliers.

12.8 Process Approach

A process is a set of interrelated or interacting activities that uses resources to transform inputs into outputs. The process approach systematically identifies and manages the linkage, combination, and interaction of a system of processes within an organization, as depicted in Fig. 12.3, linking the various parts of ISO 13485:2003 in a generic process flow. The QMS documentation will reflect the actual process flows of the particular organisation.

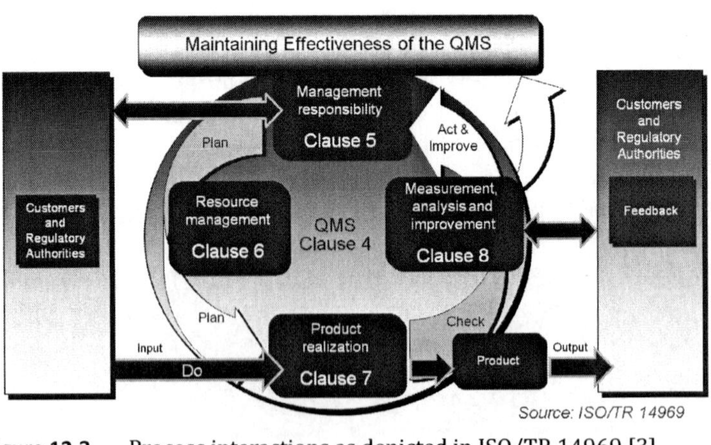

Figure 12.3 Process interactions as depicted in ISO/TR 14969 [3].

The process model of the Plan–Do–Check–Act cycle is used in the ISO13485:2003 standard to link Clauses 4 to 8 of the standard (Fig. 12.4). It is used to show how the requirements of customers and regulatory authorities can be meet.

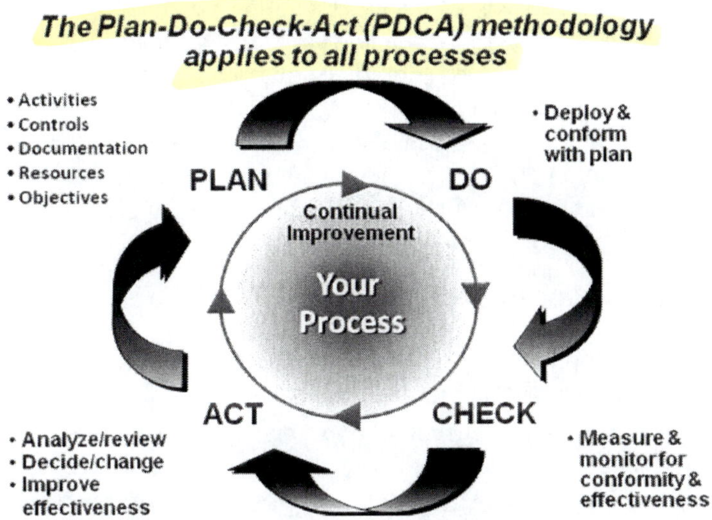

Figure 12.4 PDCA for your processes.

The process approach considers the importance in understanding and meeting requirements by looking at processes in terms of the value that they can add, in measuring the performance of processes, determining if that process is effective and by the use of the objective measurement of processes to improve that process.

12.9 Planning the Implementation

The implementation process begins with the assumption that the decision to implement has already been taken. Best practice traces back the origin of the decision to implement and the underlying causes or views, such as supply chain requirement, regulatory requirement, or desire to improve performance, reduce waste, etc.

Some initial general steps for a successful implementation effort would include knowing how to interpret the ISO 13485:2003 requirements for your system, ensuring team members are knowledgeable on the current system, arranging management commitment, and developing a comprehensive project plan which includes monitoring steps. Where needed training should be provided to staff to enhance their knowledge and to boost their commitment which is crucial to the successful implementation and continuing compliance to the requirements of the standard.

Key elements would include promoting awareness, performing a critical gap analysis and following effective implementation of course getting ready for continually improving the system, where regulatory requirements allow.

The ultimate assessment and verification of the first implementation is in a round of internal audits followed by a management review concluding the effectiveness of the QMS.

12.10 Scope, Exclusions and Non-Applicability

ISO 13485:2003 can be applied to any organisation who wishes to demonstrate the ability to provide medical devices and/or related services that meet customer and regulatory requirements ISO 13485:2003. ISO13485:2003 can be applied irrespective of type or size. Providing it is permitted in the regulatory requirements that apply to the organisation that is implementing ISO13485:2003 exclusions are permitted. Organisations can exclude design and development controls, Clause 7.3 but the justification for the exclusions must be clearly documented in the organisations quality system and must be an appropriate exclusion for any regulatory system being followed. Other clauses can be excluded if they are not applicable, e.g. sterilisation if the manufacturer does not produce sterile medical devices.

12.11 Document Control

To be efficient and effective, an organisation has to manage how to ensure that those working within that organisation carry out the process in a consistent way. This includes both large and small organisations. In a large organisation, this means that tasks are completed in the same systematic way. Large organisations or those with complicated processes will benefit significantly with the adoption and implementation of an appropriate quality management system.

Section 4.2 of ISO13485:2003 describes the requirements for documents and records that are used to support the quality management system, which very often is divided into four tiers with their own types of documentation (Fig. 12.5).

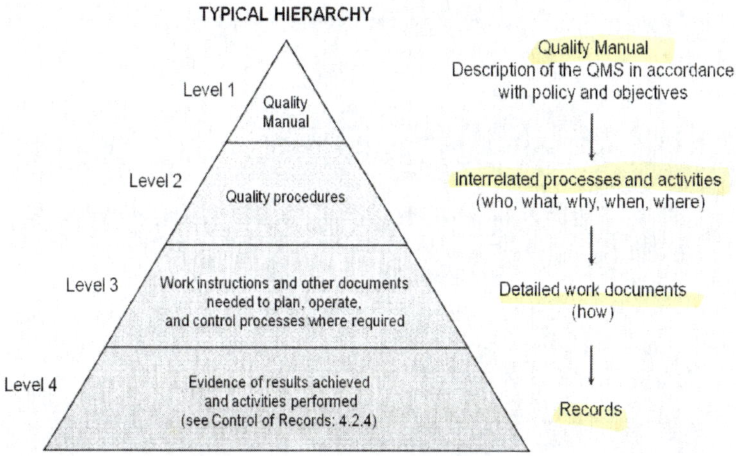

Figure 12.5 Typical four-tier quality management system setup.

12.12 Record Completion and Control

Quality records are an important part of any quality management system and especially in ISO13485:2003 as they are the evidence that that activities that are required as part of the quality management system have been completed. Requirements for records are referenced in at least 50 places within the standard, but many organizations will have the need for records for other aspects of the quality management system due to the nature of the business.

12.13 Management Responsibility

The emphasis in Clause 5 is on the role of top management of the organisation within the quality management system in ensuring that the system remains effective and is maintained and that customer and regulatory requirements are met by the organisation.

Top management has to ensure that the organisations quality policy is defined and that this is linked to the quality objectives of the organisation. A management representative is appointed by top management.

Reviews are conducted at planned intervals and in the standard the aspects of the quality management system that should be considered at these reviews are defined.

12.14 Resource Management

It is important for any organisation to have adequate resources to be able to meet the customer and regulatory requirements and these needs to ensure that the requirements of the products are met. These should include the effective initiation of the resources and their continued maintenance to support the processes of the quality management system. It is the role of top management to ensure that the appropriate resources are available.

There are many aspects to resources they can be people, infrastructure, work environment, information, suppliers and partners, natural and financial resources. Even if these resources are outsourced they have to be managed by the organisation like the processes that are within the organisation.

12.15 Product Realisation

Product realisation includes all the processes that bring the product or service to the customer. These include planning, understanding customer requirements, communicating with customer, the design and development of the product or service, purchasing of the materials and services, production/manufacturing, delivery of the products/service and calibration of any equipment that is used.

12.16 Risk Management [4, 5]

The only place where risk management is identified within ISO 13485:2003 is under the planning of product realisation. Risk management is a requirement throughout product realisation.

The requirements for risk management must be documented and records of the risk management must be retained. It ultimately forms the basis of the decision to place a product on the market or to refrain from it, depending on the outcome of the final risk to clinical benefit evaluation (Fig. 12.6).

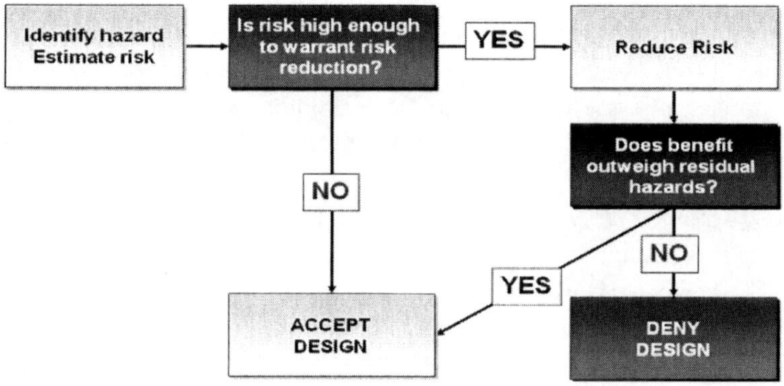

Figure 12.6 Essential steps in risk management.

There is a standard which gives guidance on risk management: ISO 14971:2007 Medical Devices — Application of Risk Management to Medical Devices. Further guidance on how to integrate risk management throughout the entire QMS can be found in GHTF guidance from Study Group SG3.

12.17 Design and Development

The design and development process includes all aspects of the process of bringing the product or service from the original concept of the idea and ensuring that is in line with the user and regulatory requirements through to that product or service that is available to customer and then how any changes to that design are managed.

In order to do this, there are various aspects that are identified within the requirements of ISO 13485:2003. These are:

(i) Planning
(ii) Inputs
(iii) Outputs
(iv) Review
(v) Verification
(vi) Validation
(vii) Control of change

12.18 Purchasing and Supplier Control [6]

The management of suppliers and the materials or services received from those suppliers is critical to the organization and the quality of the product and service supplied by the organization to their customers.

The GHTF has published guidance on the Control of Products and Services Obtained from Suppliers. The guidance describes the process of establishing controls for products and services obtained from suppliers. This typically comprises six phases as follows:

(i) Planning
(ii) Selection of potential supplier(s)
(iii) Supplier evaluation and acceptance
(iv) Finalization of controls
(v) Delivery, measurement and monitoring
(vi) Feedback and communication, including corrective action and preventive action process

When an organization outsources the process, they still remain responsible for that process. They must ensure that the processes remain suitable and effect as part of the quality management system. They need to ensure that that the product requirements are not effected as a result of outsourcing that process as the manufacturer is responsible for the product throughout the time the product is being managed by the subcontractor. For example, if the design process is being out sourced the business that is outsourcing the process would need to have involvement in defining the design inputs to ensure that the customer and regulatory requirements are met. Other key processes that may be outsource or subcontracted are sterilization or distribution

12.19 Production and Service Provision

The standard clearly calls out to plan and carry out provisions under controlled conditions, including availability of information describing product characteristics, availability of documented procedures, work instructions, and reference standards, use of suitable equipment and use of measuring and monitoring devices. As for controlled environments used, there is no clear guidance, but applied conditions should be found suitable in the process risk assessment and appropriate to the final use of the device.

Clearer requirements are provided on the validation need for the processes for production and service provision (usually following a master validation plan approach), identification and traceability, customer property including drawings and IP, and the preservation of the product.

For many medical devices, ensuring that the device is stored and handled so that the performance of the device is maintained is important. Preservation of products covers many perspectives including storage at the defined temperature, making sure the product remains sterile, protection of fragile products. In order to be able to do this, the organisation has to understand the requirements specific to the product, for example, what temperature range the product should be stored at and how the product should be protected if it is fragile. Any special storage conditions have to be controlled and recorded. What this means is that the area where the product is stored it need to be known to be capable of maintaining that temperature range throughout whether is it a refrigerator or freezer or a walk-in freezer and it has to have been qualified to show that it maintains the temperature range throughout.

12.20 Monitoring and Measuring, Including Internal Audits and Management Review

The quality management system needs to be implemented to a high level before internal audits are conducted. Of course, to conform to ISO 13485:2003, an internal audit program must be operational, helping the organization investigate any quality problems and verify solutions are effectively implemented. Periodic audits also keep the quality awareness level of staff high and foster improved internal communications.

The internal audits are expected to cover all areas and all shifts, auditing some areas more often based on previous results, whilst increasing audit frequency for changed or high-risk areas. ISO 19011 can serve as guidance.

Based on the internal audits and further management information, top management arranges the management review to come to a supported conclusion towards the (continuing) effectiveness of the QMS as well as to ensure continuing suitability. The standard identifies minimum requirements to be taken into the review including also any new or revised regulatory requirements for any country the company sells products or provides service to. Records of such reviews are kept, including action lists and their follow up activities.

12.21 Control of Non-Conforming Product

Non-conforming product needs to be identified and controlled to prevent its unintended use or delivery. Controls and responsibilities need to be defined in a documented procedure that should arrange for action taken to eliminate the detected non-conformity and for the authorization of non-conforming product's use, release or acceptance by concession. Such acceptance of non-conforming product by concession can only be signed off if regulatory requirements, including a dedicated risk assessment, are met and the identity of the person authorizing the concession is identified and recorded.

12.22 Analysis of Data

The intent of this section is to stimulate the manufacturer to collect and analyze data on the quality system, both from the inside (e.g. production inspections), as well as from external sources which include complaint handling and more active ways of post market surveillance. It further supports the demonstration of the suitability and effectiveness of the QMS. In many cases, a selection of the analysed data might well be used to stimulate quality awareness and motivate staff to further improve quality and efficiency.

12.23 Improvement: Corrective Action and Preventive Action

Following the documented procedure for corrective action and recording the results of the action taken will allow quick identification of any findings in one area. This can potentially help the remaining areas to avoid a similar problem (and reduce the number of reported non-conformities in ISO 13485:2003 certification assessments). The correction is the immediate remedy to a non-conformity, e.g. clearing an uncontrolled messy area. The corrective action, which follows the root cause analysis (e.g. using the five-why method), is the sum of measures that will ensure the same non-confirming situation does not re-occur. A different part of the improvement system are the preventive actions, which in a similar way work to ensure a non-conforming situation does not occur, but based on rationales and other input, not stemming from an existing non-conformity.

Clear distinction should be made between cases where some non-conforming situation was found, where correction and or corrective action to prevent reoccurrence are warranted, and the cases where no non-conformity was found but where preventive action can prevent a non-conformity from happening at all.

12.24 Purpose and Goal of ISO 13485:2003 Certification

Formal certification is achieved only through external (third party) assessment by a Certification Body. Certification can only be achieved after correct preparation for the initial audit, which is a two-stage event comprising a readiness review followed by a complete in-depth audit of all applicable areas of the standard.

Benefits of certification include expanded access to world markets, the improved ability to bid for contracts, the use as a market differentiator. The display of the certification mark (e.g. a symbol granted by the certification body which usually is a combination of the registrar's logo and ISO13485) and the evidence of independent audits by professional, independent certification bodies designated by an accreditation agency can help to provide a much greater trust in the company's ability to provide a consistent high quality product or service.

These benefits clearly outweigh the barriers to certification such as the difficulty to identify and create new processes for the system, development of the necessary documented procedures and instructions and the resistance by some employees to change (and process measurements) that are found in most organisations.

12.25 Achieving Certification and Continuing to Maintain Certification

For an organization to be ready for certification, it is important that they have fully implemented an ISO13485:2003 QMS and are using the system. When the QMS is being assessed for certification, the certification body considers two aspects:

(i) Are all the requirements included in the QMS? This will be completed by the review of the QMS as it is documented and by review of the internal audits and management reviews that have taken place. This is often called a stage 1 assessment or document review.

(ii) The second stage of the certification process is to show the effectiveness of the processes that have been put in place to meet the requirements of the standard. During this assessment, the organisation has to demonstrate the continual improvement of the quality management system. This is stage 2 of the assessment.

An organisation needs to be sure that they are ready to demonstrate both of these aspects. Often organisations try to complete the process too quickly and do not have sufficient evidence of the working of the QMS to demonstrate compliance.

Other pitfalls are as follows:

(i) There is insufficient awareness throughout the organisation.

(ii) Top management have not been sufficiently involved to show that they are taking top management responsibility seriously.

(iii) There has been insufficient training throughout the organisation to understand what is required.

(iv) The requirements especially related to Clauses 6 and 7 have not been related to the products or services that the organisation is manufacturing or delivering.

(v) Internal audits have not been completed of the whole QMS.

(vi) Appropriate metrics and measures have not been put in place for the analysis of data.

Once an organisation has received its assessment and achieved certification to ISO1345:2003, this is not the end of the process. The continuing process of maintaining certification begins as part of the continual improvement process.

Becoming certified to ISO13485:2003 is a significant achievement for an organisation and is a cause for celebration. When the celebrations are over, it is important for everyone in the company to realise that maintaining the effective implementation of the quality management system is just as important. This includes understanding that it is a continuous process that everyone is committed to and involved in to ensure that the requirements of the quality management system continue to be met.

References

1. ISO 13485:2003 — Medical Devices — Quality Management Systems — Requirements for Regulatory Purposes.
2. ISO/TC 210 N382 — Explanation of Differences between ISO 13485:2003 and ISO 9001:2008.
3. ISO /TR 14969:2004 — Medical Devices — Quality Management Systems — Guidance on the Application of ISO 13485: 2003.
4. GHTF SG3/N15R8/2005 — Implementation of Risk Management Principles and Activities within a Quality Management System.
5. ISO 14971:2007 — Medical Devices — Application of Risk Management to Medical Devices.
6. GHTF/SG3/N17:2008 Quality Management System — Medical Devices — Guidance on the Control of Products and Services Obtained from Suppliers.

Chapter 13

ISO 14971: Application of Risk Management to Medical Devices

Tony Chan[a,b,c] **and Raymond K. Y. Tong**[d,e]

[a]*Virginia Tech, 21520 Yorba Linda Blvd. Suite G288, Yorba Linda, CA 92887, USA*
[b]*US Co-Chair, ISO TC 210 JWG1 Risk Management*
[c]*US Expert Member, IEC TC 56 WG4 Dependability Management*
[d]*Hong Kong Polytechnic University, Hung Hom, Hong Kong*
[e]*Asia Regulatory Professional Association (ARPA)*

chant@vt.edu, tchan@agsm-inc.com, k.y.tong@polyu.edu.hk

13.1 Introduction

The development of ISO 14971 was not carried out in a vacuum but instead was shaped by precedent activities in the European Union (EU) to establish risk management standards quite early in the 1990s. The first step made by the EU was the publication in 1997 of a European Standard, EN (European Norm) 1441 on Risk Analysis for Medical Devices. The framework focused on using a specific set of methods called Failure Mode and Effect Analysis (FMEA), for medical device risk analysis. ISO adopted this European Standard in 1997, when it essentially duplicated its publication under the title "*Medical Device — Risk Analysis*," ISO 14971-1. This standard was useful for prioritizing activities but remained incomplete because of its focus on the particular use of a single approach,

Handbook of Medical Device Regulatory Affairs in Asia
Edited by Jack Wong and Raymond K. Y. Tong

ISBN 978-981-4411-21-9 (Hardcover), 978-981-4411-22-6 (eBook)
www.panstanford.com

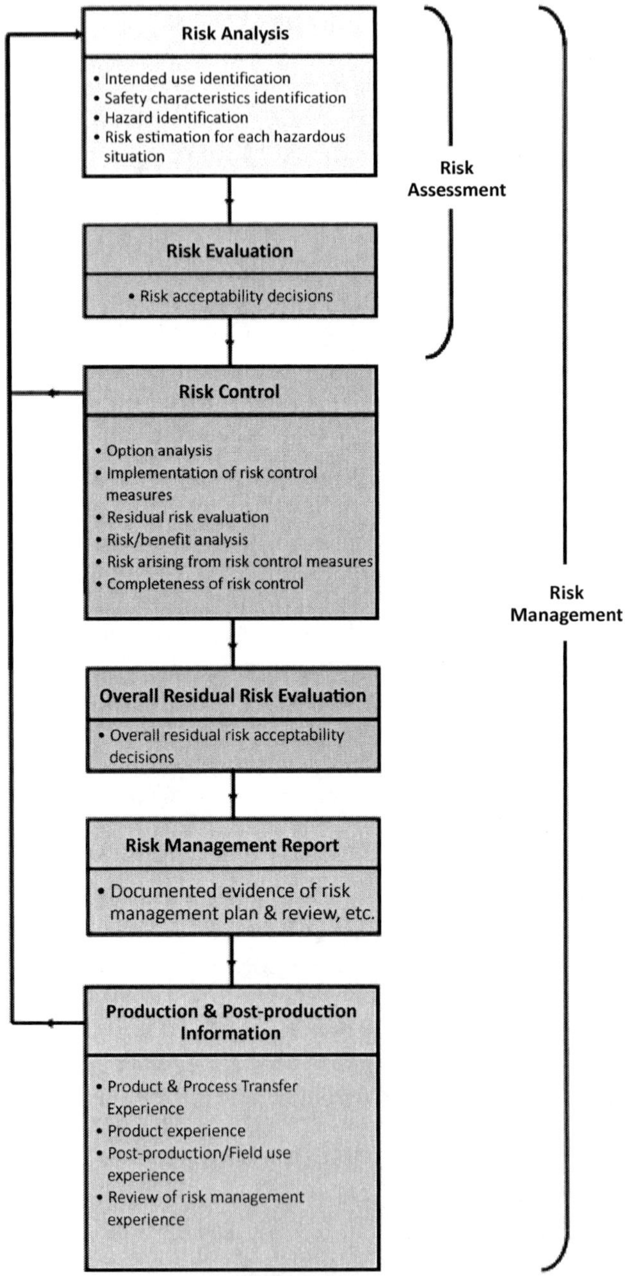

Figure 13.1 ISO 14971 Risk Management Process.

namely FMEA. Thus, a working group was formed to incorporate risk management practices already defined in the IEC 60601 Standard Series, a set of standards focusing on medical electrical equipment, into its new international standard, designated as ISO 14971, in 2000. This standard then replaced the ISO/IEC 14971-1 standard and was recognized as both a European-harmonized standard (GHTF SG3/N15R8:2005 [1]) and an FDA-recognized standard. It emphasized a more complete risk management framework, shown in Fig. 13.1.

The ISO 14971 Standard includes all the basic principles of risk management that are applicable to medical devices. It specifies the steps required for identifying hazards, estimating risk, evaluating risk, and controlling risk. A medical device manufacturer's risk management process must include these steps. The new standard has two important aspects that deserve special mention. First, the standard expands the scope and potential approaches to the risk management process that enables manufacturers to satisfy the essential requirements of the medical device directives of the EU. These directives have similar authorities in the EU as the US Code of Federal Regulations in the United States. Essential requirements are necessary elements for protecting the public interest in the EU, are mandatory for product compliance before they are put into commerce and must be applied as a function of the hazards inherent to a given product.

Second, the standard deemphasized the use of FMEA, which is recommended only if it fulfills appropriately the particular risk analysis task under study; many other analytical approaches are acknowledged to potentially be suitable to achieve the same end. The expanded scope of the standard emphasizes management responsibilities. The standard stipulates that management responsibility is the initial and key requirement. More precisely, management must incorporate the following tasks:

(1) defining policies for determining acceptable risk
(2) ensuring the provision of adequate resources, including the identification of a risk management team
(3) ensuring the assignment of trained personnel to perform risk assessment and management activities
(4) reviewing the results of risk management activities at defined intervals to ensure the effectiveness of the risk management process

The expanded scope also mandates implementation of the following records:

(1) risk management plan
(2) risk management file
(3) risk management report
(4) production and post-production information

These requirements are interesting because they draw attention to the fact that risk management rests on more than having a framework, but also on a human dimension where the activities of people must be directed and organized. Currently, the ISO 14971 Standard has just gone through a second edition that incorporated only minor changes from the initial edition; however, the volume of explanation of the stipulated framework in the second edition has increased almost three-fold (from 22 pages to 65 pages). The ISO 14971:2007 *"Application of Risk Management to Medical Devices"* [2] stipulates an expectation of a risk management framework that considers the total lifecycle of the product. It includes a risk management process, and defines executive responsibilities, personnel qualifications for performing risk management activities, and the documentation needed to provide a record of risk management activities. Some limitations in the document are still perceived by some to exist. For example, it does not provide guidance with respect to clinical decisions that may be a significant part of the risk/benefit analysis. In fact, the EU is currently challenging the committee on the sufficiency of the guidance with regard to risk/benefit analysis. In addition, some readers of the standard can develop the false impression that it only addresses the design control elements of a quality management system because manufacturing only appears once in the text although it is in fact mentioned a further twenty times in the annexes of the document which are provided for explanations but not requirements.

In summary, the ISO Standard provides a framework to the medical device manufacturers for effective management of the risks associated with the use of their products and within which experience, insight, and judgment are applied systematically to manage these risks. It also helps practitioners to identify processes by which they can identify hazards associated with a medical device, estimate and evaluate the risks associated with these hazards, control these risks, and monitor the effectiveness of that control.

13.2 The Foundation of a Risk Management (RM) Framework: Policy, Plan, Team, Process, and Documentation

The foundation of an RM framework consists of five elements: (1) policy, (2) plan, (3) team, (4) process, and (5) Documentation.

13.2.1 Policy

A risk management policy is essential to a company that operates on RM. This policy should take into account of relevant international, national, or regional standards and regulations. It should define how to determine acceptable risk and include the review of results of risk management activities at defined intervals. The review ensures the continuing suitability and effectiveness of the RM process. Moreover, the policy should be established before or at the time of implementation of the RM process. The RM process should not begin without such policy in place.

13.2.2 Plan

The company should establish a risk management plan for every product based on its risk management process. This plan [1] should

(a) identify and describe the product
(b) define a scope
(c) state verification activities
(d) indicate roles and responsibilities of the allocated resources
(e) define intervals for review
(f) specify criteria for risk acceptability
(g) record the plan changes and its revision

13.2.3 Team

A description of each of the RM team members' roles and responsibilities should be defined and recorded. It is a part of the evidence to demonstrate sufficient resource is allocated for risk management activities.

13.2.4 Process

A medical device company should establish a process describing how, what, and when risk management activities are carried out during the entire product life cycle (See Fig. 13.1 and Section 13.3). At the broadest level, the RM process consists of a four-part, continuous-management process: (1) analyze risk, (2) evaluate risk, (3) control risk, and (4) get feedback from both production and post-production information. The next section describes the details of each major activity of the process.

13.2.5 Documentation

Documentation can be electronically stored records or paper records. It provides objective evidence for regulatory compliance as well as for legal purposes. The documentation should include policy, procedures, plans, and records of all risk management activities during the entire product life cycle.

13.3 The RM Process

13.3.1 Analyze Risk

This initial task involves the following steps:

(a) Familiarize yourself with the product.

It is important to understand thoroughly the requirements of developing a product before the start of any risk management activities. The background understanding of requirements, such as marketing, performance, functional, regulatory, legal, etc., would provide a firm foundation for those who are engaged in the risk management activities.

(b) Understand intended purpose and use.

In addition to aforementioned requirements, the intended purpose and use of a product provide a boundary and scope for the subsequently risk management activities. Understanding the medical purpose, anatomy and/or organs of body affected, patient profile, user profile, and application environment of the product forms the basis to initiate hazard identification and for carrying out further risk management activities.

(c) **Identify hazards and hazardous situations.**

In the framework of the Standard, hazard is defined as the potential source of harm; harm is physical injury or damage to the health of people, property, or the environment. Thus, one should focus on identifying the immediate source or a situation(s) that causes the hazard that results in harm, i.e., the hazard or hazardous situation. It is also beneficial to distinguish that a failure may not cause harm or directly cause harm.

(d) **Estimate risk.**

Once a hazard or hazardous situation is identified, its consequence or severity of harm and probability of occurrence of harm need to be estimated. The consequence or severity of harm of a hazard or hazardous situation could be assessed directly and immediately. However, the probability of occurrence of harm may be an indirect assessment since the harm is related to the hazard and the hazard is related to the product. The risk level of a hazard or a situation(s) that initiate the hazard would then be estimated based on the probability of occurrence and severity of that harm posed by the hazard or the hazardous situation.

13.3.2 Evaluate Risk

This subsequent activity after risk analysis is to make an acceptability decision. Consequently, there are many actions need to be taken depending upon the level of risk on each of the identified issues. Generally, there are three kinds of actions. First, the risk could be accepted without further actions. Second, the risk is so high that control measures must be taken to reduce it to an acceptable level. Lastly, the risk is at a marginally acceptable or unacceptable level. It requires further investigation, either conduct a risk/benefit analysis before making accept or reject decisions, or implement further risk control measure(s) to reduce the risk to an acceptable level.

13.3.3 Control Risk

After the initial risk analysis and evaluation, risk control measures may be deemed necessary to maintain, reduce or eliminate the risk. In the framework of the Standard, risk has two components: the probability of occurrence of harm and the severity of that harm. Therefore, a risk control measure could either affect the probability of occurrence of the harm or the severity of that harm. Generally, it is much easier to work on maintaining or minimizing the occurrence aspect of the harm. It would take relatively much more resources and efforts in reducing or eliminating the severity of harm. In fact, risk control is aiming at controlling the identified hazards and the hazardous situations that are causing harm.

The Standard is very specific about how risk should be controlled. It stipulates an Option Analysis [1] that requires a hierarchy of priority order when approach to risk control measures. Risk control measure(s) should be considered in the following priority order:

(a) inherent safety by design (the most preferred risk control measure)
(b) protective measures in the product or in the manufacturing process
(c) information for safety (the last resort for risk control measure)

It is indispensable to ensure the implementation of these risk control measures have taken place as well as to demonstrate their effectiveness after implementation. Objective evidence of implementation and demonstration of effectiveness of these measures should be documented.

In practice, risk analysis, risk evaluation, and risk control are steps of an iterative process. These activities may happen at least three times in a product development process. Initial risk is analyzed, evaluated for acceptance the first time and then risk control measures are considered as necessary for each hazard and hazardous situation. Then, residual risk needs to be analyzed and evaluated for acceptance as related to each individual hazard after the control measures are applied. This process continues until the residual risk is judged acceptable. Finally, a review of the overall residual risk, i.e., the accumulation of all the residual risks posed by each individual hazard after effective control measure(s) is applied, should take place. This is when a company decides whether a product is safe for use.

If an individual residual risk or the overall residual risk [1] is judged unacceptable using the policy or criteria pre-established by the company and further risk control is impractical, the company may gather and review data and literature on the medical benefits of the intended purpose and use of the product to determine if they outweigh the residual risk. If the evidence does not support the conclusion that the medical benefits outweigh the residual risk, then the risk remains unacceptable. The project should be cancelled or the product needs redesign. If the medical benefits outweigh the residual risk, then the company should document all the evidence to support the acceptability decision. This iterative process should continue until all individual residual risk and the overall residual risk are judged acceptable before the commercialization of a product.

13.3.4 Feedback from Production and Post-Production Information

In this part of the risk management process, the focus is on information received after all risk control measures are deployed. When considering the entire product life cycle, the company should establish and maintain a systematic process. It could be a well-developed information system, to review information gained about the product after development. This information should include information from design and process validation, product transfer, design to production, vendor to company, company to vendor, outsourced activities, production activities, field use, etc. The information should be evaluated for possible relevance to safety [1] especially the following:

(a) if previously unrecognized hazards are present
(b) if the estimated risk(s) arising from a hazard is no longer acceptable
(c) if the original assessment is otherwise invalidated

If any of the above conditions is satisfied, the results of the evaluation should be fed back as an input to the risk management process. A review of the appropriate steps of the risk management process for the product should be considered. If there is a potential that the residual risk(s) or its acceptability has changed, the impact on previously implemented risk control measures should be evaluated.

The above four risk management activities are integral parts of a continuous process improvement within a management system. Certain activities may be initiated out of the aforementioned order.

They are useful if applied appropriately, especially early in the product development process.

13.4 Conclusion

RM is about focusing on the number of safety issues to the vital few that will make a difference. A comprehensive RM framework helps a company gain confidence that it understands those risks that really matter to avoid unacceptable and unexpected crises or surprises. The framework also helps the company know how to avoid, eliminate, or contain the causes or drivers of those significant risks that may cripple the business if they were neglected. It also provides a basis for measuring, comparing, controlling, monitoring, and preventing those risks that have the potential to exhibit significant negative impact to the company.

In conclusion, RM is a disciplined, structured, and scientific approach that provides a proactive business strategy to enable a company to manage and prevent potential crisis and create a sustainable strategic advantage while maximizing shareholder value. Through the RM process, a company is better able to protect and secure its value, guard its growth potential, and hedge against market, capital, operational, and financial volatility.

13.5 Case Study — An Example to Illustrate Risk Management on a Medical Device: Functional Electrical Stimulation System for Walking

Functional electrical stimulation (FES) is generally referred to as an artificial electrical stimulation of a muscle that has diminished nervous control, with the aim of providing muscular contractions and producing functionally useful movements. The FES is a technique that uses bursts of short electric pulses to generate muscle contractions by stimulating motor-neurons or reflex pathways.

A FES system for walking consists of a main unit, a control sensor, and adhesive surface electrodes connected with wires (Fig. 13.2). The surface electrodes are located on the surface of the skin, above a targeted muscle or nerve. With regard to the lower limbs, drop-foot is a common clinical feature of those who have suffered from stroke, which is characterized by the inability to dorsiflex the foot during the swing phase of gait. People affected tend to have a labored and unsafe gait, and compensatory movements such as hip hiking and limb circumduction may occur. The intended use of an FES drop-foot stimulator system is to correct the problem of drop-foot by stimulating the ankle dorsiflexors or the common peroneal nerve to achieve toe clearance (Fig. 13.3). The stimulation of the hemiplegic leg can be controlled by a heel-switch worn on the hemiplegic side. When the switch is on the hemiplegic side, stimulation is initiated by a heel off and terminated by a heel strike. The effectiveness of the system is to save effort in walking, increase the patient's ability to walk, and reduce spasticity.

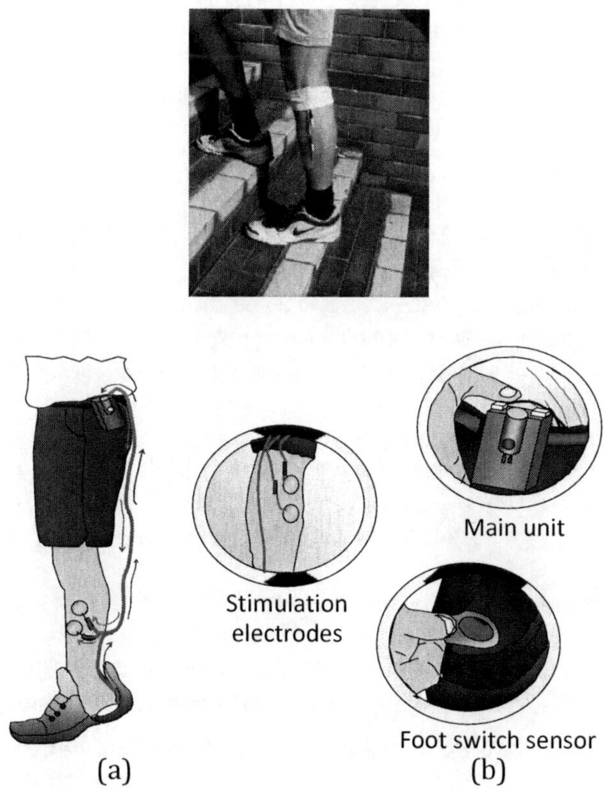

Figure 13.2 Using FES for walking.

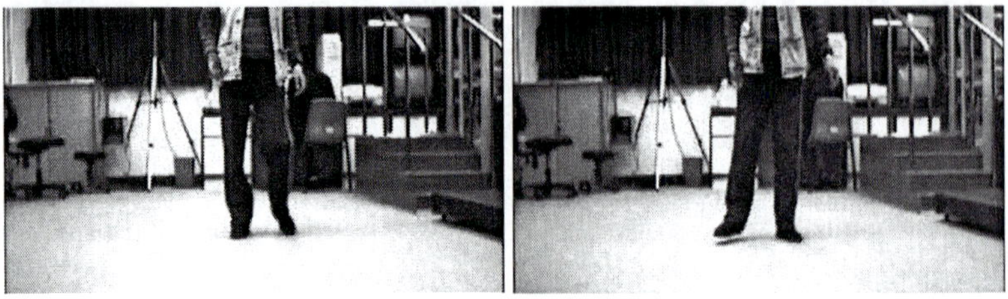

(a) (b)

Figure 13.3 Right hemiplegic stroke patient: (a) without FES and drop foot on the right side; (b) with FES system to correct drop foot problem.

13.5.1 Risk Management Process

Step 1: Intended use/intended purpose

- For the particular medical device or accessory being considered, the manufacturer shall describe the intended use/intended purpose and any reasonably foreseeable misuse. They should also have a list of all those qualitative and quantitative characteristics that could affect the safety of the medical device and, where appropriate, their defined limits.

The intended use of the FES drop-foot stimulator system is to correct the problem of drop-foot by stimulating the ankle dorsiflexors or the common peroneal nerve to achieve toe clearance. The timing of stimulation is controlled by a heel-switch worn on the hemiplegic side. Electrical stimulation is initiated by a heel off and terminated by a heel strike in every walking step on the hemiplegic side.

The FES system only can be applied on stroke patients with drop foot problem by a trained clinician/rehabilitation engineer. The patients must be trained by the clinician/rehabilitation engineer before they can take the device back home for training and daily use.

The FES stimulation parameters are 40 Hz with adjustable pulse width of the stimulation pulse (100–500 us) and the maximum stimulation intensity is 100 mA. These parameters are safe and they are currently use in clinical/hospital for rehabilitation with FES.

Step 2: Identification of known or foreseeable hazards

- The manufacturer shall compile a list of know or foreseeable hazards associated with the medical device in both normal conditions and fault conditions.

Example of Hazards

1. Surface stimulation electrodes are placed on the wrong position on the skin and cause injury.
2. There are three connection ports on the FES main unit and they are connected wrongly: one is connected to the stimulation electrodes, another one is for foot switch and last one is for computer data transfer.
3. The output electrical stimulation is too high and cause injury.
4. Patient pressed or turned wrong button to change the FES parameters, which causes injury.
5. There is skin allergy to the surface electrode.

Step 3: Estimation of risks for each hazard

- ISO14971: For each indentifies hazard, the risk(s) in both normal and fault conditions shall be estimated using available information or data. The hazard is combined with the hazard severity and the probability of occurrence (Tables 13.1 and 13.2).

Estimated Risk = (Estimated hazard Severity) × (Estimated Probability of Occurrence)

Each manufacturer is free to define his own category system (Tables 13.1 and 13.2) and has to recorded these in the risk management file.

Table 13.1 Example of five qualitative severity levels (ISO 14971:2007 Table D.3)

Common terms	Possible description
Catastrophic	Results in patient death
Critical	Results in permanent impairment or life-threatening injury
Serious	Results in injury or impairment requiring professional medical intervention
Minor	Results in temporary injury or impairment not requiring professional medical intervention
Negligible	Inconvenience or temporary discomfort

Table 13.2 Example of semi-quantitative probability levels (ISO 14971: 2007 Table D.4)

Common terms	Examples of probability range
Frequent	$\geq 10^{-3}$
Probable	$<10^{-3}$ and $\geq 10^{-4}$
Occasional	$<10^{-4}$ and 10^{-5}
Remote	$<10^{-5}$ and $\geq 10^{-6}$
Improbable	$<10^{-6}$

Step 4: Risk Evaluation

- For each identified hazard, the manufacturer shall decide the criteria in the management file to consider whether the estimated risk(s) is needed to have risk reduction or not (Tables 13.3 and 13.4).

Table 13.3 Estimation of risks for each hazard

Hazards	Severity	Probability
R1. Surface stimulation electrodes are placed on the wrong position	Serious	Remote
R2. The three connection ports on the FES main unit are connected wrongly with wires	Minor	Probable
R3. The output electrical stimulation is too high	Serious	Remote
R4. Patient pressed or turned wrong button to change the FES parameters	Serious	Probable
R5. Skin allergy to the surface electrode.	Minor	Occasional

Table 13.4 Risk evaluation

Qualitative severity levels

Semi-quantitative probability levels	Negligible	Minor	Serious	Critical	Catastrophic
Frequent					
Probable		R2	R4		
Occasional		R5			
Remote			R1, R3		
Improbable					

Key

Unacceptable risk
Investigate further risk reduction
Insignificant risk

Step 5: Risk Control

- The manufacturer shall identify risk control measure(s) that are appropriate for reducing the risk(s) to an acceptable level. Risk control shall use the following in the priority order listed:

(1) inherent safety by design
(2) protective measures in the medical device itself or in the manufacturing process
(3) information for safety

R2, R3, R4, and R5 are using inherent safety by design to reduce the risk and R1 are using information for safety.

Step 6: Implementation of risk control measure(s)

- The manufacturer shall implement the risk control measure(s) selected in step 5.

Implementation of risk control measure(s) (Table 13.5)

R1: A qualified trained clinician/rehabilitation engineer shall provide information sheet and taught the patients on how to place the stimulation electrode correctly.

Table 13.5 Table with risk mitigation measures

Semi-quantitative probability levels	Qualitative severity levels: Negligible	Minor	Serious	Critical	Catastrophic
Frequent					
Probable					
Occasional					
Remote		R5	R4		
Improbable		R2	R1, R3		

Key

Unacceptable risk
Investigate further risk reduction
Insignificant risk

R2: The connection ports are designed only one plug can fit in one socket for all the three ports (Fig. 13.4).

R3: The system use standard 9 V battery and the circuit can only generate maximum 100 mA. And the stimulation pulse width can be changed by the clinician through an FES program software only.

R4: Patient can only change the stimulation amplitude in a limited range, and all the parameters are pre-programmed by the clinician.

R5: Biocompatible electrode for clinical use on surface electrical stimulation shall be used. They will receive the biocompatible standard.

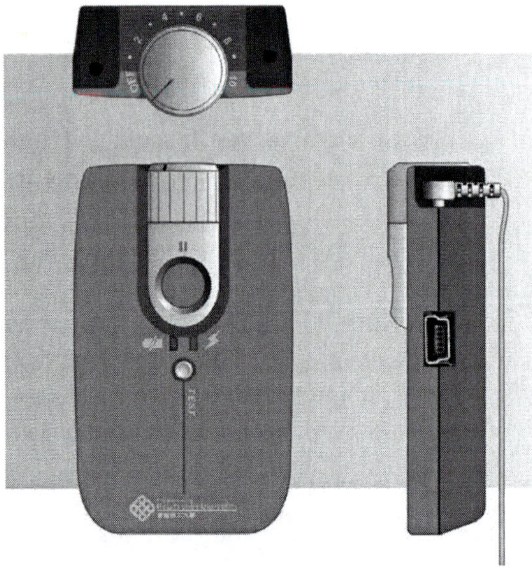

Figure 13.4 The connection ports are designed only one plug can fit in one socket. And the patient can only adjust the stimulation intensity in the limited range on a knob from 0 to 10.

Step 7: Residual risk evaluation

- Any residual risk that remains after the risk control measure(s) are applied shall be evaluated using the criteria defined in the risk management plan. If the residual risk does not meet the criteria, further risk control measures shall be applied.

  The residual risk is judged acceptable for the FES system.

References

1. GHTF (2005). SG3/N15R8:2005 Implementation of risk management principles and activities within a Quality Management System, Global Harmonization Task Force.
2. ISO 14971:2007 — Application of Risk Management to Medical Devices.
3. ISO/IEC Guide 51:1999 — Safety Aspects — Guidelines for their inclusion in standards.

Part 3

Harmonization of Medical Devices in Asia

Chapter 14

Medical Devices in the World Health Organization

Adriana Velazquez Berumen[a] and Jack Wong[b]

[a]*HSS/EHT/DIM, World Health Organization,*
20 via Appia, 1211 Geneva, Switzerland
[b]*Asia Regulatory Professional Association (ARPA)*

velazquezberumena@who.int, speedxquality@yahoo.com

The World Health Organization (WHO) is the directing and coordinating authority for health within the United Nations system. It is responsible for providing leadership on global health matters, shaping the health research agenda, setting norms and standards, articulating evidence-based policy options, providing technical support to countries and monitoring and assessing health trends.

The World Health Assembly approved 13 "core functions" for strategic objectives in 2006, the number 11 is to improve access to effective, quality and safe medical products.

The medical devices unit of the WHO had been hosted in the Essential Health Technologies unit since 2006. Then in 2012, with the dissolution of the Health Technologies Department, the medical devices unit became part of the Essential Medicines and Health Products Department under the Health Systems and Innovation cluster.

Handbook of Medical Device Regulatory Affairs in Asia
Edited by Jack Wong and Raymond K. Y. Tong

ISBN 978-981-4411-21-9 (Hardcover), 978-981-4411-22-6 (eBook)
www.panstanford.com

The World Health Assembly recognized that medical devices are indispensable for health care delivery under prevention, diagnostics, treatment and rehabilitation. In response to the WHA60.29, the health technologies resolution that was approved by all 194 member states in 2007, it has been developing four major activities:

1. **Assessing the global situation on medical devices**
   - The first-ever global Baseline Country Survey on Medical Devices was launched in February 2010. Respondents from 146 countries identified the key areas requiring support; in 2011, 171 countries responded. This survey contains information about the health technology policies, lists of medical devices for reimbursement, and focal points in the regulatory agency, in the health technology management, and in the health technology assessment, if they have any of them. It also includes the census of health care facilities and of five major medical equipment for diagnosis or treatment, such as nuclear magnetic resonance (NMR), radiotherapy or positron emission tomography (PET) scanners.
   - All the information is available on the Internet in the country profiles as well as statistical analysis and maps in the Global Health Observatory in the WHO web page.
2. **Strengthening capacity**
   - In 2011, the WHO launched the *Medical Device Technical Series*. These reference documents provide those in low-resource settings with information and guidance they can adapt to their particular situation. Eight reference documents have been printed that include needs assessment, procurement, donations, maintenance, inventories, health technology assessment, and steps on how to develop policies on medical devices at the country level.
   - The Global medical devices information system will be an online clearing house, requested by the World Health Assembly Resolution WHA60.29 on Health Technologies, in providing evidence based, impartial information on medical devices, tailored to different levels of care and health interventions.

- The Core Medical Equipment Fact Sheets provide technical information on the devices most commonly used in health care facilities.
- The e-Documentation Centre is a centralized repository of more than 300 WHO documents and resources in various languages that relate to health technologies. These are all available on the website.

3. Encouraging innovation

- Medical devices currently on the market do not meet all of the global health needs. The Priority Medical Devices Project proposes a research agenda to inform innovators how best to address this gap
- The Compendium of Innovative Health Technologies showcases medical devices that address health concerns in low-resource settings, in order to promote dialogue between biomedical engineers, ministries of health, donors, innovators, manufacturers and end users. The compendium and the call were done in 2010 and 2011; a new update is available and a 2013 call has been launched.

4. Fostering partnerships

- The WHO Medical Devices Unit coordinates the activities of non-governmental organizations, academia, professional societies, governments, health professionals and WHO Collaborating Centres, in reference to medical devices.
- In September 2010, over 300 participants from around the world gathered in Bangkok, Thailand, for the first WHO Global Forum on Medical Devices, building on three years of intense activity that followed the adoption of the first resolution on health technologies by the World Health Assembly in May 2007. The Second WHO Global Forum on Medical Devices will take place in 2013 and will address regulations, innovations and access to medical devices.
- The WHO, APEC, and AHWP discussed the training strategy and potential needs. The team agreed to work together to generate a "Pilot Medical Device Regulatory Awareness Workshop" and develop a "Joint 5 years training strategy/roadmap".

- WHO is looking into the regulatory convergence and harmonization as a way to increase access to safe and effective medical devices, uptake of core essential medical devices, dissemination of innovation to help target global health concerns.
- WHO has become official observer of IMDRF, International Medical Devices Regulators Forum, which will be following on the implementation of the GHTF documents.
- WHO is working in the update of regulation guidelines, tools, norms and standards and particularly in capacity building.
- WHO encourages that the Biomedical Engineering programmes and curricula worldwide addresses regulations of medical devices, this will then prepare the professionals that are in Academia, research and development, industry or in health care services to be aware of the importance of medical devices regulation, from registration, premarket approval, standards, requirements, to post market surveillance, adverse event reporting through continuous technovigilance monitoring safe and effective use of medical equipment for the well being of the population.
- WHO has been now an official observer of the IMDRF.
- A global action plan is now being developed to follow a five-year strategy and invite all stakeholders to participate in order to increase access to safe, appropriate, and affordable medical devices, particularly to the population in need.

Chapter 15

Asian Harmonization Working Party

Saleh Al Tayyar

Asian Harmonization Working Party
Saudi Food & Drug Authority, Riyadh, Saudi Arabia
AHWP-Chair@sfda.gov.sa

15.1 Introduction

The Asian Harmonization Working Party (AHWP) has been established as a non-profit organization. Its goals are to study and recommend ways to harmonize medical device regulations in the Asian and other regions and to work in coordination with the Global Harmonization Task Force, APEC, and other related international organizations aiming at establishing harmonized requirements, procedures, and standards. The AHWP is a group of experts from medical device regulatory authorities and the medical device industry. Membership is open to those representatives from the Asian and other regions who support the above-mentioned goals.

Handbook of Medical Device Regulatory Affairs in Asia
Edited by Jack Wong and Raymond K. Y. Tong

ISBN 978-981-4411-21-9 (Hardcover), 978-981-4411-22-6 (eBook)
www.panstanford.com

15.2 Future Directions

Organize awareness education, training, and seminars for medical device regulators and industry in the area of regulatory requirements (such as Essential Principles of Safety and Performance of Medical Devices; Classification Rules and risk-based management approach) and premarket review processes. One possibility is to tap the availability of Global Harmonization Task Force (GHTF) Study Group (SG) resource persons on business trips or visits to Asia:

- Define the scope and deliverables and tasks of the Technical Committee, including the conduct and frequency and venue of meetings;
- Seek budgetary and strategic support for AHWP activities and programs;
- Establish an effective communication network and presence among participating Asian economies through scheduled AHWP meeting, e-mails, correspondence, and Internet-based access site;
- Plan for the next AHWP Meeting;
- Work toward enlarging the base of participating economies so as to maximize the benefit of the GHTF harmonization process to Asia.

I am honored to write on behalf of the Asian Harmonization Work Party (AHWP) an introductory note to the *Handbook of Medical Device Regulatory Affairs in Asia*, as part of the Asia Regulatory Professional Association (ARPA) initiative.

This handbook is in line with Asian Harmonization Working Party scope and objectives to harmonize Medical Device Regulation among member economies. The AHWP is a nonprofit organization that was formed by a group of regulators in Asia Pacific around 1996–1997. It aims to develop techniques to harmonize medical device regulations in Asia and other regions, to work in coordination with the Global Harmonization Task Force (GHTF), Asia-Pacific Economic Cooperation (APEC), and other related international organizations aiming at establishing harmonized requirements, procedures, and standards.

The AHWP is planning to organize awareness education, training, and seminars for medical device regulators and industry in the area of regulatory requirements (such as Essential Principles of Safety and Performance of Medical Devices; Classification Rules and Risk-Based Management Approach) and premarket review processes.

The *Handbook of Medical Device Regulatory Affairs in Asia* is intended to give an overview of the medical device regulatory systems in the United States, European Union, Australia, and Japan. It also looks at regulatory frame work in the AHWP member economies, (i.e., China, Hong Kong, India, Indonesia, Jordan, Korea, Malaysia, the Philippines, Saudi Arabia, Singapore, Chinese Taipei, Thailand, the United Arab Emirates (Abu Dhabi), Vietnam, Laos, Cambodia, Brunei Darussalam, Myanmar, South Africa, Yemen, Pakistan, Kuwait, and Chile).

The handbook touches base on important and controversial issues in medical device regulations such as medical device clinical trials, labeling, and language complexity in relation to the intended use, labeling compliance, and access of medical device in developing countries.

A tremendous effort has been made to cover various topics related to medical devices to allow regulatory staff from various levels to benefit from this handbook and consider it one of their main references. Medical Device Safety and Related Standards have also been discussed in this handbook. The handbook also looks at the harmonization of medical devices and examines efforts and contributions by the AHWP, ASEAN, APEC, and GHTF to the medical device harmonization.

The handbook is well structured and organized. The contributions by highly distinguished experts in the field of medical device regulation from all over the world make this book rich in knowledge and an important reference. I hope regulators in developing countries will find it beneficial to them and use it as a tool for benchmarking and guidance in setting up and/or improving their medical device regulations.

In conclusion, I would like to thank everyone who contributed to the development of this handbook.

Chapter 16

Asia-Pacific Economic Cooperation

Lindsay Tao
Corporate Director,
Regulatory Government Affairs at Johnson & Johnson
ltao@jnj.its.com

16.1 Introduction

APEC is the premier forum for facilitating economic growth, cooperation, trade and investment in the Asia-Pacific region. APEC is the inter governmental grouping of 21 members as listed below, which account for approximately 40.5% of the world's population, approximately 54.2% of world GDP and about 43.7% of world trade.

The Asia-Pacific Economic Cooperation (APEC) works in three broad areas to meet the Bogor Goals of free and open trade and investment in the Asia-Pacific by 2010 for developed economies and 2020 for developing economies.

Handbook of Medical Device Regulatory Affairs in Asia
Edited by Jack Wong and Raymond K. Y. Tong

ISBN 978-981-4411-21-9 (Hardcover), 978-981-4411-22-6 (eBook)
www.panstanford.com

Table 16.1 List of member economies constituting APEC

Date of entry	Member states	
1989	Australia	Indonesia
	Brunei Darussalam	Japan
	Canada	Republic of Korea
	The Philippines	Malaysia
	Singapore	New Zealand
	Thailand	The United States
1991	People's Republic of China	Chinese Taipei
	Hong Kong	
1993	Mexico	Papua New Guinea
1994	Chile	
1998	Peru	Vietnam
	Russia	

Known as APEC's "Three Pillars," APEC focuses on three key areas:

- trade and investment liberalization
- business facilitation
- economic and technical cooperation

The outcomes of these three areas enable APEC Member Economies to strengthen their economies by pooling resources within the region and achieving efficiencies. Tangible benefits are also delivered to consumers in the APEC region through increased training and employment opportunities, greater choices in the marketplace, cheaper goods and services and improved access to international markets.

16.1.1 Trade and Investment Liberalization

Trade and Investment Liberalization reduces and eventually eliminates tariff and non-tariff barriers to trade and investment. Protectionism is expensive because it raises prices of goods and services. Thus, trade and investment liberation focuses on opening markets to increase trade and investment among economies, resulting in economic growth for APEC member economies and increased standards of living for all. This goal is also now furthered by APEC's Regional Economic Integration agenda, which includes work on model measures for bilateral and regional trade agreements and an examination of the prospects for a Free Trade Area of the Asia-Pacific.

16.1.2 Business Facilitation

Business Facilitation focuses on reducing the costs of business transactions, improving access to trade information and aligning policy and business strategies to facilitate growth, and free and open trade. Essentially, Business Facilitation helps importers and exporters in Asia Pacific meet and conduct business more efficiently, thus reducing costs of production and leading to increased trade, cheaper goods and services and more employment opportunities due to an expanded economy. APEC's Structural Reform agenda addresses this area: It focuses on reforming domestic policies and institutions that adversely affect the operation of markets, and the capacity of businesses to access markets and to operate efficiently.

16.1.3 Economic and Technical Cooperation

Economic and Technical Cooperation (ECOTECH) is dedicated to providing training and cooperation to build capacities in all APEC member economies to take advantage of global trade. This area builds capacity at the institutional and personal level to assist APEC member economies and its people gain the necessary skills to meet their economic potential.

APEC is a unique forum, operating on basis of

- ***non-binding*** commitments, open dialogue and equal respect for views of all participants
- decisions by consensus; commitments undertaken on ***voluntary basis***
- individual and collective action

APEC Chair rotates annually — host economy (Peru, 2008; Singapore, 2009; Japan, 2010; the United States, 2011; Russia, 2012).

APEC operates at policy level and working level as shown in Fig. 16.1.

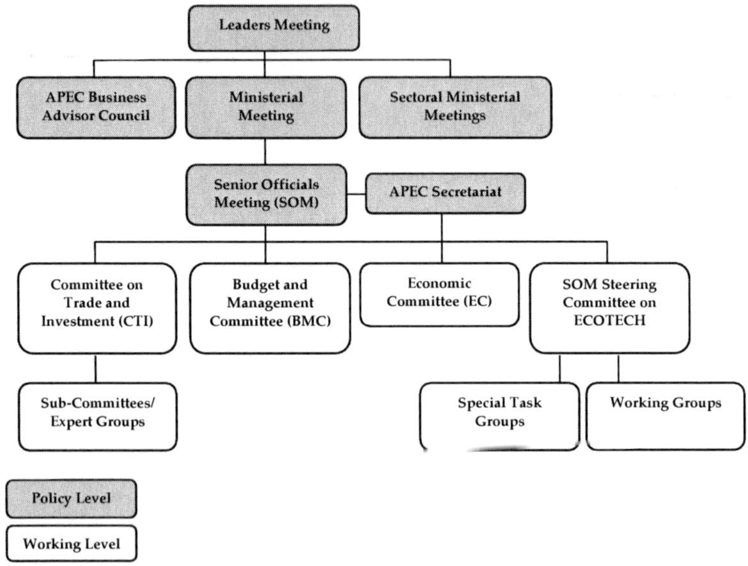

Figure 16.1 Structure of APEC.

16.2 APEC LSIF: Life Sciences Innovation Forum (Reports to Committee on Trade and Investment)

Life sciences innovation is critical to growth and socio-economic development as healthy people produce healthy economies. Efficient and effective delivery of patient focused products and services can improve a population's longevity, wellness, productivity and economic potential. Established by APEC leaders in 2002, the Life Sciences Innovation Forum (LSIF) has since grown to become APEC's leading initiative on health and health sciences innovation.

It is a tripartite forum that engages representatives from the highest levels of government, industry and academia to create the right policy environment for life sciences innovation. The LSIF brings together scientific, health, trade, economic, and financial considerations to address the challenges of infectious and chronic disease and ageing populations. Guiding principles include transparency, meaningful dialogue with stakeholders and recognition of due process. The LSIF forum also acknowledges that capacity building is critical to successful implementation.

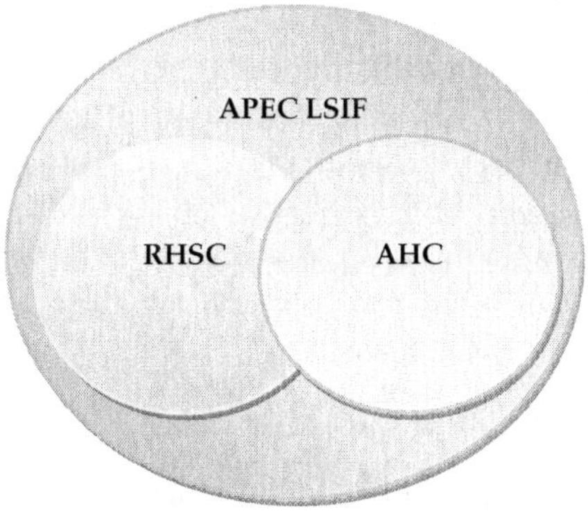

Figure 16.2 Operational model.

The APEC Life Science Strategic Plan, which was approved by APEC ministers in 2004, provided recommendations for collective action and an implementation schedule. The Strategic Plan also provides recommendations for strengthening the innovative life sciences sector in the APEC region, placing particular emphasis on boosting region-wide levels of investment in research and development for health innovation. In the strategic plan, regulatory harmonization was highlighted: Toward this end, leaders also recognized that "**Harmonization of standards... according to international best practices**...will give the APEC region a competitive edge and expand opportunities for the rapid development of innovation."

In 2007, the LSIF was tasked to undertake a multidisciplinary study on the role of and returns to economies from investment in health innovations that address health and related economic and fiscal challenges facing the region. It was also mandated to establish frameworks for public-private sector partnerships to better utilize resources to meet health needs.

The LSIF has developed an Enablers of Investment Checklist, a voluntary guidance tool for policy makers in each APEC economy to assess their investment environment for life sciences innovation. Singapore volunteered to fill out the implementation of the Checklist in 2009.

Based on a series of seminars held in 2008–2009 that dealt with ways to combat the increase in counterfeit medical products, the LSIF has developed an Anti-Counterfeit Medical Product Action

Plan. The objective is to share best practices in the detection and prevention of counterfeits to both regulatory authorities and industry professionals, and to build capacity at the economy level to combat the threat.

A series of regional seminars for government regulators on the issue of harmonization of medical device regulation were held in 2008 and 2009 (Malaysia and Canada). The objective was to help regulators of medical devices in APEC economies develop robust regulatory systems. The seminars highlighted the benefits to patients, regulators, and industry and to global and regional trade when economies implement a medical device regulatory system based on harmonization standards and procedures. Industry representatives were invited to participate. The training programs were closely coordinated with the medical devices Global Harmonization Task Force (GHTF) and two regional working parties: the Asian Harmonization Working Party and the Latin American Harmonization Working Party.

Workshops aimed at strengthening drug regulatory authorities' capacity to harmonize regulatory practices relating to drug development in clinical trials, and to good clinical practice/clinical research, were also held in Thailand in 2009.

The APEC Harmonization Center (AHC) was launched in Seoul, Korea, in June 2009. The AHC is an important step toward harmonizing regional regulatory priorities. An LSIF Regulatory Steering Committee has also been created to advance the harmonization agenda. The AHC has since organized a series of events, including an "APEC Harmonization Center Biosimilar Workshop" in September 2009. The workshop focused on the opportunities and challenges of biological medicines, regulatory issues for Biosimilars and the regulatory landscape for Biosimilars. A "Good Manufacturing Practice Pharmaceutical Validation Workshop," was also held by the AHC in December 2009 and drew over 450 participants.

16.3 APEC LSIF/RHSC: Regulatory Harmonization Steering Committee

Regulatory harmonization is identified by the LSIF as strategic imperative and by its significant contribution to the life science innovation.

The LSIF has sponsored successful series of workshops on anti-counterfeiting, clinical trial evaluation and GCP inspection, ICH quality guidance, and harmonization of medical device regulatory approaches based on the GHTF over the years. However, despite the progress made, the recognition that the LSIF has not been used to its full potential in promoting a more strategic and effective approach within the APEC region as a driver of regulatory harmonization and cooperation has been due to

- insufficient engagement of regulatory authorities in LSIF process
- clear articulation of how LSIF can take best advantage of strengths to achieve stated objectives in a more strategic and coordinated fashion
- diversity of APEC region and lack of well-established network of subject matter experts have made effective interactions with harmonization initiatives such as ICH challenging

In August 2007, LSIF VI in Lima, series of recommendations were made to address these issues, notably the support for the establishment of the APEC Harmonization Center (AHC) and creation of a Regulatory Harmonization Steering Committee (RHSC).

The RHSC's goal is to promote a more ***strategic***, ***effective***, and ***sustainable*** approach to harmonization within the APEC region by

- ***proactively*** identifying and prioritizing projects seen to be of greatest value
- providing direction to the AHC on projects and activities that best meets these needs
- enhancing the effectiveness of interactions with international and regional harmonization initiatives
- promoting the establishment of APEC networks of technical experts and repository of reference materials
- supporting mechanisms for the sharing of regulatory information and best practices
- seeking, in partnership with the AHC, to establish/strengthen linkages with harmonization initiatives, training organizations and other key players in efforts to promote ***complementary*** actions and most effective use of resources
- undertaking activities in accordance with a strategic plan to be developed by the SC

- ensuring products within the remit of SC: *medical life science products* (notably drugs and devices)

The RHSC consists of eight regulatory authorities (the United States, Canada, China, Japan, Thailand, Korea, Chinese Taiwan, and Peru), two official regulatory observers (Singapore and Mexico), four industry representatives (two from the device industry and two from the pharmaceutical industry), three official observers (PhRMA, AdvaMed, and RDPAC), and one academic representative (director of AHC).

The objective of the RHSC is to provide leadership on a strategic approach on regulatory convergence in APEC region. The RHSC developed strategic frameworks aiming at achieving regulatory convergence in APEC region by 2020 and was endorsed by APEC economies in 2011. It also identified priority regulatory work areas at

- good review practice
- multi-regional clinical trial
- supply chain integrity
- biologics
- combination products
- advanced therapies

Regulatory authorities take championship of these priority working areas and develop projects supporting the achievement of strategic framework.

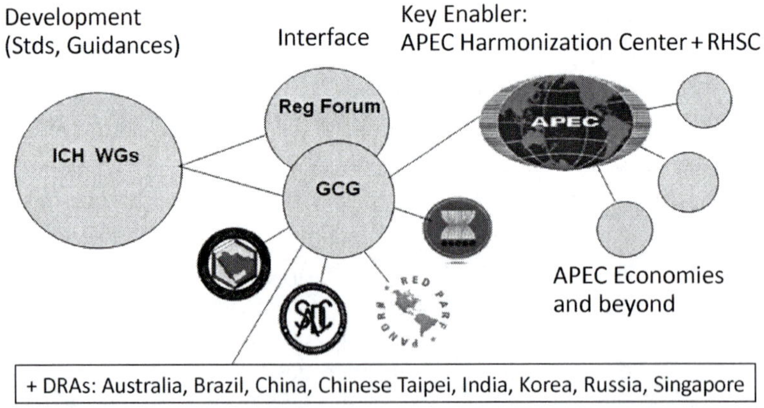

Figure 16.3 Building a better harmonization model.

Reference

1. Life Sciences Innovation Forum, Retrieved January 2012, from http://www.apec.org/Groups/Committee-on-Trade-and-Investment/Life-Sciences-Innovation-Forum.aspx.

Chapter 17

Harmonization of Medical Device in ASEAN

Petahn McKenna
ASEAN Regulatory Affairs Manager,
Johnson & Johnson Medical Singapore
PMCKENN1@its.jnj.com

17.1 Introduction

17.1.1 Medical Device Market in ASEAN

ASEAN (Association of Southeast Asian Nations) was founded on 8 August 1967, aimed at accelerating economic growth, social progress, and cultural development among its members, and to promote regional peace.

ASEAN has 10 member states, including Indonesia, Singapore, Malaysia, the Philippines, Thailand, Brunei Darussalam, Cambodia, Vietnam, Laos and Myanmar. With a combined population of approximately 600 million and a combined gross domestic product (GDP) of approximately $2.9 trillion, the ASEAN region represents a sizable market for medical devices with considerable potential. In

Handbook of Medical Device Regulatory Affairs in Asia
Edited by Jack Wong and Raymond K. Y. Tong

ISBN 978-981-4411-21-9 (Hardcover), 978-981-4411-22-6 (eBook)
www.panstanford.com

comparison, the population of the European Union is 500 million and a GDP of $14.7 trillion [1]. The average life expectancy of the ASEAN population is increasing, and consequently, there is a growing demand for better healthcare. Tied to this is an expectation to implement tighter regulatory controls for therapeutic products.

17.1.2 Medical Device Regulatory Environment in ASEAN

The respective Ministries of Health from each ASEAN member state are facing increasing pressure to implement regulatory requirements applicable to the therapeutic products supplied in their respective countries. Patients and surgeons now demand higher standards of healthcare, and the local industry strives to participate in globalized trade where the absence of a regulatory framework would put them at a disadvantage. From the regulator's perspective, increased regulatory requirements provide increased protection for the public against substandard medical devices by ensuring that the devices meet internationally recognized standards for safety, quality and efficacy. It is also in the interest of the local government and trade associations to ensure that locally manufactured medical devices will not face international trade restrictions and technical barriers when compared to global competitors.

The status of medical device regulation in the 10 ASEAN member states varies considerably: Singapore, Indonesia, Thailand, Vietnam, the Philippines and Myanmar have implemented mandatory regulatory requirements, whereas medical device registration is currently voluntary in Malaysia. Brunei, Cambodia and Laos are currently developing their requirements.

17.2 ASEAN Medical Device Directive and Harmonization

As part of the ASEAN Consultative Committee on Standards and Quality (ACCSQ), the Medical Device Product Working Group (MDPWG) was established to implement specific measures to facilitate harmonization of medical device regulations in ASEAN. Such measures include

- developing a common submission dossier template for product approval in ASEAN
- formalizing of a post-marketing alert system for defective or unsafe medical devices

Both of these goals have been addressed in the ASEAN Medical Device Directive (AMDD), developed by the MDPWG through cooperation of all ASEAN member countries, with input from industry and international regulatory bodies, including the Global Harmonization Task Force (GHTF), Asian Harmonization Working Party (AHWP) and World Health Organization (WHO).

Equivalent to the European Medical Device Directive adopted in the European Union (EU), the AMDD represents a harmonized set of regulatory requirements for medical devices by which medical device companies can demonstrate that a medical device meets the Essential Requirements for safety and performance. The AMDD itself will not be recognized as legislation; however, all member countries will be required to harmonize their regulatory requirements with the provisions of the AMDD. The AMDD states that "Member States shall undertake all necessary measures to ensure that only medical devices which conform to the provisions of this Directive and its Annexes and Appendices may be placed in the markets of Member States."

The following sections describe the provisions of the AMDD, with specific attention to the definition of a medical device, medical device classification system, Common Submission Dossier Template (CSDT), and ASEAN post-marketing alert system.

17.2.1 Provisions of the AMDD

The AMDD largely focuses on pre-market regulatory requirements that a company must adhere to before placing a medical device on the market. In contrast, post-market regulatory requirements apply to medical devices which have been granted approved for supply by the applicable regulatory authority. The AMDD's 18 articles, which are generally based on those of the GHTF, are as follows:

1. General provisions
2. Definition and scope of medical devices (including *in vitro* diagnostics (IVDs))
3. Essential requirements of safety and performance of medical devices

4. Classification of medical devices (A–D) according to level of risk
5. Conformity assessment of medical devices
6. Registration and placement on market
7. Registration of persons responsible for placing medical devices on the markets of member states
8. Technical documents for medical devices (e.g. CSDT, Declaration of Conformity)
9. Relevant technical standards (ISO, etc.)
10. Labelling
11. Product claims
12. Post-marketing alert system
13. Clinical investigation
14. Institutional arrangements
15. Safeguard clauses
16. Confidentiality
17. Special cases
18. Implementation

17.2.2 Definition of a Medical Device

The AMDD applies to all products covered by the "definition of a medical device." The definition includes (but is not limited to) medical instruments, machines, *in vitro* diagnostic (IVD) products and software which are intended to be used for human beings for a medical purpose. Critically, for a product to meet the definition of a medical device, it must not achieve its primary intended purpose by pharmacological, immunological or metabolic means. A drug product may be included as a component of the medical device, but can only act to support the medical device achieve its primary indication.

The definition of a medical device according to the AMDD also includes "Accessories", defined as another article which is intended to be used together with a "parent" medical device to enable that medical device to achieve its intended purpose. According to the AMDD, accessories are regulated independently, and according to the same regulations as the parent medical device. This means that the accessory may have a different risk classification to the medical device.

17.2.3 Medical Device Classification

The AMDD is aligned to the GHTF model of four medical device classes, defined according to potential risk to the patient.

Class	Risk level
A	Low risk
B	Low-moderate risk
C	Moderate-high risk
D	High risk

A set of classification rules is provided within the AMDD to guide Member states and medical device companies in classifying their medical devices into one of the above categories.

The AMDD sets out that any member state that reclassifies or differs in its interpretation of the classification rules shall notify the ASEAN Medical Device Committee (AMDC).

17.2.4 Common Submission Dossier Template

The AMDD sets out the requirements for all Member States to adopt and implement common technical documents, including the ASEAN CSDT.

The CSDT outlines the standard data which must be included in a submission to register a medical device with a regulatory authority, as follows:

- executive summary
- essential principles and methods used to demonstrate conformity
- device description
- summary of design verification and validation
- preclinical and clinical data (if necessary)
- device labelling
- risk analysis
- manufacturer information

The purpose of the CSDT is to provide a template to guide manufacturers and device sponsors to collate documentation which will be sufficient to demonstrate conformance to the Essential Principles of Safety and Performance of Medical Devices.

The CSDT largely aligns with the Summary of Technical Documentation (STED) published by GHTF, with some key differences such as the Device Description section, which contains the following additional items: potential adverse effects and alternative therapies. The benefit of the alignment between the CSDT and STED is that when adopted by ASEAN member countries, 80–90% of the documentation submitted to the US Food and Drug Administration can also be used to complete the submissions for the local ASEAN Market, thereby reducing time in preparing the submission dossier. This alignment also provides regulators of member countries with a level of confidence that products which have been approved in countries where the STED has been adopted, that product conforms to the same standards as the ASEAN Member countries.

The standard language for documentation submitted in the CSDT will be English.

17.2.5 Post-Market Alert System

ASEAN Member states are required to record and evaluate all information brought to their attention regarding any malfunction or deterioration of a device, or inadequacy in the labelling or the instructions for use which might lead to or might have led to the death of a patient or user or to a serious deterioration in their state of health, or any technical or medical reason which may have lead to a systematic recall of devices of the same type. The AMDD encourages member states to work with the applicable medical device company throughout the evaluation.

Furthermore, following the evaluation, member states are required to immediately inform the other member states of the incidents referred to above.

17.2.6 AMDD Status

The first version of the AMDD was presented in January 2008 and has been developed throughout subsequent MDPWG meetings. The official deadline for all ASEAN members to comply with the AMDD is 2015. However, the date on which each country will be able to comply will depend on the priorities and resources of the local government.

17.2.7 Future of ASEAN Harmonization

In addition to the development of the AMDD, other points of focus of the MDPWG include the following [2]:

- exploring the feasibility of an abridged approval process for medical devices which regulators of benchmarked countries or recognized regulators have approved
- exploring the feasibility of adopting a harmonized system of placement of medical devices into the ASEAN markets, based on a common product approval process

To date, work on these projects has not commenced; however, similar to the AMDD, they present immense potential to the advancement of the medical device industry in ASEAN.

References

1. ASEAN Community in Figures, 2010, ASEAN Community in Figures (ACIF) 2010 Jakarta, ASEAN Secretariat — Retrieved April 2011, from http://www.aseansec.org/publications/ACIF2010.pdf.
2. Objectives and Scope of the ACCSQ-MDPWG, MDPWG website [Online], retrieved 16 January 2012, from http://accsq-mdpwg.org/index.php?option=com_content&view=article&id=19&Itemid=60.

Chapter 18

Regulatory Affairs Professionals Society

Sherry Keramidas and Zachary Brousseau
Regulatory Affairs Professionals Society®
skeramidas@raps.org, zbrousseau@raps.org

18.1 Introduction

Founded in 1976, the Regulatory Affairs Professionals Society (RAPS) is the largest international organization of and for healthcare product regulatory professionals. RAPS is headquartered in suburban Washington, DC, with offices in Europe and Asia, and chapters and affiliates worldwide, and can be found online at www.RAPS.org. It helped establish the regulatory profession and continues to promote its identity and prestige, operating outside the political arena as a neutral, non-lobbying organization.

RAPS members help ensure the safety, effectiveness and availability of the full range of healthcare products, including medical devices, pharmaceuticals, biologics and biotechnology products, and nutritional products, as well as some foods and cosmetic products. They work in a variety of employment settings, including the companies that make and sell healthcare products; the regulatory agencies that oversee them, such as the US Food and Drug Administration (FDA), the European Medicines Agency (EMA), the

Handbook of Medical Device Regulatory Affairs in Asia
Edited by Jack Wong and Raymond K. Y. Tong

ISBN 978-981-4411-21-9 (Hardcover), 978-981-4411-22-6 (eBook)
www.panstanford.com

Singapore Health Sciences Authority, Japan's Pharmaceuticals and Medical Devices Agency (PMDA) and Ministry of Health, Labour and Welfare (MHLW), Taiwan Food and Drug Administration and others; academic institutions; clinical research organizations; and other companies and organizations where regulatory expertise is needed. RAPS members and regulatory professionals in general, play a myriad of vital roles throughout the lifecycle of healthcare products, from research and development to manufacturing to compliance and postmarketing.

RAPS supports these individuals and the organizations that employ them by providing integrated solutions with products and services that meet the shared needs of regulatory professionals worldwide, as well as the unique local needs of different countries and employment settings. This includes education and training, professional standards, research, knowledge-sharing, publications, networking, career development opportunities and other valuable resources. It also provides Regulatory Affairs Certification (RAC), the only post-academic professional credential to recognize regulatory excellence (www.RAPS.org/rac).

18.2 Importance in Today's Global Environment

Around the world, patients, healthcare providers, and payers increasingly demand safer, more effective healthcare products, improved outcomes, more-affordable treatments, advanced diagnostic tools, and better adherence to treatments. In the current global business environment, regulatory requirements dominate biopharmaceutical and medical device development and lifecycle management. Regulatory professionals today are engaged beyond just submission and compliance. They play integral roles throughout the product lifecycle (Fig. 18.1) and are increasingly engaged in critical business functions, including organizational and business strategy, health technology assessment, comparative effectiveness research, and even bridging the gap between regulation and reimbursement.

RAPS' research shows that together, business and strategy occupy more than 28% of regulatory professionals' time, and more are pursuing business education. These trends underscore the regulatory profession's important position at the intersection of business, emerging healthcare technologies, and government regulation.

Regulatory professionals have a unique ability to adapt to changes in science, technology, manufacturing, business, economics, and regulatory processes. The role of the regulatory professional today is more complex and demanding than ever.

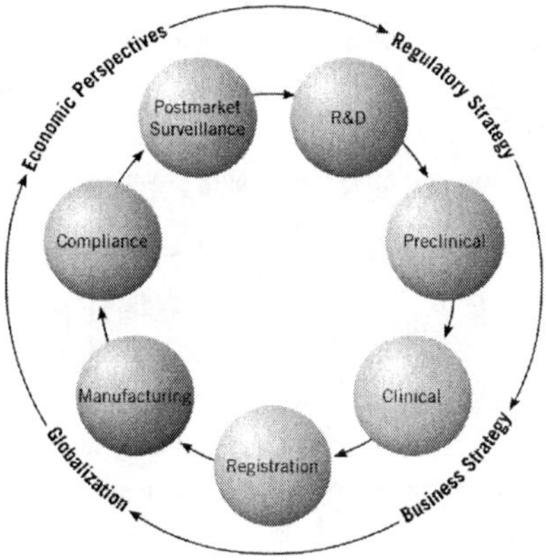

Figure 18.1 The healthcare product lifecycle.

18.3 The Global Regulatory Community

RAPS represents 25,000 professionals in the local and global regulatory communities from 90 countries. At the local level, RAPS has 14 chapters in North America, one in Switzerland, and one in Israel, as well as 15 affiliates throughout the world, including Brazil, Germany, India, Taiwan, and the United Kingdom (Fig. 18.2). RAPS chapters and affiliates host local educational and networking events throughout the year.

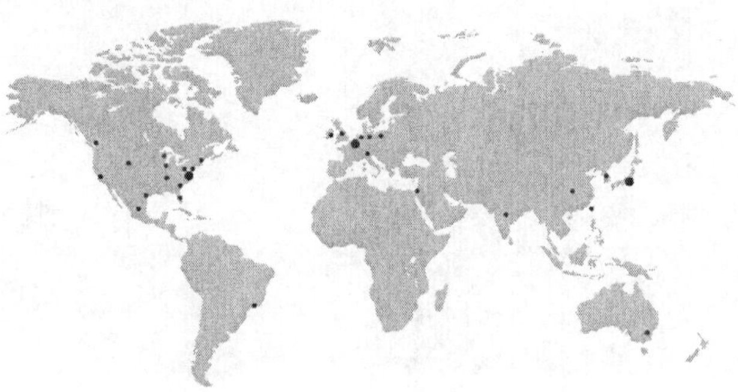

Figure 18.2 RAPS offices, chapters and affiliates.

RAPS connects regulatory professionals around the world to the global regulatory community. Through face-to-face meetings, networking events, and RAPS' online community, Regulatory Exchange (connect.RAPS.org), professionals interact with one another and their broader community to converse, exchange ideas, ask questions, or weigh in on the latest developments in healthcare and regulation. The RAPS global network also allows members to find other RAPS members based on geographic location, regional interests, or the types of products with which they may be involved.

18.4 Building Knowledge and Competencies

RAPS strives to meet regulatory professionals' needs for knowledge, skills and competencies across all career levels and geographies. It offers a range of high-quality regulatory education and training options, including workshops, webcasts, online courses and certificate programs, and the organization's annual conference (www.RAPS.org/education-amp-training).

RAPS' annual flagship conference, dubbed The Regulatory Convergence, is the largest annual gathering exclusively for the regulatory profession (Fig. 18.3). It provides a critical opportunity for regulatory professionals and thought leaders from industry, regulatory agencies, academia and other stakeholder organizations to come together to learn, network, and exchange ideas.

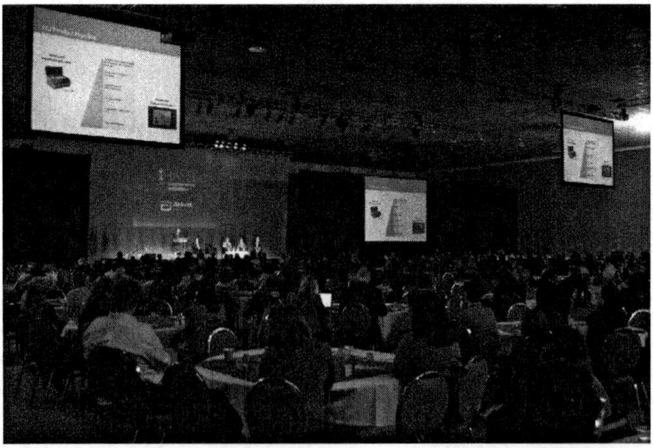

Figure 18.3 RAPS annual conference, San Jose, CA, USA.

At this annual gathering, expert presenters cover the latest regulatory developments and implications across a range of healthcare topics in biologics and biotechnology, clinical, compliance, electronic intervention, health-related foods, medical devices and *in vitro* diagnostics, pharmaceuticals, and regulatory business.

Attendees hear from top officials from agencies including the US FDA, the EMA, the European Commission, China's State Food and Drug Administration, Japan's PMDA and MHLW, the Korea Food and Drug Administration, Health Canada, Brazil's Anvisa, and other regulators from around the globe.

RAPS also hosts regular workshops, meetings and webcasts covering important topics of interest to the regulatory community.

RAPS Online University (RAPS.org/onlineu) provides self-paced continuing education for regulatory professionals, making quality regulatory study available worldwide. Online University courses reflect the real-world environment of the regulatory profession. The competency-based learning is designed by regulatory experts, around the specific responsibilities of regulatory professionals and delivered through RAPS' proprietary learning platform for desktop and iPad. Online University offers more than 35 courses covering regulatory essentials, clinical, medical devices, pharmaceuticals and quality, with many more courses in development.

Online University students may also earn a regulatory affairs certificate by completing customizable curricula of courses pertaining to the medical device and/or pharmaceutical industries. Certificates may be earned in pharmaceuticals or medical devices, or students may choose a dual certificate that covers both areas.

18.5 The RAC Credential

Regulatory Affairs Certification® (RAC) is the only post-academic professional credential for the healthcare product regulatory field. The credentialing exam and credential maintenance criteria are developed, managed, and administered by the Regulatory Affairs Certification Board (RACB) and supported by RAPS. Since its inception in 1990, more than 7,000 professionals in 35 different countries have earned the RAC.

RAC-credentialed professionals are among the current and rising leaders in the regulatory profession. They work in all parts of the world and in many settings, including industry, government and academic organizations.

Earning the RAC demonstrates regulatory knowledge, critical thinking skills and professional commitment. Professionals with the credential are highly valued by employers, and RAPS' own research shows that those with the RAC earn 6% more than their peers without the credential.

Candidates for the RAC credential sit for one of the four versions of the exam — the RAC (US) covering US regulations, the RAC (EU) covering European regulations, the RAC (CAN) covering Canadian regulations, and the RAC (General Scope), which covers general regulatory responsibilities and international standards. The computer-based exam is administered worldwide and intended for regulatory professionals with three to five years of regulatory experience.

Once earned, the RAC is maintained through continuing professional development and activities, such as attending or speaking at meetings and conferences, writing for professional publications, self-paced distance education, university coursework, earning additional certifications, or professional leadership and involvement. Recertification is required every three years.

18.6 Professional Knowledge and Standards

RAPS develops the standards for knowledge, competency, and ethics for the regulatory profession.

Every two years, RAPS conducts the largest, most comprehensive study of the regulatory profession, the RAPS Global Scope of Practice & Compensation Survey. RAPS has conducted this research for more than 20 years, and the data collected help regulatory professionals benchmark their compensation against others in the field and better understand the range of responsibilities of their regulatory peers. This information also helps RAPS support the development of the profession and create effective tools to support regulatory professionals' career development.

The Scope of Practice research has uncovered a number of important developments over the 20-plus years it has been conducted. Results have shown increased movement of professionals across product lines and expanded involvement in combination products over time, as well as a move away from country-specific specialization as more professionals now have multinational or global responsibilities.

The results have revealed strong similarities in the scope of practice of professionals around the world, regardless of where they live and work. And in the past decade, the increased involvement of regulatory professionals in business and strategic decision making was identified through the Scope of Practice research.

RAPS also initiated and supported the development of a code of ethics for the regulatory profession. Following a series of surveys and focus groups held over two years, a task force of volunteers was convened in 2003 to craft the Code of Ethics for Regulatory Affairs Professionals.

The task force identified eight fundamental principles guiding regulatory professionals in their professional endeavors: duty, competence, objectivity, integrity, honesty, courage, fairness and respect. These core values of the profession are detailed in the full code, available from RAPS.

18.7 News and Information

Since its inception in 1996, RAPS' *Regulatory Focus* (RF) has been the flagship publication for regulatory professionals around the world (Fig. 18.4). It provides readers an in-depth picture of the global regulatory environment with features and views from regulatory experts and professionals in the field.

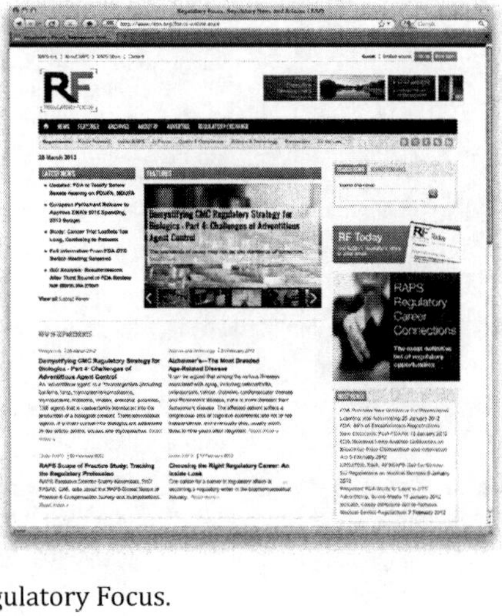

Figure 18.4 Regulatory Focus.

In 2012, RF moved to an all-digital format, available online at www.regulatoryfocus.org, allowing RAPS to offer more timely information and articles, increased accessibility, and greater depth and breadth of regulatory resources connected with the topics of interest to readers. RF publishes free online regulatory news and content, as well as features and other information available exclusively to RAPS members. In addition, RF is accessible via mobile application for the iPhone and iPad, and applications for Android devices will be available in late 2012.

RAPS publishes numerous books and materials to address specific needs of regulatory professionals at all levels, involved in all product lines and across the full product lifecycle, including the highly regarded Fundamentals of Regulatory Affairs series of reference books, as well as books covering a range of specific regulatory, medical device and pharmaceutical topics. All are available from the RAPS Store (RAPS.org/store).

Chapter 19

Expediting Innovation in Singapore with Regulatory Knowledge

Patricia Ho and Jui Lim

Singapore Stanford Biodesign, 61 Biopolis Drive #01-02, Proteos, 138673 Singapore

ssbenquiry@scei.a-star.edu.sg

One of the most positive developments for the medical device industry in Singapore has been, in recent years, the recognition by innovators, clinicians, engineers, and economic planners of the regulatory approval process' centrality in bringing innovation to the benefit of patients. The recognition that medical technology innovation cannot exist without the regulatory approval process is, in the first instance, founded on ethical and medical grounds, but it also drives economic considerations as embodied by the following questions: "How do we maximize the effect of R&D investments?," and "how do we reduce the attrition rate in medical device development?" This recognition has spurred into action the panoply of programs now available in Singapore that raises awareness of, and builds capabilities in, the regulatory approval process. We believe that there is heuristic value in the Singapore experience, and this chapter will outline these programs, highlighting for illustrative purposes the Singapore-Stanford Biodesign Program [1].

Handbook of Medical Device Regulatory Affairs in Asia
Edited by Jack Wong and Raymond K. Y. Tong

ISBN 978-981-4411-21-9 (Hardcover), 978-981-4411-22-6 (eBook)
www.panstanford.com

Conjointly with Singapore's efforts to raise the profile of "regulatory" knowledge in medical device development, there has been an equally concerted effort to bring clinicians, engineers, and business people together to form multidisciplinary teams. These efforts correctly acknowledge the complexity of medical device commercialization, as too often good ideas lay dormant for want of technical expertise to actualize the idea, or projects without prior financial due diligence lead to the attrition of projects and consumed resources gone to waste.

Programs are now available from the Ministry of Health, the Ministry of Trade & Industry, and the Prime Minister's Office, either directly or through their organizations and statutory boards, such as the National Research Foundation (NRF), the Standards, Productivity, and Innovation Board (SPRING Singapore), the Health Sciences Authority (HSA), the Economic Development Board (EDB), the National Medical Research Council (NMRC), and the Agency for Science, Technology, and Research (ASTAR). These programs emphasize medical device development using a multidisciplinary approach that is compliant with quality and regulatory requirements.

Some of the more energetic and forward-thinking of these programs are those initiated by ASTAR. Through its Health and Lifestyle (H&L) Office, ASTAR makes sizeable (S$500,000 to S$2,000,000) grant calls that require for each qualifying application, two co-principal investigators, one clinician and one engineer. There are separate grant calls for diagnostic device projects and therapeutic device projects. For all project applications, a regulatory section must be completed, forcing applicants to consider the type of device they are developing, and its regulatory requirements, including the associated timeline and budgetary implications of that device. Writing a research grant is now comparable to writing a business plan [3].

In addition to making grant calls for medical device development, ASTAR, through its H&L Office holds bi-monthly forums aimed to bring clinicians, engineers, business people, and regulators together to discuss selected clinical themes. Regulatory courses and talks are also organized at a regular cadence, conducted by practitioners in the industry. At the time of writing this chapter, ASTAR is even evaluating the possibility of offering diploma and/or degree courses in regulatory affairs.

Other government agencies are following suit, especially grant funding agencies, which now require in their applications the commercialization plans that acknowledge both quality and regulatory requirements. Elsewhere, the HSA has recently announced a multi-year plan to roll out a new approval process for medical devices, which further raises the importance of regulatory knowledge. This has been matched by a vigorous and regular outreach effort to keep all stakeholders informed of the HSA's requirements, which has had the effect of raising awareness of "regulatory" importance for and relevance to medical devices. At the National University of Singapore, the Medical Engineering Research and Commercialization Initiative (MERCI) was set up, comprising engineers and doctors from industry, to provide early inputs on issues relating to quality and regulatory matters to contemplated medical device development projects [2].

In 2009, EDB and ASTAR teamed up to advance efforts to train Singaporean innovators as a way of strengthening its medical device industry. Through a joint venture with Stanford University's Biodesign Program, the Singapore-Stanford Biodesign (SSB) Program was born and launched in 2010 [1].

19.1 The Biodesign Innovation Process

SSB, like its older sibling in the United States, is predicated on the belief that innovation can be taught, rather than it being a sudden, ineluctable, unpredictable, and random "bright idea." This belief has now been fully articulated as the "Biodesign Process" and validated by the phenomenal output of technologies and start-up companies that have emanated from this "Process."

The "Biodesign Process" begins by forming teams of people with differing backgrounds (medical doctors, engineers, and business backgrounds) to identify unmet clinical needs, brainstorm and design novel solutions for these needs, and then develop business proposals to commercialize these innovations. SSB is based on the three-stage innovation process as shown in Fig. 19.1. In this chapter, this approach to innovation will be introduced as an example of how information, such as the regulatory knowledge provided in the other chapters of this book, helps expedite innovation.

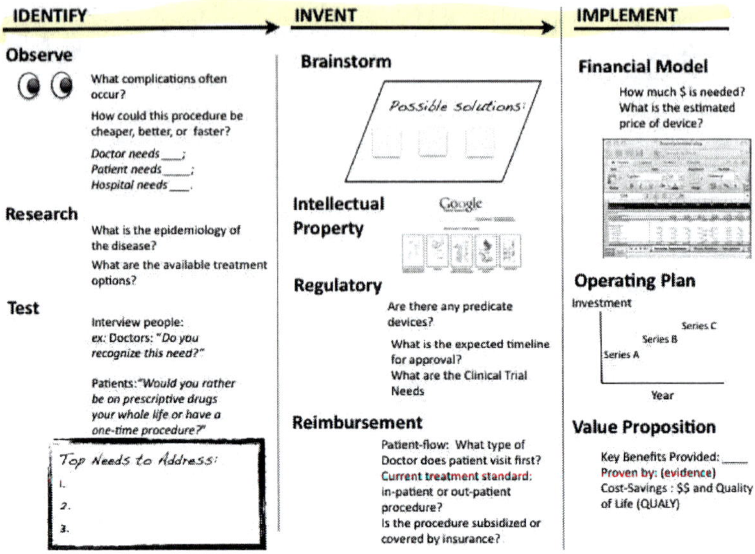

Figure 19.1 The three-stage innovation process used to train innovators.

19.1.1 Identify

In the first stage of the innovation process, our students are tasked with searching for unmet needs by way of full clinical immersion. They observe procedures and treatments with an eye to identifying the shortcomings with current procedures and their implements. Literature reviews are performed concurrently to understand the state of the art and its complications. Students interview the relevant clinician-operators to obtain deeper understanding of any particular problem and associated need. All observed problems are then ultimately re-expressed as a need statement, a written statement concisely defining the need. This may be further refined over multiple iterations. This stage of defining the need statement to address is the fulcrum of the innovation process. Thereafter, our students evaluate their list of need statements, effectively triaging them to arrive at a shortlist of the top needs. The parameters of this triage are a deep understanding of the disease process, the treatment options, the market, and the stakeholders involved.

19.1.2 Invent

After they have shortlisted the top needs, our students, in this second stage, begin to draw and design various possible solutions to address a selected clinical need. Innovators also begin to acknowledge and utilize country-specific regulatory information, such as contained in this book.

After concluding with some possible designs, a patent search is done, to see whether or not such solutions already exist and if the innovator has the freedom to operate. With each possible design, regulatory pathways are evaluated. Does a predicate device exist? Early on, the innovator may wish to eliminate device concepts that, for example, foreshadow an arduous and expensive regulatory process, in favor of equally effective device concepts that may undergo expedited approval. Patient flow is examined to see if the invention would be disruptive to current patient flow, which would affect key stakeholders. Understanding patient flow and key stakeholders helps the innovator discern whether the intended users would be willing to adopt this proposed technology versus existing technologies, and if so, at what price range. Doctors may not wish, for instance, to accept such technologies that may decrease their number of patients or commoditize their expertise. The commonly used example of the Scribner Shunt highlights the issues that may arise with a successful novel invention. The Scribner Shunt, a device used in hemodialysis that allows for the blood to be filtrated outside of the body, radically changed the standard of treatment and patient flow [4]. Prior to this invention, maintenance dialysis for irreversible kidney failure was not done and end-stage kidney disease was fatal. With its introduction, the device allowed for the treatment of irreversible chronic renal failure. To deliver this new treatment, the first outpatient dialysis centers were introduced with specialized nurses and technicians, replacing clinics and nephrologists. Now that chronic hemodialysis had become possible, the expenses of treatment largely increased, and certain issues, such as reimbursement and who should be allowed treatment, arose. With key stakeholders identified, the innovator can identify prices of existing treatments, how to increase physician adoption, possibilities for government subsidies and insurance coverage, and determine an estimated price for their device.

This "invent" stage helps innovators avoid the problem many failed startups face of leaping from the identification phase to implementation, only to find there is no market or that regulatory hurdles are too steep.

19.1.3 Implement

By the time this final stage is reached, the student may have repeated the previous two stages, refining the need statement and subsequent prototypes, before selecting a final concept. This third stage focuses on creating the strategy to execute successful production and commercialization. Financial models are built to estimate the amount of funding needed and the associated funding period. Regulatory issues again take center stage. To address regulatory issues such as assessing the requirements for regulatory approvals and consultation with regulatory authorities and consultants may take place at this stage. This helps the innovator with strategic decisions, such as determining the requirements for pursuing regulatory approval in one market and deciding if they are capable of leveraging the data and approval to expedite regulatory approval in another market. Potential animal and clinical trials are designed. Again, as in the invent stage, the innovator must examine the flow of patient care, whether the device will be accepted by the user community, and how the device will be sold and distributed. By the end of this final stage, innovators are left with an estimated cost and time needed to bring their device to market, followed by a proposed sales and distribution strategy.

19.2 The Innovator's Resource

SSB was founded in 2010 as a collaboration among the Singapore Agency for Science Technology and Research (A*STAR), Singapore Economic Development Board (EDB), and Stanford University. In its current form, SSB consists of a fellowship and class, to train approximately 36 people annually on the innovation process who are expected to become leaders in the medical device innovation industry. Although it is primarily a training program, SSB is also interested in creating a resource for innovators to use, to help expedite the innovation process and increase the number of successful innovations in Asia.

Unlike many of the organizations participating in the regulatory harmonization efforts, SSB is unique as it is neither a governmental regulatory agency nor a part of industry. This resource SSB is in the process of compiling will serve as a first-stop for entrepreneurs, guiding them on who the country's regulatory authority is, how healthcare is distributed and paid for, and how their inventions can be protected. These entrepreneurs often lack the funding and resources large multinational companies have, to identify and hire credible consultants early on in the process. SSB hopes to encourage more entrepreneurs to come to Asia by filling their gaps of knowledge, helping to guide them in their early-stage decisions. The resource for innovators focuses on Regulatory, Reimbursement, and Intellectual Property (IP), with personal vignettes and case studies showcasing various experiences.

For example, most innovators are less familiar with knowing, for example, that the regulatory authority in Singapore is the Health Sciences Authority (HSA). Figure 19.2 provides a general sample checklist for innovators to use as to understand the regulatory basics in Singapore. Similar checklists will hopefully be provided for other countries and topics such as reimbursement and IP as well.

- ☐ Is the innovation a medical device?
  - o What is the intended purpose of the device? What is its primary mode of action?
  - o Where to Look: HSA website, Health Products Act 2007
- ☐ Classify the Device
  - o Follow the rules noted in HSA's Guidance Document on Classification
  - o Where to Look: GN-13-R1 Guidance on Risk Classification of General Medical Devices and the Singapore Medical Devices Register (SMDR)
- ☐ Prepare Product Registration Application
  - o For class A device, see if the device is exempt from product registration
  - o Prepare the submission dossier based on the ASEAN Common Submission Dossier Template (CSDT)
  - o Where to Look: HSA GN-15-R3 Guidance on Medical Device Product Registration, GN-17 Guidance on Preparation of Product Registration Submission for General Medical Devices using the ASEAN CST, and GN-22 Guidance to the List of Medical Devices Exempted from Product Registration
- ☐ Determine the Appropriate Regulatory Pathway
  - o Has the device been evaluated or approved in at least one of the GHTF member countries?
  - o Where to Look: GN-15-R3 Guidance on Medical Device Product Registration
- ☐ Submit Product Registration Application
  - o Use the online Medical Device Information and Communication System (MEDICS)
  - o Where to Look: GN-15-R3 Guidance on Medical Device Product Registration
- ☐ Consult Regulatory experts or consult with a regulator within HSA.

Figure 19.2 Checklist for innovators for Singapore regulatory approval.

Other areas of regulatory useful for innovators to know include upcoming or new regulations, estimated regulatory approval times and fees, and what country-specific considerations an innovator should be aware of. For example, when dealing with Japan's PMDA, the innovator could benefit from knowing one key success factor would include arranging a meeting with the PMDA, with a consultation fee of thousands of dollars, price-dependent on the type of consultation.

Intertwined with regulatory issues are other areas important for innovators to understand, which SSB strives to provide resources for. In the reimbursement section, SSB hopes to provide a general overview of healthcare distribution and financing, medical device procurement, subsidization, and grants. For example, an innovator interested in entering China would benefit from the knowledge that the National Development & Reform Commission (NDRC) is responsible for price supervision policies for medical devices, while the Ministry of Human Resources and Social Security is in charge of Urban Employee and Residents Basic Medical Insurance and other medical insurance findings. Equipped with this knowledge, the innovator can further investigate the specific government agencies to understand how prices of devices are determined to assess the affordability of their proposed device. Further, they should know whether the local government will provide a subsidy for the device, whether it be on a list of subsidized devices or simply partially paid for up to a certain amount. If I had a new device, would I sell the price through tender? Is the model of consignment often seen in hospitals? Which types of hospitals are most frequented, and would they be able to afford the care I am proposing? These are some of the questions many innovators ask, yet the answers are currently not provided in a one-stop resource of information.

As with regulatory and reimbursement issues, Intellectual Property is another section with country-specific knowledge SSB hopes to highlight for innovators. Innovators must understand the basics of the legal system, prevailing attitudes, and forms of available protection. This will help the innovator go about protecting and maximizing the value of their invention. The innovator faces questions such as, how do I protect my product's reputation and patents, avoiding the potential of counterfeits more easily available and at a discounted price? How long would it take for the country's authority to grant the patent after submitting an application? With the answers, the innovator is able to plan his timelines accordingly, to maximize efficiency while executing regulatory and intellectual property strategies.

19.3 Current Direction

Innovators are becoming increasingly interested in innovating for Asia, as they see the potential in creating cutting-edge technology for the growing middle-class in emerging markets. These devices often must be priced competitively, limiting the technological capability or quality of the products. Entrepreneurs with little or no prior to the medical device environment in Asia arrive, struggling to find the correct contacts to answer the questions as they subject their ideas to the innovation process. With the helpful collaborations from people in government authorities and industry, SSB hopes to compile this resource for innovators to cultivate the hunger to innovate for Asian markets and expedite the innovation process.

References

1. Singapore Stanford Biodesign (2010). *What the Program Is About.* Singapore Stanford Biodesign. Retrieved March 8, 2012, from http://www.ssb.a-star.edu.sg/about-program.html.
2. MERCI (n.d.). *NUS's Medical Engineering Research and Commercialization Initiative (MERCI).* Special Feature: Singapore Medtech Innovations & Initiatives. Retrieved March 20, 2012, from http://www.medtechsingapore.com/pdf/Universities_A_Source_of_Innovation_in_the_Medtech_Sector.pdf.
3. A*STAR (3 April 2012). *Grants & Sponsorships.* Agency for Science, Technology, and Research. Retrieved March 8, 2012, from http://www.a-star.edu.sg/tabid/136/default.aspx.
4. Christopher R. Blagg. The Early History of Dialysis for Chronic Renal Failure in the United States: A View from Seattle. *American Journal of Kidney Diseases*, **49**(3) (March 2007), 482–496.

Part 4

Medical Device Regulatory System in the United States and the European Union

Chapter 20

United States Medical Device Regulatory Framework

Carole C. Carey

U.S. Food and Drug Administration, Center for Devices and Radiological Health, 10903 New Hampshire Ave., Silver Spring, Maryland, USA

carole.carey@fda.hhs.gov

20.1 Introduction

The United States Food and Drug Administration (USFDA), well known as the FDA, is an agency within the U.S. Department of Health and Human Services (HHS). The FDA is a science-based, regulatory and public health agency. Its statutory mandate is to ensure that the nation's food supply is safe and wholesome, products that emit radiation are safe, and medical products marketed in the United States are safe and effective. Furthermore, the FDA also regulates mammography facilities as well as cosmetics and tobacco products. The FDA does not regulate medical practice. State law regulates medical practice. The FDA's regulatory authority extends to the 50 States, the District of Columbia, Puerto Rico, Guam, the Virgin

Handbook of Medical Device Regulatory Affairs in Asia
Edited by Jack Wong and Raymond K. Y. Tong

ISBN 978-981-4411-21-9 (Hardcover), 978-981-4411-22-6 (eBook)
www.panstanford.com

Islands, American Samoa, and other US territories. The medical device industry is a highly regulated segment of the US economy. A report, *Medical Device Industry Assessment, Updated March 24, 2010,* (International Trade Administration, US Department of Commerce), [http://ita.doc.gov/td/health/medical.html] points to the United States as the leader in the manufacturing of medical devices and the largest medical devices market in the world. It is roughly 42% of the world's total, with an estimated value at more than US$100 billion in 2008. The report also noted that over the past decade, the value of exported and imported medical devices steadily increased. Shown in Table 20.1 is the medical device sector trade flow in 2007 and 2008 based on the North American Industry Classification System (NAICS) code.

Table 20.1 Medical device sector trade flows by NAICS code in billions of US dollars

NAICS code	Description	2007 exports	2008 exports	2007 imports	2008 imports
334510	Electro-medical apparatus	7.2	8.08	6.8	7.22
334517	Irradiation apparatus	3.1	3.34	3.6	3.72
339112	Surgical and medical instruments	8.8	9.98	8.8	9.14
339113	Surgical appliances and supplies	6.8	7.39	7.3	9.01
339114	Dental equipment and supplies	1.1	1.22	1.2	1.28
339115	Ophthalmic goods	1.3	1.39	3.3	3.26
	Total	**28.3**	**31.4**	**31.0**	**33.63**

In this chapter, we will focus on the regulatory management and supervision of medical devices. The learning objective is to provide students and other interested individuals a concise overview of the US regulatory framework, as well as to introduce the general regulatory requirements, premarket and postmarket, necessary to legally market medical devices in the United States. Since the majority of device submissions are classified in Class I and Class II, there is more effort to clarify the premarket notification 510(k) clearance process and the general regulatory controls mandatory to all classes (I, II, and III).

20.2 The FDA Center for Devices and Radiological Health

In the United States, the FDA's Center for Devices and Radiological Health (CDRH) is responsible for regulating medical devices and radiation-emitting products (medical and non-medical). Within CDRH, the Division of Mammography Quality and Radiation Programs ensures that a mammography facility must meet the Mammography Quality Standards Act (MQSA) certification in providing quality mammography services, and are inspected. The USFDA CDRH evaluates new medical devices for safety and effectiveness before they are marketed; and monitors products already on the market, so that unsafe and ineffective products are kept out of the market. In addition, the USFDA CDRH regulates companies that design, manufacture, repackage, relabel, and/or import medical devices into the United States.

To learn more about the Center's mission, vision, and shared values as well as strategic planning, transparency, and innovation initiatives, the following Web site provides comprehensive information:

http://www.fda.gov/AboutFDA/CentersOffices/OfficeofMedicalProductsandTobacco/CDRH/ucm300639.htm

20.3 Total Product Life Cycle Approach

CDRH's regulatory paradigm in managing medical devices is based on risk. That is, the higher the risk of harm to humans, the greater the level of regulatory control. Further, the integrated systematic approach of Total Product Life Cycle (TPLC) is applied in the regulatory oversight of medical devices. Figure 20.1 is a schematic representation of CDRH's Total Product Life Cycle (TPLC) model, a "cradle to grave" concept. It depicts the interconnection of the continuing stages throughout the different lifecycle phases; beginning from the initial design concept, prototype, premarket testing, clinical study, manufacturing, marketing, to widespread use, and finally to obsolescence of the "old" technology. An attribute of TPLC is the required interaction among stakeholders. The sharing of important information on device experience and lessons learned from a product's life cycle are applied to the development of the next phase, and ultimately in the design of the next generation or future products.

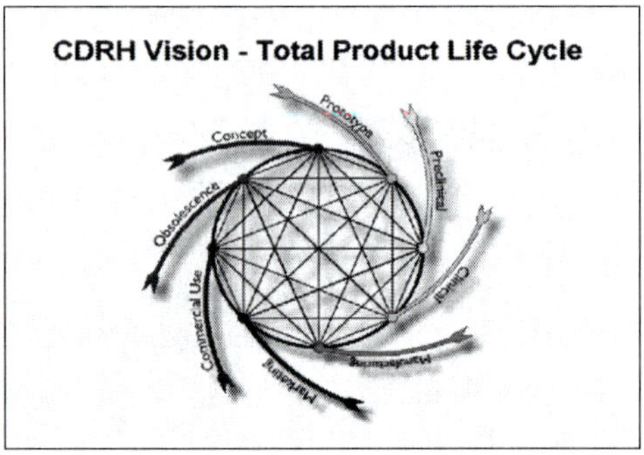

Figure 20.1 FDA's Center for Devices and Radiological Health Model of Total Product Life Cycle (TPLC).

20.4 Legislation and Device Laws

The 1968 mandate of the Radiation Control for Health and Safety Act (RCHSA) required safety standards for electronic products that give off radiation, such as microwave ovens, x-ray equipment and others. People should not be exposed to harmful levels of radiation from these products. A few years later, on May 28, 1976, President Gerald Ford signed into law the Medical Device Amendments to the US Federal Food, Drug, and Cosmetic Act (FD&C Act). This was the result of a US Senate finding that faulty medical devices had caused 10,000 injuries, including 731 deaths. The statute established Federal regulatory controls for medical devices. It granted FDA the authority to require premarket testing and submissions of safety and effectiveness information for FDA review.

20.4.1 FDA Law vs. FDA Regulations vs. FDA Guidance

Federal laws establish the legal framework within which FDA operates. The FD&C Act is a federal law enacted by Congress in 1938 giving authority to the USFDA to oversee the safety of food, drugs, and cosmetics. The FD&C Act has been amended many times. For instance, it was amended in 1976 as described above to incorporate into law the Medical Device Amendments Act.

Based on the laws set forth in the FD&C Act and other federal laws, the FDA develops regulations. This process is known as "notice and comment rulemaking." Hence, FDA regulations are also federal laws and are commonly referred to as Title 21 Code of Federal Regulations (CFR). The CFR represents all current regulations and the volumes are published annually. There are nine volumes; the volume that contains the medical device and electronic product regulations is Part 800-1299.

On the other hand, FDA guidance is not law. Guidance describes the agency's current thinking on regulatory issues. Guidance is not legally binding on the public or the FDA but is a very practical and useful regulatory tool for FDA staff and regulated industry. Guidance facilitates the regulatory process by providing more information on the interpretation of medical device regulations. The CDRH Office of Device Evaluation and Office of *In Vitro* Diagnostic Device Evaluation and Safety develop guidance documents to articulate safety and effectiveness requirements on specific device types. The guidance documents provide consistency and predictability, which helps manufacturers gather appropriate non-clinical and clinical data, plan, and submit an organized and well-thought out marketing application.

More information on FDA laws, regulations, and guidance is available at http://www.fda.gov.

20.5 The Regulatory Environment for Bringing a Medical Device to Market

Anyone who wishes to commercially distribute in the United States medical devices or electronic products that emit radiation must comply with applicable US laws and regulations, even if the product is authorized for marketing in another country. At present, the FDA does not recognize regulatory marketing approvals from other countries. However, it will evaluate all safety and effectiveness information submitted to it in the premarket application, including foreign clinical data.

Comprehensive information about the Center for Devices and Radiological Health and the regulation of medical devices can be found at http://www.fda.gov/MedicalDevices.

It is also important to know that device regulatory topics discussed in this chapter are accessible from the FDA Medical Devices homepage, under Medical Device Topics, "Device Advice: Comprehensive Regulatory Assistance" http://www.fda.gov/MedicalDevices/DeviceRegulationandGuidance.

20.6 Regulatory Considerations to Market and Keep Devices in Distribution

20.6.1 Definition of Medical Devices

Section 201(h) of the FD&C Act defines the term "device" as "an instrument, apparatus, implement, machine, contrivance, implant, *in vitro* reagent, or other similar or related article, including a component part, or accessory which is recognized in the official National Formulary, or the United States Pharmacopoeia, or any supplement to them, intended for use in the diagnosis of disease or other conditions, or in the cure, mitigation, treatment, or prevention of disease, in man or other animals, or intended to affect the structure or any function of the body of man or other animals, and which does not achieve any of its primary intended purposes through chemical action within or on the body of man or other animals and which is not dependent upon being metabolized for the achievement of any of its primary intended purposes."

The definition above determines whether the product is a medical device and provides a clear distinction between a medical device and other FDA regulated products such as drugs or biologics. In such cases, another FDA Center is responsible for the regulation of the product.

You may also find the definition of a medical device by entering in the Search box "medical device definition" at http://www.fda.gov/MedicalDevices/DeviceRegulationandGuidance.

20.6.2 Classification of Medical Devices

The FD&C Act also requires FDA to classify all devices intended for human use into one of three regulatory categories (Class I, Class II, and Class III). The tiered classification is based on risk. Appropriate level of regulatory control necessary to assure safety and effectiveness of each device increases according to its classification. Some examples of Class I devices are battery-powered ophthalmic electrolysis units and protective restraints. Examples of Class II devices include blood pressure monitors, oximeters, and electrocardiographs. Further, in an effort to reduce regulatory burden, the FDA judged most Class I devices and some Class II devices exempt from submitting a Premarket Notification (510(k)) application (discussed below). Examples of Class I Exempt devices include tongue depressors, elastic bandages, and manual stethoscopes. Examples of Class II Exempt devices are radiologic tables and biofeedback devices. Class III devices have the highest risk and the most stringent regulatory controls. Examples of Class III devices are implantable cardiac pacemakers, hip joint acetabular metal cemented prostheses, and heart valves.

Often used in the surgical setting are kits or trays consisting of two or more separate types of finished devices packaged together for the convenience of the user and often referred to a convenience kit. The device classification of the kit is based on the highest classification of the devices that are provided in the kit.

CDRH makes available to the public several medical device databases under Tools and Resources at http://www.fda.gov/MedicalDevices/DeviceRegulationandGuidance/Databases.

The publicly available product classification database (Fig. 20.2) provides a means for conducting a simple and advanced search. It contains the medical device name, the associated three-letter product code unique to CDRH and identifies the device class as well as the type of premarket submission. Other information also includes the device definition, the regulation description, any applicable recognized consensus standard, and other important regulatory information about the generic device type.

http://www.accessdata.fda.gov/scripts/cdrh/cfdocs/cfPCD/classification.cfm

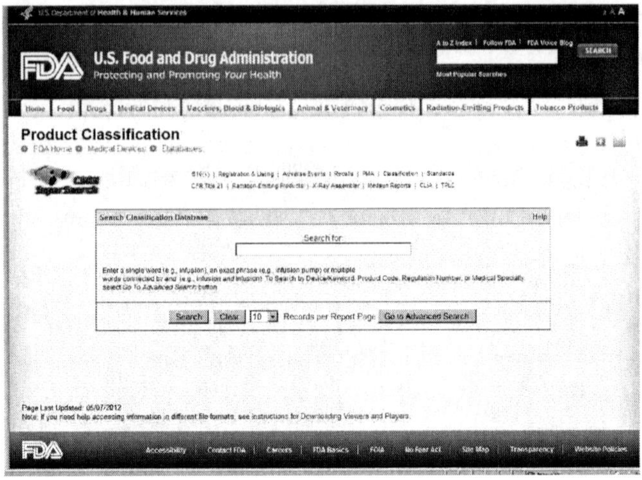

Figure 20.2 Screen shot of the Product Classification search database.

All classes of medical devices are subject to general regulatory controls.

The FD&C Act requires baseline controls necessary for marketing, proper labeling and monitoring performance once a device is on the market. All devices must comply with the following General Controls:

- Adulteration and Misbranding
- Establishment Registration and Medical Device Listing
- Premarket Notification (510(k)), unless exempt
- Labeling requirements
- Quality System Regulation/Good Manufacturing Practices (GMP)
- Medical Device Reporting (MDR)

More information is available at http://www.fda.gov/MedicalDevices/DeviceRegulationandGuidance/Overview.

20.6.3 Adulteration and Misbranding

Medical devices are subject to the adulteration and misbranding provisions of the FD&C Act. In Section 501, a device is considered to be adulterated if it includes any filthy, putrid, or decomposed substance, or if it is prepared, packed, or held under unsanitary conditions. The misbranding provisions of various aspects of drug and device labeling requirements are covered in Section 502. An example of misbranding violation is if a device labeling is false and misleading, or if it does not bear adequate directions for use, warnings, etc.

Particulars are available at http://www.fda.gov/MedicalDevices/DeviceRegulationandGuidance/Overview/GeneralandSpecialControls/ucm055910.htm.

20.6.4 Establishment Registration and Medical Device Listing

Manufacturers (both domestic and foreign) and initial distributors (importers) of medical devices must register their establishments with the FDA and are required to pay a fee and register annually. The initial registration and/or device listing information must be submitted within 30 days of an establishment beginning an activity or placing a device in commercial distribution. Afterwards, the fee-based registration information must be submitted every year even if no changes have occurred between October 1 and December 31 of each year. Device listing must also be reviewed at the same time. However, device listing updates may be submitted at any time without additional fees. The registration process is done electronically.

In addition, foreign manufacturers must also designate a US Agent. Most establishments that are required to register are also required to list the devices that are made in those facilities, as well as activities that are performed on those devices. If a device requires 510(k) clearance or PMA approval before being marketed in the United States, the manufacturer must wait until the FDA has granted the clearance or approval to market the device. Note that Registration and Listing is not a marketing authorization, certification or license to market a device in the United States. However, one should be aware that in some regulatory systems in the world, the term "Registration" may be equivalent to marketing authorization to sell and distribute a device.

More information on the required fees, how to register, payment process, US agent, and other important reminders about registration and listing can be found at http://www.fda.gov/MedicalDevices/DeviceRegulationandGuidance/HowtoMarketYourDevice/RegistrationandListing.

20.6.5 Premarket Notification (510(k))

Two of the most common pathways in successfully bringing a medical device to market are described in this chapter: (1) Premarket Notification (510(k)) clearance (21 CFR Part 807 Subpart E), and (2) Premarket Approval (PMA) process (21 CFR Part 814).

The Section 510(k) of the FD&C Act requires device manufacturers to notify FDA, at least 90 days in advance, of their intent to market a medical device in the United States. The 510(k) regulatory process requires manufacturers to demonstrate "substantial equivalence," that is, the proposed (or new) device is at least as safe and effective as a predicate device. The predicate device is a legally marketed device that has previously been cleared to market through the 510(k) program and serves as a comparator to which substantial equivalence is claimed. A predicate device cannot be in violation of the Act. A substantial equivalence determination or request for additional information is usually made within 90 days upon receipt of a 510(k) submission.

Special Controls

All Class I and Class II devices, unless exempt, require submission of a 510(k) application and are subject to General Controls. Exempt devices are only exempt from a 510(k) submission but are subject to the requirements of other applicable General Controls (Registration and Listing, Labeling, GMP). Additionally, Class II devices must meet the requirements for Special Controls since General Controls alone are insufficient to assure safety and effectiveness of Class II devices. Examples of Special Controls include special labeling requirements, patient registries, mandatory performance standards, and postmarket surveillance studies. Class II Special Controls Guidance Documents have been written for some device types (e.g., bone sonometers, percutaneous transluminal coronary angioplasty (PTCA) catheters) or systems (e.g. full field digital mammography system and instrumentation for clinical multiplex test systems). All available medical guidance documents, including Special Controls guidance documents are searchable at the following site: http://www.fda.gov/MedicalDevices/DeviceRegulationandGuidance/GuidanceDocuments

20.6.5.1 Kits

For a kit to be marketed in the United States as described in the classification section above, the submission must identify all devices provided in the kit and document the marketing status of each device in the kit by including the Kit Certification for 510(k)s. Certain convenience kits that meet the criteria in the Convenience Kit Interim Regulatory Guidance are under enforcement discretion and do not require a 510(k). If a 510(k) is not required, it is recommended to maintain this information in your files.

The Guidance documents pertaining to convenience kits are

- Convenience Kits Interim Regulatory Guidance
- Sterilized Convenience Kits for Clinical and Surgical Use

There are special considerations for medical device kit that include gloves and/or sutures. Kit manufacturers and assemblers should assure that the gloves and/or sutures in their kits are cleared for marketing in the US additional guidance and other requirements for medical gloves are available in Guidance for Medical Gloves.

20.6.5.2 Predicate device and substantial equivalence

For purposes of seeking to market a device in US interstate commerce, the first step is to confirm that the product is a medical device according to the definition discussed in the section above. The next step is to determine which regulatory pathway is required. If the appropriate market application is determined to be through the 510(k) clearance regulatory process, the manufacturer must demonstrate that the proposed device is *at least as safe and effective*, that is, *substantially equivalent* to a *legally marketed* device (21 CFR 807.92(a)(3)) that is not subject to PMA. The legally marketed device to which equivalence is drawn is also known as the "predicate" device. Most often devices recently cleared under 510(k) are selected as the predicate to which equivalence is claimed. However, any legally marketed 510(k)-cleared device may be used as a predicate.

Demonstration of substantial equivalence does not imply the new and predicate devices must be identical. Substantial equivalence is established with respect to intended use, design, energy used or delivered, materials, chemical composition, manufacturing process, performance, safety, effectiveness, labeling, biocompatibility, standards, and other characteristics, as applicable.

A device is substantially equivalent if, in comparison with a predicate, it

- has the same intended use as the predicate; **and**
- has the same technological characteristics as the predicate; **or**
- has the same intended use as the predicate; **and**
- has different technological characteristics and the information submitted to FDA;
  - does not raise new questions of safety and effectiveness; **and**
  - demonstrates that the device is at least as safe and effective as the legally marketed device.

A device may not be marketed in the United States until the submitter receives a letter declaring the device substantially equivalent and "clears" the device for commercial distribution.

Details may be found at http://www.fda.gov/MedicalDevices/DeviceRegulationandGuidance.

Of the note are the lists of topics that appear on the left side of the screen (Fig. 20.3) as they provide a detailed explanation of regulatory topic of interest, often in a tutorial fashion. For example, from the Device Regulation and Guidance Web site, the link to Premarket Submissions will then lead to the Premarket Notifications (510(k)) site. Below is an example of the Premarket Notification 510(k) screen with subtopics on the left hand side such as Submission Process, 510(k) Forms, How to Find a Predicate Device, How to Prepare a Traditional 510(k), Abbreviated 510(k) or Special 510(k) and many more topics.

Additionally, an excellent resource for identifying predicate device(s) and other important regulatory information about a legally marketed device such as product code, regulation number, description, and others is to make use of publicly available search engines under Medial Device Databases, namely: Product Classification, Premarket Notifications (510(k)), etc. A more recently added database is the TPLC (Total Product Life Cycle) database that integrates premarket and postmarket data about a device.

(http://www.fda.gov/MedicalDevices/DeviceRegulationand Guidance/Databases)

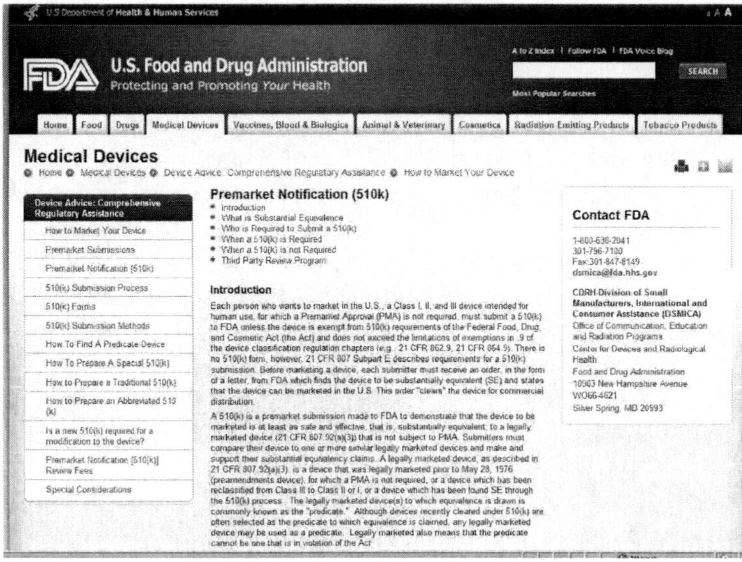

Figure 20.3 Screenshot of the Device Regulation and Guidance Web site and Premarket Submissions.

20.6.5.3 Planning and assembling the 510(k) submission process

In the Code of Federal Regulation, 21 CFR 807 Subpart E, describes requirements for a 510(k) submission. The Office of Device Evaluation (ODE) and the Office of *In Vitro* Diagnostic Device Evaluation and Safety (OIVD) within CDRH are responsible for review of 510(k) applications. Within the offices, Divisions and Branches are organized into sub-units according to medical scientific disciplines and specialties. The pool of *scientific reviewers* is multidisciplinary that include engineers (electrical, software, biomedical, mechanical, etc.), physicians, physicists, microbiologists, chemists, material scientists, statisticians and others who perform and evaluate the safety and effectiveness of 510(k) applications and other regulatory submissions such as clinical investigations under the Investigational Device Exemption (IDE) regulation (discussed below). The scientific reviewer recommends whether a new device is found substantially equivalent (SE) or not substantially equivalent (NSE).

The 510(k) submission process begins when the application is received in the CDRH Document Mail Center, date stamped, entered into the internal FDA database and assigned a unique document control number that is referred to as the 510(k) number. It begins with the letter "K" and is followed by 6 numeric digits. Having a general understanding of the next steps, (i.e., what happens to the document after the log-in procedure) is helpful knowledge to acquire before preparing the 510(k) application. It is recommended that a 510(k) application be administratively complete in order for the scientific review to proceed. The Web link below explains in more detail the routing process: Division Acceptance and Review, Scientific Reviewer Assignment, FDA Requests for Additional Information, Issuance of the Decision Letter, and Request the Review Status of the 510(k) submission.

(http://www.fda.gov/MedicalDevices/DeviceRegulationandGuidance/HowtoMarketYourDevice/PremarketSubmissions/PremarketNotification510k/ucm070201.htm)

When writing the 510(k) submission, it is critical to clearly identify and articulate the "*indications for use*," for which, a substantially equivalent determination is sought. CDRH will include the indications for use in the clearance letters for devices found to be substantially equivalent to a legally marketed predicate device. The confusion between the agency and the 510(k) submitter is minimized if not eliminated.

Furthermore, it is very important to understand the different forms associated with premarket notification and comply with the applicable requirements. This would facilitate the preparation time and prepare a well-organized submission that meets the essential administrative elements. An incomplete submission package may result in FDA "*refuse to file*" your application.

Following is the list of the forms:

- 510(k) Pre-Review Form
- Exempt Device Review Form
- Screening Checklist for Traditional/Abbreviated Premarket Notification [510(k)] Submissions
- 510(k) Format Guidance
- 510(k) Review Template

- Premarket Notification [510(k)] Status Request and Response (PDF-419 KB)
- 510(k) Review Template Instructions
- 510(k) Cover Sheet Memorandum
- 510(k) "Substantial Equivalence" Decision Making Process
- Standards Data Form for Abbreviated 510(k)s
- Sterile Devices in Premarket Notification [510(k)] Submissions
- Description of 510(k) "Substantial Equivalence" Decision-Making Process (Accessible Text)
- Premarket Notification Class III Certification and Summary
- Premarket Notification Truthful And Accurate Statement
- Premarket Notification 510(k) Statement
- Required Elements for a Declaration of Conformity to a Recognized Standard

Moreover, in the premarket phase, it is vitally important for an applicant to consider the Quality Systems (QS) regulation in planning and during the 510(k) process. Class II, Class III, and certain Class I devices are subject to design control requirements of the QS regulation during the design phase of product development. The topic is discussed further in Section 20.6.9.

20.6.6 Premarket Approval (PMA)

For new, more innovative, non-substantially equivalent devices, the pathway to market is the PMA (21CFR Part 814) route. These devices are the Class III high risk devices, usually those that support or sustain human life, implanted in the body, or pose a significant risk of illness or injury. This regulatory process is more involved and includes submission of clinical data to support medical device claims. In addition to meeting applicable General Controls and Special Controls, a PMA application is required. The regulatory time to review the PMA and for FDA to make a regulatory decision is 180 days.

Details can be found at http://www.fda.gov/MedicalDevices/DeviceRegulationandGuidance/HowtoMarketYourDevice/PremarketSubmissions/PremarketApprovalPMA.

20.6.7 Investigational Device Exemption (IDE)

An IDE allows the investigational device to be used in a clinical study in order to collect safety and effectiveness data. In some cases, clinical data may be required to support a 510(k) submission. The studies must be conducted under the principles of medical device Good Clinical Practices (GCP). The GCP refer to the regulations and requirements that must be complied with while conducting a clinical study. These regulations apply to the manufacturers, sponsors, clinical investigators, institutional review boards, and the medical device. The primary regulations address the following important areas: Investigational Device Exemption (21CFR 812); Protection of Human Subjects (i.e., informed consent) (21CFR 50); Institutional Review Boards or IRB (21CFR 56); Clinical Investigators' Financial Disclosure (21CFR 54); Good Laboratory Practice or GLP for Nonclinical Laboratory Studies (21 CFR 58); and Design Controls of the Quality System Regulation (21CFR 820).

Before a significant risk (SR) IDE study can begin, the FDA and the IRB must review and approve the study. The regulatory time for FDA to review the IDE and make a determination is 30 calendar days or it is deemed approved. A non-significant risk (NSR) IDE study only requires IRB approval before the study can begin but must still comply with the abbreviated requirements of the IDE regulation.

Under the Pre-IDE Program, manufacturers are encouraged to have early dialogue with FDA staff on specific aspects of the IDE application before they submit an official IDE application. An added benefit for early interactions is the "heads-up" on the new device investigational technology and/or clinical protocol that this provides to FDA. The CDRH Office of Device Evaluation conducts the primary review of the IDE submission. The Bioresearch Monitoring Program within the CDRH Office of Compliance oversees the IDE enforcement of good clinical practices.

Details can be found at

http://www.fda.gov/MedicalDevices/DeviceRegulationandGuidance/HowtoMarketYourDevice/InvestigationalDeviceExemptionIDE

20.6.8 Labeling

Labeling includes labels on the device as well as descriptive and informational literature that accompany the device. The general labeling requirements for medical devices are specified in 21 CFR Part 801. These regulations specify the minimum requirements for all devices. There are additional requirements needed for specific categories of devices such as labeling for *in vitro* diagnostic device, IDE devices, radiation-emitting products and natural rubber (latex).

20.6.9 Quality System (QS) Regulation/Good Manufacturing Practices (GMP)

Device manufacturers must comply with the FDA Quality System Regulation (21 CFR Part 820). The regulation includes requirements related to the methods used in the facilities and controls used for designing, purchasing, manufacturing, packaging, labeling, storing, installing and servicing of medical devices in order to conform to current good manufacturing practices (GMP). FDA inspects manufacturing facilities to assure compliance with the QS requirements. Certain types of devices are exempt from GMP. However, exemption from GMP requirements does not exempt manufacturers from keeping complaint files or from general requirements concerning records. IDE clinical studies are exempt from GMP, except for the Design Controls that provide the requirement for procedures to control the design of the device in order to ensure that the specified design requirements are met.

The International Organization for Standardization (ISO) developed and published ISO 13485:2003. It is the international standard relating to Quality Management Systems for organizations involved in the manufacture of Medical Devices. Although there are few substantive differences between the FDA Quality System Regulation and the ISO 13485:2003, there are no conflicting requirements.

For more information on the FDA Quality System (QS) regulation, please refer to Quality Systems at http://www.fda.gov/MedicalDevices/DeviceRegulationandGuidance/PostmarketRequirements/QualitySystemsRegulations.

20.6.10 Medical Device Reporting (MDR)

Reporting of adverse events is a mandatory postmarketing requirement for medical devices. Firms who have received complaints of device malfunctions, serious injuries or deaths associated with medical devices are required to notify FDA of the incident. User Facilities (e.g., hospitals, nursing homes) are required to report suspected medical device related deaths to both the FDA and the manufacturers. They report medical device-related serious injuries only to the manufacturer unless the manufacturer is unknown. In such instances, the serious injury is reported to FDA.

The MDR regulation is contained in 21CFR Part 803. These regulations allow a mechanism for FDA and manufacturers to identify and monitor significant adverse events involving medical devices. The objectives of the regulation are to detect and correct problems in a timely manner. Under the Medical Device Reporting program, incidents in which a device may have caused or contributed to a death or serious injury must to be reported to the FDA. Further, certain malfunctions must also be reported. Currently, CDRH has an electronic medical device reporting program, eMDR. At present, participation in the eMDR program is voluntary.

For more detailed information on postmarket requirements, i.e., reporting adverse events, postmarket surveillance studies, and post-approval studies, go to http://www.fda.gov/MedicalDevices/DeviceRegulationandGuidance/PostmarketRequirements.

How to report a medical device problem: http://www.fda.gov/MedicalDevices/Safety/ReportaProblem.

20.6.11 User Fees

Under the 2002 Medical Device User Fee and Modernization Act (MDUFMA), the FDA began to collect user fees for certain medical device applications, such as 510(k)s, PMAs and Premarket Reports. Additionally, the 2007 reauthorization allowed FDA to collect fees for other types of submissions: 30-day notices, requests for information regarding classification (513g), annual fees for periodic reporting on Class III devices and establishment registration. Small business may be eligible for reduced or waived fees.

For more information on how a firm may qualify for small business and be eligible for substantially discounted rates as well as information on the latest reauthorization of the medical device user fees, go to the medical devices homepage and enter in the search box "user fees."

(http://www.fda.gov/MedicalDevices/DeviceRegu-lationand Guidance)

20.7 Summary

The set of laws in the 1938 FD&C Act, 1968 RCHSA, 1976 Medical Device Amendments, Title 21 Code of Federal Regulations and other statutes, regulations, policies remain the underpinnings for the current US medical devices regulatory framework to protect public health. The USFDA CDRH is the regulatory authority that regulates medical devices in the United States. If a product is labeled, promoted, or used in a manner that meets the definition of a medical devices defined in section 201(h) of the FD&C Act, it will be regulated as a medical device and is subject to premarketing and postmarketing regulatory controls (QS Regulation/GMP and MDR). Foreign companies that manufacture medical devices and/or radiation-emitting products that are imported into the United States must comply with applicable US regulations before, during, and after their import into the United States or its territories. It is important to recognize that the same safety and effectiveness standards apply to all medical devices intended for marketing and distribution in the United States or its territories irrespective of the origin of manufacture.

Figure 20.4 is a simple guide in deciding if a 510(k) or a PMA regulatory route would be the appropriate means to bring a new medical device to the US market. Note that the 510(k) process requires a predicate device as discussed in the Premarket Notification section above.

The FDA Medical Devices Web site (http://www.fda.gov/MedicalDevices) is very rich in information and the main source of all published information regarding the regulation of medical devices in the United States. It is intended to be an intuitive content management based-format display of information that links to more specific locations.

The starting point to get information on how to market a medical device is "Device Advice: Comprehensive Regulatory Assistance." (http://www.fda.gov/MedicalDevices/DeviceRegulationand Guidance)

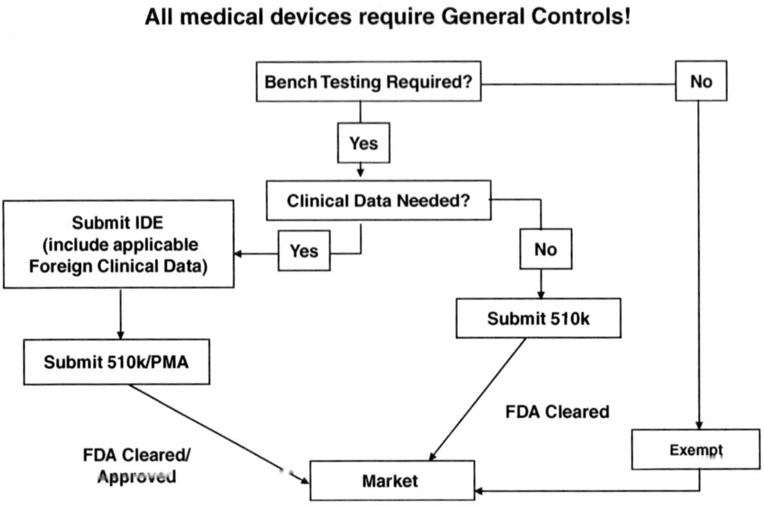

Figure 20.4 Two most common pathways to market a new medical device, a 510(k) or PMA route.

References

1. Center for Device and Radiological Health (2012), Food and Drug Administration. Division for small Manufacturers, International and Consumer Assistance 10903 New Hampshire Avenue WO66-4621 Silver Spring, MD 20993.
2. Device Advice is an on-line comprehensive regulatory assistance. Available: http://www.fda.gov/MedicalDevices/DeviceRegulationandGuidance/.
3. CDRH Learn is a Web-based tutorial consisting of a series of training modules. The different modules describe many aspects of medical device and radiological health regulation, covering both premarket and postmarket issues. Some modules are also available in Spanish and Chinese Mandarin. Available: http://www.fda.gov/Training/CDRHLearn/.
4. Medical Devices Web site. Access to more information concerning other medical device topics, including current program initiatives, device clearances and approvals, recalls and alerts, public databases, and others; Available at http://www.fda.gov/MedicalDevices/.

5. Health Industries: Medical Device Industry Web site. U.S. Department of Commerce, International Trade Administration report, "Medical Device Industry Assessment Updated March 24, 2010. Available April 17, 2012, at http://ita.doc.gov/td/health/medical.html.

Chapter 21

European Union: Medical Device Regulatory System

Patricia Teysseyre

Johnson & Johnson Medical Asia Pacific,
No. 2, International Business Park,
#07-01, Tower One, The Strategy, 609930 Singapore
pteyssey@its.jnj.com

Disclaimer

The regulatory information contained in this chapter is intended for market planning and is subject to change frequently. Translations of laws and regulations are unofficial.

21.1 Glossary of Terms

AIMD	Active Implantable Medical Devices Directive 90/385/EEC
BBP	Benzyl butyl phthalate
CE	European Conformity
CEN	European Committee for Standardization
CENELEC	European Committee for Electrotechnical Standardization
CMR	Carcinogenic, Mutagenic and Toxic to reproduction
COCIR	European Coordination Committee of the Radiological, Electromedical and Healthcare IT Industry
DBP	Dibutyl Phthalate
DEHP	Di-(2-ethylhexyl) phthalate

Handbook of Medical Device Regulatory Affairs in Asia
Edited by Jack Wong and Raymond K. Y. Tong

ISBN 978-981-4411-21-9 (Hardcover), 978-981-4411-22-6 (eBook)
www.panstanford.com

EC	European Community
EDMA	European Diagnostic Manufacturers Association
EEA	European Economic Area
EEC	European Economic Community
EFTA	European Free Trade Association
EMIG	European Medical Devices Industry Group
ETSI	European Telecommunications Standards Institute
EU	European Union
EUCOMED	European Medical Devices Technology Industry Association
EUROM VI	European Medical Technology Industry
FSCA	Field Safety Corrective Action
GHTF	Global Harmonization Task Force The GHTF will evolve in 2012 into the International Medical Device Regulators' Forum (IMDRF)
IAF	International Accreditation Forum
IEC	International Electrotechnical Commission
ISO	International Standards Organization
IVD	*In-Vitro* Diagnostics Medical Devices Directive 98/79/EC
MD	Medical Device
MDD	Medical Device Directive 93/42/EEC
MDEG	European Medical Devices Expert Group
MEDDEV	Medical Devices Guidance Document
NANDO	New Approach Notified and Designated Organizations information system: database operated by the European Commission that catalogs all the notified bodies and the directives that the organizations technically are qualified to review.
NB	Notified Body
NB-MED	Co-ordination of Notified Bodies Medical Devices on Council Directives 90/385/EEC, 93/42/EEC and 98/79/EC
NBOG	Notified Body Operations Group
PMS	Post-Market Surveillance
STED	Summary Technical Documentation for Demonstrating Conformity to the Essential Principles of Safety and Performance of Medical Devices
TEAM-NB	European Association for Medical Devices of Notified Bodies
UDI	Unique Device Identifier

21.2 European Union: History and Structure

The European Community as of 2011 comprises 27 countries, which represent 830 million people (Table 21.1). The medical device market is estimated to be of €62 billion.

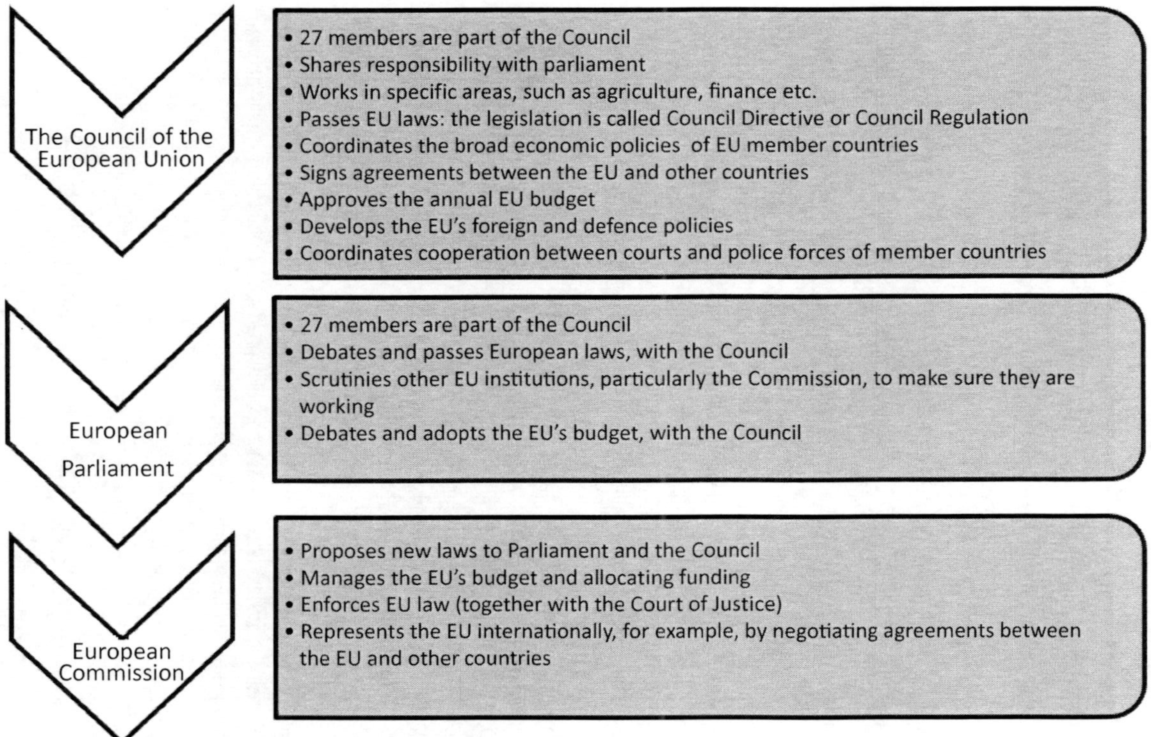

Figure 21.1 Structure of the European institutions.

Table 21.1 List of member states of the European Union

Year of entry into the EU	Member states
1958	Belgium, France, Germany, Italy, Luxembourg, the Netherlands
1973	Denmark, Ireland, the United Kingdom
1981	Greece
1986	Portugal, Spain
1995	Austria, Finland, Sweden
2004	Czech Republic, Cyprus, Estonia, Hungary, Latvia, Lithuania, Malta, Poland, Slovak Republic, Slovenia
2007	Bulgaria, Romania

The European Union member countries facilitate the free movement of goods and humans. The structure of the European Institutions is illustrated in Fig. 21.1. Medical devices bearing the CE mark are considered to be cleared in the European Union market. The European Economic Area (EEA) was established on 1 January 1994 following an agreement between the member states of the European Free Trade Association (EFTA) and the European Community: Iceland, Liechtenstein and Norway are allowed to participate in the EU's Internal Market without a conventional EU membership. In exchange, they are obliged to adopt all EU legislation related to the single market, for Medical Devices for instance. One EFTA member, Switzerland, has not joined the EEA; CE marking of Medical Devices is, however, recognized in Switzerland by means of a Mutual Recognition Agreement (MRA) between the EU and Switzerland. CE marking is now also in place in Turley, following the Ankara Agreement between EU and Turkey. Mutual acceptance between Turkey and EFTA is arranged in an agreement between these parties based on CE marking.

The next country currently in the process of entering the EU is Croatia, expected to be member in 2013.

21.3 New Approach — Global Approach Concepts

As Foodstuffs, Chemicals and Pharmaceuticals were already regulated in EU, a new legislative and technical frame has been created in 1985 for the other products circulating in the EU countries.

The New Approach concept [8] is a legislative-technical frame for harmonization in Europe: it is to link industrials and regulators for harmonization for the elaboration of Directives and Technical Standards.

Using the New Approach for market access results in most of the cases by having a product recognized by a European Conformity (CE) mark. However, among the Directives (around 20; Table 21.2) which adopt the New Approach, some did without the CE mark like the Directive 94/62/EC on waste and packaging.

The New Approach concept (Fig. 21.2) was established in 1985 and resulted in the elaboration of European Directives, which are based on the following principles:

- Only products fulfilling the essential requirements may be placed on the market and put into service.
- Harmonized standards, the reference numbers of which have been published in the Official Journal and which have been transposed into national standards, are presumed to conform to the corresponding essential requirements.
- Application of harmonized standards or other technical specifications remains voluntary, and manufacturers are free to choose any technical solution that provides compliance with the essential requirements.
- Manufacturers may choose between different conformity assessment procedures provided in the applicable directive.

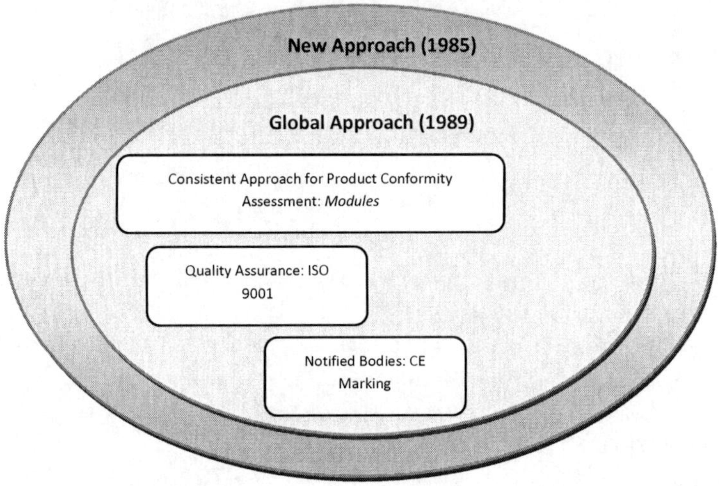

Figure 21.2 New Approach: Global Approach Diagram.

The Global Approach concept was issued in 1989 and introduced the following points:

- Modules for each development phase of the product (design/prototype/manufacture) were established for the conformity assessment, defining criteria for use and designation of bodies operating these procedures.
- The use of European standards relating to quality assurance (EN ISO 9000 series), which by now includes ISO 13485 for the medical device industry.
- Accreditation systems and use of inter-comparison techniques were promoted in member states.
- Mutual recognition agreements concerning testing and certification.
- Programs to minimize the differences between member states and industrial sectors (quality infrastructures: calibration/metrology, testing laboratories, certification/inspection/accreditation bodies).
- Mutual recognition agreements with third countries to facilitate the cooperation and technical assistance programs.

Table 21.2 List of European directives

Directive reference	Subject of directive
90/396/EEC	Appliances burning gaseous fuels
2000/9/EC	Cableway installations designed to carry persons
89/106/EEC	Construction products
2004/108/EC	Electromagnetic compatibility
94/9/EC	Equipment and protective systems in potentially explosive atmospheres
93/15/EEC	Explosives for civil uses
90/396/EEC	Gas appliances
95/16/EC	Lifts
2006/95/EC	Low Voltage Equipment
2006/42/EC	Machinery safety
2004/22/EC	Measuring instruments
93/42/EEC	**Medical devices**
90/385/EEC	**Medical devices: Active implantable**
98/79/EC	**Medical devices: *In vitro* diagnostic**

92/42/EEC	New hot-water boilers fired with liquid or gaseous fluids (efficiency requirements)
90/384/EEC	Non-automatic weighing instruments
94/62/EC	Packaging and packaging waste
89/686/EEC	Personal protective equipment
97/23/EC	Pressure equipment
1999/5/EC	Radio and telecommunications terminal equipment
94/25/EC	Recreational craft
87/404/EEC	Simple pressure vessels
88/378/EEC	Toys safety

Regulations address essential safety and performance principles. Detailed technical requirements and characteristics are provided by voluntary product standards developed by national and international expert groups (see ISO TR 16142:1999). The international reference standard for medical device quality systems requirements is ISO 13485.

21.4 Harmonized Standards and Presumption of Conformity

A standard stands for an agreed understanding of key words and terminology and methods, which, when applied by the manufacture, ensure a common global level of safety of medical care to patient.

The formal definition of a standard is: standards are documented agreements containing technical specifications or other precise criteria to be used consistently as rules, guidelines or definitions of characteristics, to ensure that materials, products, process are fit for their purpose. Standards can:

- Provide reference criteria that a product, process or service must meet;
- Provide information that enhances safety, reliability and performance of products, processes and services;
- Assure consumers about reliability or other characteristics of goods or services provided in the marketplace [16].

Harmonized standards are European standards prepared in accordance with the General Guidelines agreed between the

Commission and the European standards harmonization, and follow a mandate issued by the Commission after consultation with the member states.

Conformity with a national standard that transposes a harmonized standard, whose reference has been published, confers a presumption of conformity with the essential requirements of the applicable New Approach directive that is covered by such a standard.

References (such as titles, identification numbers) of harmonized standards are published in the Official Journal for the directive in question. Member states must publish the reference of the national standard that transposes a harmonized standard. The application of harmonized standards, which give a presumption of conformity, remains voluntary. Thus, the product may be manufactured directly on the basis of the essential requirements.

For getting information about standards under review or creation and for acquisition of the published standard, the manufacturer has to apply and buy them from the standard organizations at the European level (Table 21.3) or at the national level.

Table 21.3 List of committees for standardization

Committee name	Scope
CEN	CEN is the European Committee for Standardization. It contributes voluntary technical standards which promote free trade, the safety of workers and consumers, environmental protection, exploitation of research and development programs, and public procurement.
CENELEC	CENELEC is the European Committee for Electrotechnical Standardization and is responsible for standardization in the electrotechnical engineering field.
ETSI	The European Telecommunications Standards Institute (ETSI) produces globally applicable standards for Information and Communications Technologies (ICT), including fixed, mobile, radio, converged, broadcast and internet technologies.
IEC	IEC is the International Electrotechnical Commission. It is the world's leading organization that prepares and publishes international standards for all electrical, electronic and related technologies.
ISO	ISO is International Standards Organizatio. It is an international standard-setting body composed of representatives from various national standards bodies.

Table 21.4 List of European associations

Association name	Competences/terms of reference	Participants
MDEG	It is a group of member states, industry and other stakeholder representatives in the area of medical devices for the implementation of the directive. This group is the umbrella group for other working groups in the field and co-ordinates and oversees their activities. In closed session MDEG is a forum to discuss all issues relating to the implementation of the medical device directives with member state competent authorities. MDEG publishes MEDDEV Guidance Documents.	competent authorities, industry (trade associations), notified bodies, standardisation bodies, COM services MDEG also meets in closed sessions including competent authorities only.
NBOG	Its aim is to contribute to improvement of the overall performance of notified bodies in the medical devices sector by primarily identifying and promulgating examples of best practice to be adopted by both notified bodies and those harmonization responsible for their designation and control. They review the "recommendations" issued by the NB-MED (group where all the EU notified bodies participate) and act as a "Mirror Group" following GHTF work relating to notified bodies.	Competent authorities/designating authorities (experts), COM services (On focal points, a notified body representative can be invited to participate)
NB-MED	To share experience and exchange views on application of conformity assessment procedures with the aim of contributing to a better understanding and consistent application of requirements and procedures. To draft technical recommendations on matters relating to conformity assessment and build a consensus. To advise the Commission, at its request, on subjects related to application of the medical device directives. To consider, and if necessary, draft reports on ethical aspects of notified bodies' activities. To ensure consistency with standardization work at European level. To keep informed of harmonization activities at European level.	notified bodies, competent authorities (experts), industry, standardisation bodies, COM services
TEAM-NB	A non-profit association of 32 notified bodies under any or all of the three medical device new approach directives: 90/385/EEC; 93/42/EEC; 98/79/EC. The association aims • to improve communications with the EC Commission, Industry, competent authorities and user groups by acting as a focal point and the single voice of notified bodies, • to promote high technical and ethical standards in the functioning of notified bodies, and • to protect the legal and commercial interests of notified bodies in their vital role in the functioning of the three medical device directives	Medical Device notified bodies

(Continued)

Table 21.4 (*Continued*)

Association name	Competences/terms of reference	Participants
EUCOMED	It represents the medical technology industry in Europe. Eucomed members include both national and pan-European trade and product associations as well as medical technology manufacturers, representing around 22,500 designers, manufacturers and suppliers of medical technology used in the diagnosis, prevention, treatment and amelioration of disease and disability.	Industry representatives
EDMA	It is the trade association that represents the *In Vitro* Diagnostic (IVD) industry active in Europe. EDMA membership brings together 22 National Associations in European countries and 43 major companies engaged in the research, development, manufacture or distribution of IVD products. Through its affiliated National Associations, EDMA represents in total more than 500 companies across Europe. Since its establishment in 1979, EDMA acts in co-operation with other European and international trade associations representing medical devices, pharmaceuticals and biotechnology in general, as well as with scientific societies and patients organisations to make a real difference in health and life quality.	Industry representatives
COCIR	This non-profit trade association was founded in 1959 and represents the medical technology industry in Europe. COCIR's aim is to represent the interests and activities of its members and act as a communication channel between its members and the European institutions and other regulatory bodies. It also cooperates with other organisations on issues of common interest. COCIR seeks to promote the development of harmonized international standards and regulatory control which respect the quality and effectiveness of the medical devices and healthcare IT systems without compromising the safety of patients and users and promote the free worldwide trade of these products. COCIR encourages the use of technology in delivering cost-efficient and state of the art healthcare systems.	Industry representatives
EUROM VI- Medical Technology	European small and medium enterprises involved in medical devices for surgery (including dental), anaesthesia, respiration and inhalation, operating theatre, gas supply, sterilization, disinfection, internal and external orthopaedics, opto-medical and ophthalmology area, rehabilitation and handicaps fields, infusion and transfusion. Its objectives are to represent the European medical technology industry to promote cooperation between members but also with other European organizations; to encourage worldwide trade by being involved in harmonization of legislation, standardization, mutual recognition and certification procedures, to be a partner on works with UE Commission and Standardization Bodies; to defend European industry views on international activities.	Industry representatives
EMIG	It is a non-profit trade association, and brings together the European medical industry organizations COCIR, EUCOMED, EDMA, EUROM VI, and a few smaller once, representing a unified European industry voice where possible.	Industry representatives

21.5 European Associations

The European associations active in Europe which contribute to shape the regulatory environment and offer platforms for regulators and industry to communicate with each other and work on harmonization are shown in Table 21.4.

21.6 Overview of Medical Devices Directives

The European Directives (Table 21.5) have to be transposed into national law by each member state in order to integrate the content of these directives into laws and regulations without major modification (Changes which conflict with EU Directive are not acceptable).

Table 21.5 List of applicable directives to medical devices

Date of enforcement	Reference	Designation	Scope	Examples
1990	AIMD 90/385/EEC	Directive on Active Implantable Medical Devices	Active Implantable Medical Devices	Cardiac Pacemaker, defibrillator
1993	MDD 93/42/EEC	Medical Device Directive	Medical Devices	Sutures, syringes
1998	IVD 98/79/EC	Directive on *In Vitro* Diagnostics Medical Devices	*In Vitro* Diagnostics Medical Devices	Blood collection system, Petri dishes

The other products which do not fall under the scope of medical devices are regulated by different directives such as

- Biocides Directive 98/8/EC
- Directive for Medicinal Products 2001/83/EC, applicable to drugs
- Directive for Cosmetics Products 76/768/EEC which will be replaced by the regulation 1223/2009 to be enacted on July 2013. This change will have an impact on the medical devices directives, as cosmetics implant will be removed from cosmetics and included in medical devices

21.7 Guidelines

The interpretation of the Directives is supported by the elaboration of guidelines entitled "MEDDEV" (Table 21.6) and issued within the MDEG Group: They are elaborated through a process of consultation with competent authorities and Commission representatives, notified bodies, industry and other interested parties in the medical devices sector. They remain voluntary; however, it is anticipated that the guidelines will be followed within the member states and, therefore, ensure uniform application of relevant Directive provisions. Guidelines are subject of a regular updating process [6].

Table 21.6 Examples of MEDDEV guidelines

Scope	Title	MEDDEV reference
Application, Definitions	Borderline products, drug-delivery products and medical devices incorporating, as integral part, an ancillary medicinal substance or an ancillary human blood derivative	MEDDEV 2.1/3 rev 3
2.3: Reference to standards	Publication of titles and references of European harmonized standards under AIMD and MDD	MEDDEV 2.3/1
2.4: Classification of MD	Guidelines to the classification of medical devices	MEDDEV 2.4/1 rev.9
	Manual Borderline Classification MD	MEDDEV ver. 1.8
2.5: Conformity assessment procedure General rules	Technical documentation	MEDDEV 2.5.1/Rec5
	Reporting of design changes and of changes of the quality system	MEDDEV 2.5.2/Rec2
2.5.4: Verification of manufactured products	Homogeneous batches	MEDDEV 2.5.4/Rec1
	Verification of manufacture products for IVD directive	MEDDEV 2.5.4/Rec2
2.7: Clinical investigation, clinical evaluation	Clinical evaluation: Guide for manufacturers and notified bodies	MEDDEV 2.7.1 Rev3
	Clinical investigations: Serous adverse event reporting	MEDDEV 2.7/3
2.11: Products using materials of biological origin	Application of council Directive 93/42/EEC taking into account the Commission Directive 2003/32/EC for Medical Devices utilizing tissues or derivatives originating from animals for which a TSE risk is suspected	MEDDEV 2.11/1 rev.1
2.12: Market surveillance; vigilance	Medical devices vigilance System	MEDDEV 2.12/1 rev.6
	Appendix, list of contact points	MEDDEV 2.12/1 rev 4
	Clinical Evaluation — Post-Market Clinical Follow-up	MEDDEV 2.12/2
	Post-Marketing Surveillance (PMS) post-market/production	MEDDEV 2.12/Rec1

Note: The exhaustive list in their latest revision is available on line on the MEDDEV website.

21.8 Definitions

21.8.1 Medical Device

A "medical device" according to 93/42/EEC directive [1] as last amended in 2007/47/EC [4], means any instrument, apparatus, appliance, software, material or other article, whether used alone or in combination, including the software intended by its manufacturer to be used specifically for diagnostic and/or therapeutic purposes and necessary for its proper application, intended by the manufacturer to be used for human beings for the purpose of

- diagnosis, prevention, monitoring, treatment or alleviation of disease
- diagnosis, monitoring, treatment, alleviation of or compensation for an injury or handicap
- investigation, replacement or modification of the anatomy or of a physiological process
- control of conception

and which does not achieve its principal mode of action in or on the human body by pharmacological, immunological or metabolic means, but which may be assisted in its function by such means.

21.8.2 CE Mark

The CE mark is the proof from the manufacturer that the product is in conformity with the regulations.

CE marking attests that the products are in conformity with the essential requirements of the applicable directives and that the products were subjected to the procedure of conformity evaluation envisioned in the directives.

CE marking is affixed before marketing the product.

CE marking allows freedom of movement of the medical device in the territory of the European Union

It engages the responsibility of the manufacturer, on all aspects relative to the product.

The manufacturer must maintain the technical documentation of the device and supply it to the proper authorities.

Devices other than those used to measure and those intended for clinical investigations that are put on the market or brought into service in Europe must be CE marked.

The manufacturer chooses a procedure for CE marking, whether or not to utilize a notified body, in particular according to the class of the medical device (Fig. 21.3).

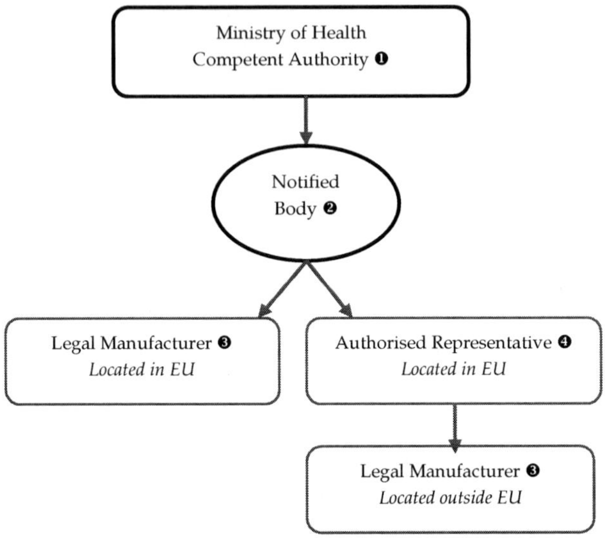

Figure 21.3 Relation between the different actors.

21.8.3 Competent Authority❶

The competent authority or regulatory authority is a government agency or other entity that exercises a legal right to control the use or sale of medical devices within its jurisdiction. It has the ability to take enforcement action to ensure that medical products marketed within its jurisdiction comply with legal requirements.
Its roles and responsibilities are as follows:

- indicates and inspects the notified bodies
- supervises the market
- centralizes and evaluates the vigilance data
- takes suitable medical measurements of police force

Following are the examples of competent authority:

- United Kingdom: MHRA (Medicines and Healthcare Products Regulatory Agency)
- France: AFSSAPS (Agence Francaise de Securite Sanitaire des Produits de Sante)

- Ireland: IMB (Irish Medicines Board)
- Germany: BfArM (Bundesinstitut für Arzneimittel und Medizinprodukte)

21.8.4 Notified Body: Conformity Assessment Body❷

A notified body (as per Medical Devices Directives terminology) is a certification organization authorized by the relevant member state's competent authority to perform conformity assessment tasks specified in the Directives.

The notified body is responsible to evaluate the conformity of the product with the essential requirements and issues the CE mark certificate.

The notified body is an organization indicated and supervised by the proper authority of the member state and must meet the criteria of Annex IX of Directive 93/42/EEC for medical devices, criteria of Annex IX of Directive 98/79/EC for *in vitro* diagnostic medical devices and criteria of Annex 8 of the Directive 90/385/CE to be notified for active implantable medical devices.

A Conformity Assessment Body (CAB from the GHTF terminology) is a body engaged in the performance of procedures for determining whether the relevant requirements in technical regulations or standards are fulfilled. A CAB is authorized to undertake specified conformity assessment activities by a regulatory authority that will ensure performance of the CAB is monitored and, if necessary, withdrawal of designation.

The manufacturer calls upon the notified body of choice: among the 76 registered notified bodies in Europe, of which 5 are in Switzerland and 1 in Australia at the time of this publication.

Nando (New Approach Notified and Designated Organisations) Information System

Notification is an act whereby a member state informs the Commission and the other member states that a body, which fulfils the relevant requirements, has been designated to carry out conformity assessment according to a directive. Notification of notified bodies and their withdrawal are the responsibility of the notifying member state.

The lists of notified bodies can be searched on the NANDO website. The lists include the identification number of each notified body as well as the tasks for which it has been notified, and are subject to regular update.

Table 21.7 Examples of notified body

Designation	Body type	Identification number
Laboratoire national d'essais/G-MED, France	LNE/G-med	0459
British Standards Institution, United Kingdom	BSI	0086
National Standards Authority of Ireland, Ireland	NSAI	0050
TÜV SÜD Product Service GmbH, Germany	TÜV	0123

21.8.5 Legal Manufacturer[3]

The legal manufacturer means the natural or legal person with responsibility for the design, manufacturing, packaging and labelling of a device before it is placed on the market under his own name, regardless of whether these operations are carried out by that person himself or on his behalf by a third party, as defined in each relevant section of the Directives: Medical Devices Directive 93/42/EEC-Article 1.2.(f), *In-Vitro* Diagnostic Devices 98/79/EC-Article 1.2.(f) and Active Implantable Medical Devices 90/385/EEC Article 1.2.(i).

The manufacturer must ensure that it is manufactured to meet or exceed the required standards of safety and performance. This includes the three phases (design/development/testing, manufacturing, packaging and labelling) that lead to a product being ready for the market. The legal manufacturer is responsible of all the operations necessary to design, manufacture, label and package the product throughout its lifecycle from design to distribution to the final customer. The legal manufacturer is responsible to choose the notified body and affixing the CE mark on the product once it is obtained. Depending on the organization, the legal manufacturer can be the design centre but not necessarily.

A manufacturer, in the meaning of New Approach, is the person who is responsible for designing and manufacturing a product with a view to placing it on the Community market on his own behalf.

The manufacturer has an obligation to ensure that a product intended to be placed on the Community market is designed and manufactured, and its conformity assessed, to the essential requirements in accordance with the provisions of the applicable New Approach directives.

The manufacturer may use finished products, ready-made parts or components, or may subcontract these tasks. However, he must always retain the overall control and have the necessary competence to take the responsibility for the product.

21.8.6 Authorized Representative[4]

The authorized representative means any natural or legal person established in the Community who, explicitly designated by the manufacturer, acts and may be addressed by authorities and bodies in the Community instead of the manufacturer with regard to the latter's obligations under this Directive as stipulated in each relevant section of each Directive: Medical Devices Directive 93/42/EEC Article 1.2.(j), *In-Vitro* Diagnostic Devices 98/79/EC-Article 1.2.(g) and Active Implantable Medical Devices 90/385/EEC Article 1.2.(j).

The manufacturer may appoint any natural or legal person to act on his behalf as an authorized representative.

For the purposes of New Approach directives, the authorized representative must be established inside the Community. The authorized representative is explicitly designated by the manufacturer, and he may be addressed by the authorities of the member states instead of the manufacturer with regard to the latter's obligations under the New Approach directive in question.

The manufacturer remains generally responsible for actions carried out by an authorized representative on his behalf.

21.9 Classification

21.9.1 Medical Devices

The EU Classification of Medical Devices is based on the risk of the device and follows the GHTF classification [14].

The classification is made based on the rules laid down in Appendix IX of the Medical Devices Directive 93/42/EEC. Annex IX classification is based on a risk assessment of the product, when used as intended. The "risk" is composed of the duration of use and the level of invasiveness, as defined by the intended purpose stated by the manufacturer (see examples in Table 21.8). The "Intended purpose" means the use for which the device is intended according to the data supplied by the manufacturer on the labelling, in the instructions and/or in promotional materials.

Medical devices are divided into four classes — **Class I, Class IIa, Class IIb, and Class III** — according to the level of risk the device as based on the following criteria [9]:

- duration of use (transient, short term, long term)
- invasiveness (invasive devices, body orifice, surgically invasive device)
- active/non-active
- implantable
- specific hazards (e.g. contact with the central nervous system, animal tissues, absorbable material, ionizing radiation, medical device with ancillary pharmaceutical substance)

Table 21.8 Examples of medical devices per class

Class	Risk	Examples
Class I	Moderate risk	Surgical instruments Non-invasive tubing to evacuate body liquids Examination gloves Hospital beds
Class Is	Moderate risk (sterile)	Sterile body liquid collection devices Sterile absorbent pads
Class Im	Moderate risk (with a measuring function)	Syringe without needle (graduated barrel) Device for measuring body temperature Non-active device for measuring intra-ocular pressure
Class IIa	Moderate–average risk	Syringe with needle Tubing intended for use with an infusion pump Non-medicated impregnated gauze dressings Short term corrective contact lenses
Class IIb	Average–elevated risk	Hemodialysers Long term corrective contact lenses Urinary catheters intended for long term use Insulin pens
Class III	Elevated risk	Neurological catheters Prosthetic heart valves Aneurysm clips Pre-filled syringe for vascular access device flushing Spinal needle Absorbable sutures

21.9.2 Active Implantable Medical Devices

The active implantable medical devices are at maximum risk: by definition they are any active medical device which is intended to be totally or partially introduced, surgically or medically, into the human body or by medical intervention into a natural orifice, and which is intended to remain after the procedure [2].

Examples of active implantable medical devices

- Implantable cardiac pacemakers
- Implantable defibrillators
- Leads, electrodes, adaptors for above examples
- Implantable nerve stimulators
- Bladder stimulators
- Sphincter stimulators
- Diaphragm stimulators
- Implantable active drug administration device

By default, all accessories to AIMDs are covered under AIMD themselves. They cannot be classified separately under the MDD.

21.9.3 *In vitro* and Diagnostics Medical Devices

The classification of *in vitro* and diagnostics medical devices is based on the risk of of usage (see examples in Table 21.9): If they are to be used by healthcare professionals, they are classified with lower risk, and thus exempt from independent pre-market approval and placed on the market based upon the manufacturer's self-declaration that the device comply with the requirements of the Directive 98/79/EC [3]. When they are of higher risk and/or intended to be used by home user for self-testing, they require a premarket design examination from a notified body.

Table 21.9 Examples of *in vitro* diagnostic medical devices per class

Class	Risk	Examples
List A including self-test	Highest Risk	Reagents, calibrators, control materials for • *Determining blood groups: e.g. ABO system, rhesus, anti-Kell* • *Detection, confirmation, quantification in human specimens of markers: e.g. HIV infection, hepatitis*
Self-tests	Interim Risk	Pregnancy tests
List B	Interim Risk	Reagents, calibrators, control materials for • *Detection, quantification in human samples of congenital infections: e.g. rubella and toxoplasmosis* • *Diagnosing hereditary disease* • *Determining human infections: e.g. Chlamydia* • *Determining tumoral marker* Software for evaluating the risk of trisomy 21 Self-diagnosis device for blood sugar measurement

(*Continued*)

Table 21.9 (*Continued*)

Class	Risk	Examples
Self-certifiable	All others, lowest risk	Instrument, intended by the manufacturer, specifically to be used for *in vitro* diagnostic procedures; Microbiological culture medium Reagents, calibrators, control materials for: • *Detection of angina pectoris, heart failure and atrium fibrillation: e.g. Hb, TSH, Gluc* • *Determining subfertility* • *Diagnosis cardiovascular disease markers: e.g. troponine, CK/CK-MB, lipidsm Km creatinine* • *Diagnosis of rheumatoid arthritis* • *Detection and differentiation of leucocytes* • *Diagnosis of allergies* Specimen containers, transport media

21.10 Conformity Assessment Procedures

Figure 21.4 shows the different steps a manufacturer has to go through from the device classification through the notified body selection to the final CE mark certificate and declaration of conformity issuance:

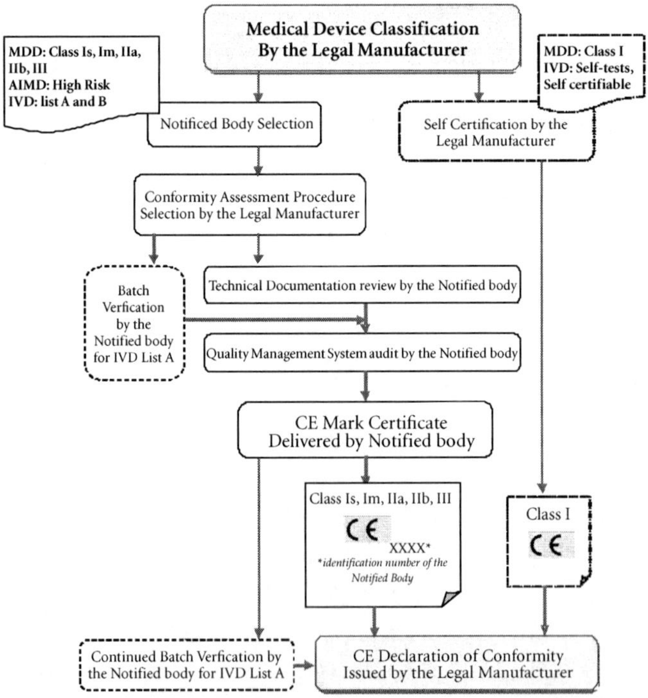

Figure 21.4 Flow chart representing steps to be followed for CE marking.

The Conformity Assessment Procedures correspond to modules described in the Medical Device Directives (Table 21.10), which the manufacturer has to follow in order to affix the CE mark on the device. The procedures may be used single or in association and are aimed to cover the Design and the production quality of the device.

The possible procedures are defined in the annexes of each Directive (Tables 21.11–21.13):

- Annex II: CE Declaration of Conformity (Full Quality Assurance)
  - Roles and responsibilities of the manufacturer
    - maintain a complete system of quality assurance including the design, manufacture and control
    - provide appropriate information about the product, and documentation about the quality system
    - maintain the design file
  - Roles and responsibilities of the notified body: quality system verification
    - study the file
    - inspect the buildings and monitoring
    - examine the design of the product for class III devices
- Annex III: CE Type Examination (Certificate by the notified body that a sample representative of production satisfied the essential requirements)
  - Roles and responsibilities of the manufacturer
    - provide the documentation about the design, manufacture, and performance of the product and a sample
  - Roles and responsibilities of the notified body
    - examine and evaluate the documentation
    - verify that the sample is manufactured in conformance with the documentation
    - perform, or subcontract suitable inspections and necessary tests
- Annex IV: CE Verification
- Annex V: CE Declaration of Conformity (quality assurance of production): approval of the production quality system by the notified body (Quality Management System with exception of design)

- Annex VI: CE Declaration of Conformity (quality assurance of the products, Quality Management System without design and manufacturing)
- Annex VII: CE Declaration of Conformity without recourse at a competent organization

Table 21.10 Overview of the relevant annexes per Directive

Title	MDD 93/42/EEC	IVDD 98/79/EC	AIMD 90/385/EEC
Internal Control of Manufacturing, EC Declaration of Conformity	VII	III	—
EC Type Examination	III	V	3
Production Quality Assurance	V	VII	5
Product Quality Assurance	VI	—	—
Product Verification	IV	VI	4
Full Quality Assurance	II	IV	2

Table 21.11 Combination of procedures for CE marking of Medical Devices as per MDD 93/42/EEC

Class I	Annex VII: Auto-certification (no intervention of a notified body)
Class Is (sterile device) **Class Im (measuring function)**	Annex II, except point 4 (Design examination) Annexes VII and IV Or Annexes VII coupled with V Or Annexes VII coupled with VI
Class IIa	Annex II, except point 4 (Design examination) Or Annexes VII coupled with IV Or Annexes VII coupled with V Or Annexes VII coupled with VI
Class IIb	Annex II, except point 4 (Design examination) Or Annexes III coupled with IV Or Annexes III coupled with V Or Annexes III coupled with VI
Class III	Annex II, including point 4 (Design examination) Or Annexes III coupled with IV Or Annexes III coupled with V

Table 21.12 Combination of procedures for CE marking of *in vitro* diagnostic medical devices as per IVD 98/79/EC

List A	Annex IV including points 4 (Design examination) and 6 (Batch verification) Or Annex V coupled with Annex VII
List B	Annex IV, except points 4 and 6 Or Annex V coupled with Annex VI Or Annex V coupled with Annex VII
Self-Test	Annex III including point 6
Others: not for self-testing	Annex III excluding point 6 (no intervention of a notified body)

Table 21.13 Combination of procedures for CE marking of active implantable medical devices as per IVD 90/385/EEC

All	Annex 2I Or Annex 3 coupled with Annex 4 Or Annex 3 coupled with Annex 5

Table 21.14 provides more practical information about how to apply and choose a conformity assessment procedure per product class: it shows the most widely used combinations and their implications and consequences in terms of Audit and Technical Documentation.

21.11 Essential Requirements

The essential requirements lay down the necessary elements for protecting the public interest: they are mandatory. Only products complying with essential requirements may be placed on the market and put into service.

Essential requirements must be applied as a function of the hazards inherent to a given product: they correspond to the technical requirements with which a device must comply in terms of safety and performance in order to be CE marked: they are to be met to demonstrate the safety and functionality of a device and are defined in the Annex I of each applicable Directives (Medical Device Directive 93/42/EEC as amended, *In-Vitro* Diagnostic Medical Devices 98/79/EC, Active Implantable Medical Device Directive 90/385/EEC as amended).

Table 21.14 Examples of most widely used conformity assessment procedures for MDD in EU at this stage

Device class		Conformity assessment procedure: quality system	Intervention of notified body in quality system	Technical documentation	CE certificate
I		Systematic procedures in place	None	Maintained on site	None
Is		Systematic procedures in place to cover provisions laid down in Annex VII and in Annex II or V	Limited to the securing and maintaining sterile conditions aspects	Maintained on site	CE Certificate of Conformance for sterility
Im		Systematic procedures in place to cover provisions laid down in Annex VII and in Annex II or V	Limited to the metrological requirements	Maintained on site	CE Certificate of Conformance for the measuring function
IIa		Annex II Full quality assurance system *Excluding Point 4 (Design)*	Audit of Quality System by notified body	Submitted upon request Can be reviewed by notified body on a statistical basis	CE Certificate of Conformance for Annex II
	Or	Annex V Production quality assurance	Audit of Quality System by notified body	Submitted upon request Can be reviewed by notified body on a statistical basis	CE Certificate of Conformance for Annex V
IIb		Annex II Full quality assurance system *Excluding Point 4 (Design)*	Audit of Quality System by notified body	Systematically reviewed by notified body	CE Certificate of Conformance for Annex II
	Or	Annex V Production quality assurance Coupled with Annex III EC Type examination	Audit of Quality System by notified body	Systematically reviewed by notified body	CE Certificates of Conformance for Annex III and Annex V
III		Annex II including point 4 Full quality assurance system	Audit of Quality System by notified body	Design Dossier Systematically reviewed by notified body	CE Certificate of Conformance for Annex II
	Or	Annex V Production quality assurance Coupled with Annex III EC Type examination	Audit of Quality System by notified body	Design Dossier Systematically reviewed by notified body	CE Certificates of Conformance for Annex III and Annex V

The essential requirements checklist is divided into the following sections:

- Safety and performance
- Design and construction
  - Chemical, physical and biological properties
  - Infection and microbial contamination
  - Construction and environmental properties
  - Devices with a measuring function
  - Protection against radiation
  - Requirements for medical devices connected to or equipped with an energy source
  - Information supplied by the manufacturer

21.12 Labelling

The labelling of medical devices in very important for the product identification and tracaebility. The Manufacturer must meet the requirements from the Annex I of the Essential Requirements of each applicable Directive:

- Annex I section 13 "Information supplied by the manufacturer" of the Medical Device Directive 93/42/EEC
- Annex I section 8 "Information supplied by the manufacturer" of the *In-Vitro* and Diagnostic Medical Device Directive 98/79/EC
- Annex 1 sections 14 and 15 of the Active Implantable Medical Device Directive 90/385/EEC

National regulations in the European Community may require the information referred to in the device label and Instructions for Use to be in their national language(s) or in another Community language when a device reaches the final user, regardless of whether it is for professional or other use (Article 4, paragraph 4 in each respective Directive (MDD, AIMD, IVD)). The use of symbols that conform to harmonized standards ensures consistency throughout the European Community and means that there is no need to translate certain information (ISO 15223-1 [13]).

21.13 Technical Documentation

The technical documentation must allow assessment of the conformity of the product with the requirements of the Directive. Its content is described in each Annex of the Directive, depending on the Conformity Assessment route chosen by the manufacturer to demonstrate conformity of the device with the provisions of the Directive.

Depending on the medical device class, a Notified body is involved for the quality system review or technical documentation review [15]. The technical documentation can be reviewed either during an audit on site by a notified body or as part of the CE certification, depending on Notify Body's practice. For instance, some notified bodies would only accept their own template as part of a CE certification; some would accept a cross-reference to the location of the evidences within the full technical documentation.

Table 21.15 provides some guidance about how to design the layout of a technical documentation for CE marking: it details the level of information which should be covered in a Technical File for low-moderate risk devices (Class I, Is, Im, IIa and IIb from MDD; List B, Self-test from IVD) and in a Design File for high risk devices (Class III from MDD; List A from IVD; AIMD). The STED (Summary Technical Documentation for Demonstrating Conformity to the Essential Principles of Safety and Performance of Medical Devices) requirements from GHTF are given as reference.

21.14 Quality Management System

A quality system implemented on the basis of the ISO 13485 [11] standard gives a presumption of conformity with the respective conformity assessment procedures with regard to the provisions in the modules that these standards cover, and provided that the quality system enables the manufacturer to demonstrate that the products fulfil the essential requirements of the directive in question. This means that the manufacturer must specifically address regulatory needs when implementing and applying a quality system, in particular:

- The quality objectives, quality planning, quality manual and control of documents must fully take on board the objective of delivering products that conform to the essential requirements;

- The manufacturer must identify and document the essential requirements that are relevant for the product and the harmonized standards to be used or other technical solutions that will ensure fulfilment of the essential requirements;
- The identified standards or other technical solutions must be used as design input, and as verification that design output ensures that the essential requirements will be met;
- The measures taken by the organisation to control production must ensure that the products conform to the identified safety requirements;
- The organisation in its measurement and control of the production process and finished products must identify and use methods which are identified in standards or other appropriate methods to ensure that the essential requirements are met; and
- Quality records, such as inspection reports and test data, calibration data, qualification reports of the personnel concerned, must be suitable to ensure the fulfilment of the applicable essential requirements.
- The manufacturer has the responsibility to implement and continuously operate the quality system in such a way that regulatory needs are respected. The notified body must ensure in its assessment, approval and continued surveillance, that this is the case.

The objective of ISO 13485 is to set out requirements for a Quality Management System that is capable of consistently providing safe and effective medical devices and consistently meeting customer requirements (including regulatory requirements).

The Quality Management System has to be evaluated by a third party [10] (notified body or general registrar) through periodic surveillance inspections (audit). The quality system certificates which are issued by a notified body have a limited validity and must be renewed every 3 years. (only exception of 5 years is Germany, which is not part of the global IAF organization) IAF is International Accreditation Forum: this is the global organization where member states discuss and review ISO accreditation rules, which they then use to supervise notified bodies issuing ISO certificates. They for instance provide a document which identifies how many audit days are needed for what size of organization, issue guidance on how many days for surveillance versus renewal versus initial audits, etc.

Table 21.15 Guideline on content of technical documentation

	Technical Documentation		
	CE Documentation		Sted
	Technical File Low-Moderate Risk	Design Dossier High Risk	
REGULATORY INFORMATION			
Sites identification and addresses:			
Manufacturer name and address	X	X	X
Authorized Representative name and address	X	X	X
Design site name and address	X	X	*If necessary*
Manufacturing site name and address	X	X	*If necessary*
Assembly Site name and address:	X	X	*If necessary*
Sterilization Site name and address	X	X	*If necessary*
Class of device and justifications	X	X	X
GMDN information	X	X	X
Notified body name and address	X	X	X
Conformity Assessment Procedure	X	X	X
Statement that no other application lodged with another notified body	X	X	
Statement on the use of material of animal origin		X	
Statement on the device including a medicinal substance		X	

	Technical Documentation		
	CE Documentation		Sted
	Technical File Low-Moderate Risk	Design Dossier High Risk	
Statement on the device including human blood derivative		X	
PRODUCT DESCRIPTION/INTENDED USE			
Intended use	X	X	X
Description of the device and its variants	X	X	X
Drawings	X	X	*If necessary*
Method of use	X	X	*If necessary*
Description of the packaging configuration	X	X	*If necessary*
Product Historic – Previous existing legislation	X	X	
COMPONENTS/MATERIALS/PACKAGING COMPOSITION			
Device Components and Materials description	X	X	X
Suppliers name and address and quality certificates	X	X	
Packaging composition	X	X	X
DESIGN VERIFICATION			
Results of Design Calculation		X	X
PRODUCT REALIZATION			

(*Continued*)

Table 21.15 (*Continued*)

	Technical Documentation		
	CE Documentation		Sted
	Technical File Low-Moderate Risk	Design Dossier High Risk	
Manufacturing description/flow chart	X	X	X
Subcontractors name	X	X	
Subcontractors quality details		X	
Method and validation of processes (e.g.: primary packaging/cleaning/disinfection/decontamination	X	X	
Quality Control: description of Incoming/In-process/Final inspections	X	X	X
Environmental controls	X	X	X
STERILIZATION			
Method/Appropriate standards	X	X	X
Sterilization Validation	X	X	X
STABILITY DATA			
Physical, chemical and functional stability (shelflife demonstration) as applicable	X	X	*Summary*
Transportation and Storage conditions if applicable	X	X	*If necessary*
RISK MANAGEMENT			

	Technical Documentation		
	CE Documentation		Sted
	Technical File Low-Moderate Risk	**Design Dossier High Risk**	
Risk Management Report – ISO 14971 requirements	X	X	*Summary*
Post-market Analysis – Complaint Data	X	X	*Summary*
Conformity when connected to other medical devices as applicable	X	X	
BIOCOMPATIBILITY			
Pre-clinical evaluation/Biocompatibility data	X	X	X
CLINICAL EVALUATION			
Scientific literature review	X	X	*Summary*
Post-market Analysis – Complaint Data	X	X	*Summary*
Clinical data assessment	X	X	*Summary*
POST-MARKET SURVEILLANCE			
Post-market Analysis – Complaint Data	X	X	*Summary*
LABELLING			
Labelling content description (Labels from all level of packaging and Instructions for Use)	X	X	X
LIST DEMONSTRATING COMPLIANCE TO STANDARDS	X	X	X
ESSENTIAL REQUIREMENTS CHECKLIST	X	X	X

21.15 Risk Management

The ISO 13485 recognizes that risk management is a key quality system element that pervades the entire life cycle of a medical device.

The ISO 14971 [12] sets for guidance related to risk management.

The manufacturer shall establish, document and maintain throughout the life-cycle an ongoing process for identifying hazards associated with a medical device, estimating and evaluating the associated risks, controlling these risks, and monitoring the effectiveness of the controls. This process shall include the following elements:

- risk analysis
- risk evaluation
- risk control
- production and post-production information

The risk/benefit analysis is the basis to be conducted to ensure a high level of protection of health and safety: its purpose is to assess the acceptable risks when weighted against benefits to the patient. The risk reduction is then the elimination or mitigation as far as possible of the risks for a safe design and construction. It addresses protection measures to be taken and information to be provided the user and patient for each residual risk.

21.16 Clinical Evaluation

The clinical evaluation corresponds to the medical assessment of a medical device: The aim is to demonstrate that the intended purpose and claim of the device are achieved and to confirm that the device is safe and performs as expected. In this aim, the conformity of the device characteristics and performances as defined in the essential requirements, needs to be assessed, based on the evaluation of the side-effects and the acceptability of the benefit/risk ratio.

Clinical data is data which is relevant to the various aspects of the clinical safety and performance of the device. This may include data from prospective and retrospective clinical investigations of the device concerned as well as market experience of the same or similar devices and medical procedures and information from the scientific literature.

Clinical data evaluation is the process by which clinical data from all selected sources (literature, results of clinical investigations and other) is assessed, analysed and deemed appropriate and adequate to establish conformity of the device with the pertinent essential requirements of the Directive as they relate to safety and performance, and to demonstrate that the device performs as intended by the manufacturer. The outcome of this process is a report which includes a conclusion on the acceptability of risks and side effects when weighed against the intended benefits of the device.

The clinical data evaluation report should be made based on the risk of the product and based on the assessment of the combination of several of the following critical evaluation:

- Relevant scientific literature currently available relating to the safety, performance, design characteristics and intended purpose of the device where the data adequately demonstrate compliance with the relevant essential requirements
- Results of existing clinical investigations issued from clinical studies
- Data from market experience of same/similar devices already regularly placed on the market
- Additional requirements of applicable standards and guidance documents
- Performance claims
- Risk analysis report

The conclusion should compile all risk/benefit assessment from each part: the rationale should be included to justify the acceptability of each remaining risk when weighted against the intended benefits from use of the device. Statements concerning the field of use of the device and its indications and contraindications, effects and side effects, should be consistent with the device labelling, including the instructions for use.

Where demonstration of conformity with essential requirements based on clinical data is not deemed appropriate, adequate justification has to be given based on risk management output and under consideration of the device/body interaction, the clinical performances intended and the claims of the device.

The clinical evaluation should be reviewed, signed and dated by a dully qualified medical practitioner or other expert (medical expert: medical director or associate).

21.17 CE Mark Certificate and Declaration of Conformity

The CE marking symbolizes the conformity of the product with the applicable European Community requirements imposed on the manufacturer.

The CE marking affixed to products is a declaration by the person responsible that the product conforms to all applicable European Community provisions, and that the appropriate conformity assessment procedures have been completed.

A CE mark certificate indicating the procedure of evaluation applied and the range of the products is established by the notified body. It is valid for a maximum of 5 years, and can be renewed. During its validity it can be amended to allow for changing products and line-extensions.

If the selected procedure utilizes a notified body, then the product labelling has to include on all levels of labelling/packaging the following symbol:

CE **XXXX**, where **XXXX** is the identification number of the notified body

In the case of self-certification (Class I, non-sterile, without a measuring function), the labelling of the product comprises the CE Symbol only:

CE

The declaration of conformity is the final step in the relevant conformity assessment procedure for all Medical Devices, which fall under the scope of one of each of the Directives and is incumbent to the Manufacturer: this is whereby the Manufacturer ensures and declares that the products concerned meet the provisions of the Directives.

The declaration of conformity is a mandatory document which must imperatively be established and signed before any product release for sale and which must be kept at regulators disposal.

A CE Declaration of conformity is established by the manufacturer whatever the class of the device. It ends any conformity assessment procedure.

21.18 Post-Market Surveillance

The post-market surveillance (PMS) is an information gathering process to ensure that any problems or risks associated with the use of a manufacturer's medical device, once freely marketed, are identified, reported to national competent authorities and corrective actions are taken to mitigate the problem or risk.

The post-market surveillance plan includes post-market clinical follow-up, reporting of serious incidents to competent authorities (Vigilance System), application of Field Safety Corrective Actions (FSCA, previously named Recall). A Field Safety Corrective Action is an action taken by the legal manufacturer to reduce a risk of death or serious deterioration in the state of health associated with the use of a medical device that is already placed on the market. Such actions should be notified via a Field Safety Notice, which is the communication of a Field Safety Corrective Action to users.

The post-market surveillance system is based on the information received from the field in the post-production phase, which is the part of the life-cycle of the product after the design has been completed and the medical device has been manufactured. The post-market surveillance system shall consist of the review and assessment for effectiveness and or further action of the following:

- Corrective and preventive actions associated with the Complaints, Medical Device Vigilance Reports and Field Safety Corrective Action activity
- The results of customer surveys
- Feedback from manufacturing plant surveillance activities
- Output reports from post-market clinical evaluation studies
- Feedback from users via sales representatives
- Reports and or interactions with regulatory authorities
- Literature reviews and media analysis where applicable
- Output from expert user/focus groups if applicable to the product platform

The post-market surveillance activities are aimed at obtaining some of the following types of knowledge or feedback:

- Detection of manufacturing problems and detection of needs for product quality improvement

- Confirmation of risk analysis
- Knowledge of performance of the device in different user populations and on ways in which the device is misused
- Feedback on indications for use, on Instructions for Use, training needed for users, use with other devices, customer satisfaction and on continuing market viability

21.19 Recent Changes of MDD 93/42/EEC and Impacts

In 2007 the European Commission issued Directive 2007/47/EC, which EU member states implemented by amending national laws implementing the Medical Device Directive (MDD) and Active Implantable Medical Devices 90/385/EEC. On 21 March 2010, the 2007/47/EC amendments came into full force and manufacturers MUST comply fully with the amended Medical Device Directive by this date.

The 2007/47/EC [7] impacts the competent authorities' roles and responsibilities: the Competent Authorities are expected to increase their communication for better co-operation, consistency and transparency; they have to take some arrangement to assess drug-device combination in a more established way. In terms of Vigilance, the measures taken to impose field safety corrective action are now subject to scrutiny by the European Commission. The Competent Authorities are allowed to request information about **ALL** Medical Devices classes, including Class I because of counterfeit/market surveillance. One authorized representative only is now allowed per Medical Device/products family in order to avoid confusing situations: the role of the Authorised Representative has been better defined as it acts as the communication interface with EU regulatory bodies and is fully responsible of regulatory compliance.

The 2007/47/EC has some impacts as well on notified bodies, as it requires Competent Authorities to increase their control of notified bodies for more consistency across the European Community. It brought greater clarity in the processes and nature of assessments and a closer scrutiny of design validation: the notified body has now to evaluate the ability of Manufacturers to produce appropriate

Technical Files (including Technical Files of Class IIa and IIb Medical Devices) and to evaluate a representative sample of a Technical File elaborated by a Manufacturer.

The changes of the Medical Device Directive 93/42/EEC as amended by the Directive 2007/47/EC are as follows:

- Classification of some Medical Devices:
    - The modifications in the annex related to the classification system bring products for the disinfection of invasive devices into Class IIb.
    - The rule for the determination of the time of contact of invasive products was modified and impacts some invasive devices.
    - Surgically invasive devices intended specifically for use in direct contact with the central nervous system are in Class III
    - Software are considered as active Medical Devices
    - Where a device is intended by the manufacturer to be used in accordance with both the provisions on Personal Protective Equipment in Council Directive 89/686/EEC and the MDD 93/42/EEC as amended, the relevant basic health and safety requirements of Directive 89/686/EEC shall also be fulfilled
- When a Manufacturer is not located in a member state, a single authorized representative must be designated in the European Union: this must be clearly defined on the product labelling and in the declaration of conformity.
- The technical documentation and solutions adopted to meet the essential requirements have to integrate the following points:
    - The Design of the Medical Device shall take into account the expected skills and knowledge of the user (reduction of use error)
    - The demonstration of conformity shall include a clinical evaluation for every class of Medical Device
    - The Software must be validated according to the state of the art

- The declaration of conformity needs to provide a clear description of the medical device(s).
- Single-use product.
    - The labelling has to be consistent throughout the European Union, using a single symbol.
    - Information must be provided as to the risks posed if the device is reused: in the instructions for use and/or on the outer packaging of the medical device.
- Identification and risk management on toxic substances:
    - Special reference is made in the Essential Requirements Checklist, Section 7.5, to phthalates and manufacturers to add suitable specific label for phthalate-containing devices.
    - Phthalates plasticizers are added to the typically rigid plastic to make it pliable (plastic softeners). Their low molecular weight makes them prone to migration from the plastic to the contained product; the PVC (polyvinyl chloride) remains the most widely used plastic in single use medical applications.
    - This applies [5] when parts of a device (or a device itself) are intended to administer and/or remove medicines, body liquids or other substances to or from the body, or devices intended for transport and storage of such body fluids or substances and when the intended use of such devices includes treatment of children or treatment of pregnant or nursing women, and when substances are classified as Carcinogenic, Mutagenic and Toxic to reproduction (CMR) Class I and II in accordance with Annex I to Directive 67/548/EEC.
    - No specific phthalates are listed in the MDD 93/42/EEC as amended; however, it can be noticed that 3 phthalates are mainly and widely considered in most of the texts (DEHP, DBP and BBP).

The changes from the 2007/47/EC which impact both the Medical Device Directive 93/42/EEC and the Active Implantable Medical Devices (90/385/EEC) concern the clinical evaluation:

- Clinical evaluation:
  - The new Directive expresses the need for clinical evidence (Essential Requirements, Section 6a) for all Medical Devices (93/42/EEC) and section 5a for Active Implantable Medical Devices (90/385/EEC).
  - The clinical evaluation is the process by which clinical data from all selected sources (information from the scientific literature, data from prospective and retrospective clinical investigations, market experience of the same or similar devices) is assessed, analysed and deemed appropriate and adequate to demonstrate that the device performs as intended by the manufacturer.

21.20 Trends

The European Commission is seeking to improve some areas in the European regulatory frame such as for the following topics:

- Designation and monitoring of the notified bodies
- Common codification and simplification of the Medical Devices Directives
- Post-market safety improvement for more consistent and timely reactions to safety issues coming from outside the European Community: implementing a better coordination with other authorities such as the United States Food and Drug Administration or the State Food and Drug Administration in China
- Clinical Safety improvement with the scrutiny of clinical evaluation and data and the strengthening of the Vigilance and post-market surveillance systems
- Transparency of the devices, with the implementation of the Summary Device Information and Unique Device Identifier for traceability of devices (UDI)
- Control the product information disclosure: enhance consistency of device information between its Instructions for Use, Internet information and marketing materials

21.21 Overview of All Interactions and Key Terminology

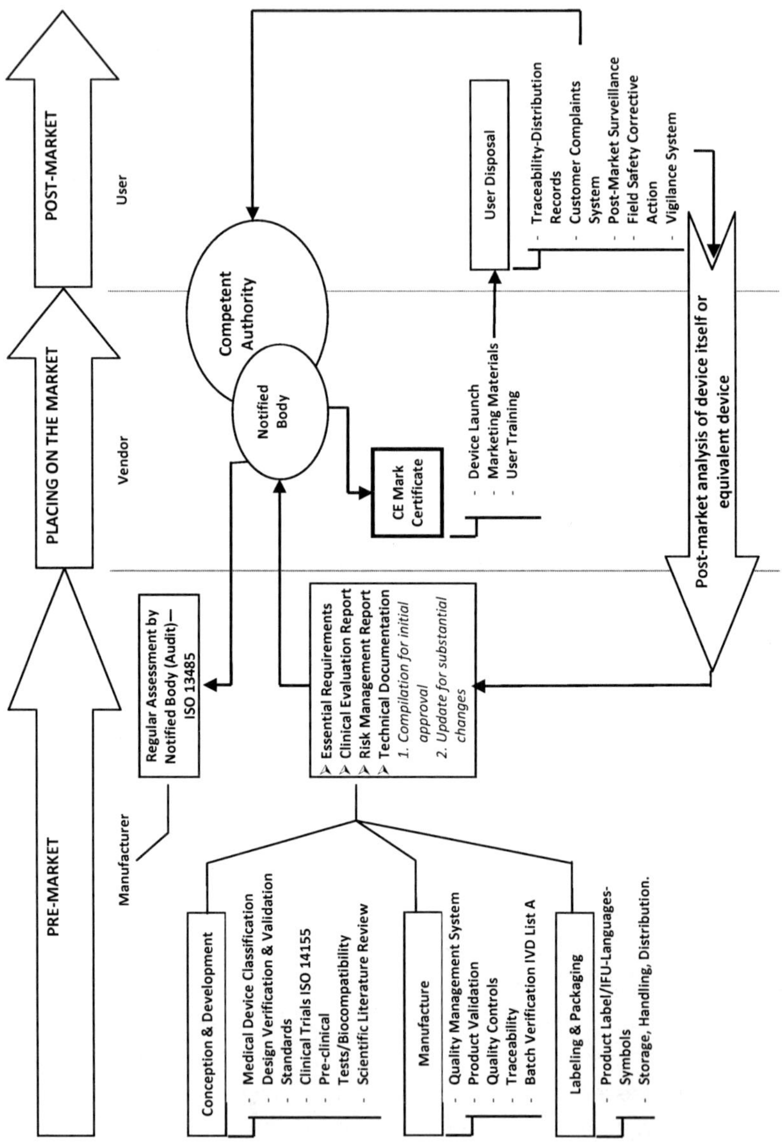

References

1. Council of the European Parliament (12 July 1993) Council Directive of 14 June 1993 concerning Medical Devices (MDD 93/42/EEC), as amended by Directive 2007/47/EC of the European Parliament and of the Council of 5 September 2007, *Official Journal of the European Communities* OJ L169 p1.
2. Council of the European Parliament (20 June 1990) Council Directive 90/385/EEC of 20 June 1990 on the approximation of the laws of the member states relating to active implantable medical devices (AIMD), *Official Journal of the European Communities* OJ L169 p1.
3. Council of the European Parliament (27 October 1998) Directive 98/79/EC of The European Parliament and of The Council of 27 October 1998 on *in vitro* diagnostic medical devices, *Official Journal of the European Communities* OJ L331 p1.
4. Council of the European Parliament (5 September 2007) Directive 2007/47/EC of the European Parliament and of the Council of 5 September 2007 amending Council Directive 90/385/EEC on the approximation of the laws of the member states relating to active implantable medical devices, Council Directive 93/42/EEC concerning medical devices and Directive 98/8/EC concerning the placing of biocidal products on the market, *Official Journal of the European Communities* OJ L247 p21.
5. EUCOMED (30 October 2009) *Guidance on the information requirements of the revised Medical Devices Directive 93/42/EEC concerning certain phthalates.*
6. European Commission Online- DG Health & Consumers — Public health Medical devices — Documents Guidelines — *Guidance MEDDEVs.* Retrieved December 2011, from http://ec.europa.eu/health/medical-devices/documents/guidelines/index_en.htm.
7. European Commission — Enterprise and Industry Directorate — General — Consumer goods — Cosmetics and Medical Devices (5 June 2009) — *Interpretative document of the Commission's services — Implementation of Directive 2007/47/EC amending Directives 90/385/EEC, 93/42/EEC AND 98/8/EC,* Brussels ENTR/F3/PBE/D(2009)19003.
8. European Commission (2000) *Guide to the Implementation of Directives based on the New Approach and the Global Approach* — Luxembourg:

Office for Official Publications of the European Communities — ISBN 92-828-7500-8.

9. European Commission DG Health and Consumer Directorate B, Unit B2 "Cosmetics and medical devices" (June 2010) MEDICAL DEVICES: *Guidance document — Classification of medical devices — guidelines relating to the application of the Council Directive 93/42/EEC on medical devices* — MEDDEV 2. 4/1 Rev. 9.
10. NBOG's Best Practice Guide applicable to MDD (July 2009) *Guidance on Notified Body's Tasks of Technical Documentation Assessment on a Representative*, NBOG BPG 2009-4.
11. ISO 13485:2003 — Medical devices — Quality management systems — Requirements for regulatory purposes.
12. ISO 14971:2007 — Medical devices — Application of risk management to medical devices.
13. ISO 15223-1:2012 — Medical devices — Symbols to be used with medical device labels, labelling and information to be supplied — Part 1: General requirements.
14. G1(PD)/N77R4 Global Harmonization Task Force — (Revision of GHTF/SG1/N15:2006) Title: Principles of Medical Devices Classification — Authoring Group: Study Group 1 of the Global Harmonization Task Force — Date: October 3, 2011.
15. Technical Secretariat NB-MED (03 February 2000) Coordination of Notified Bodies Medical Devices on Council Directives 90/385/EEC, 93/42/EEC and 98/79/EC Recommendation NB-MED/2.5.1/Rec5 — *Technical Documentation* — 2.5.1 Conformity assessment procedures; General rules.
16. World Health Organization Geneva (2003) *Medical Device Regulations Global overview and guiding principles Medical device regulations: global overview and guiding principles,* WHO Library Cataloguing-in-Publication Data ISBN 92-4-154618-2.

Chapter 22

Regulation of Combination Products in the United States

John Barlow Weiner and Thinh X. Nguyen

Office of Combination Products, Food and Drug Administration, WO32, Hub/Mail Room #5129, 10903 New Hampshire Avenue, Silver Spring, MD 20993, USA

John.Weiner@fda.hhs.gov, THUYNTT@its.jnj.com

Disclaimer

This chapter represents the views of the authors in their personal capacities. It does not represent an official statement by the US Food and Drug Administration.

22.1 Introduction

This chapter addresses the regulation of combination products in the United States. As the discussion below indicates, combination products present particular challenges. For example, issues may arise with respect to premarket data requirements and postmarket regulatory requirements, as well as associated practical considerations such as information technology needs and collaboration with other regulated entities.

The following topics are addressed: what products are considered "combination products"; the standards for determining

Handbook of Medical Device Regulatory Affairs in Asia
Edited by Jack Wong and Raymond K. Y. Tong

ISBN 978-981-4411-21-9 (Hardcover), 978-981-4411-22-6 (eBook)
www.panstanford.com

whether a product is a combination product and for determining which component of the US Food and Drug Administration (FDA) has primary responsibility for the regulation of a combination product; how to obtain a formal product classification or assignment determination from the FDA; premarket review and post-market regulatory considerations for combination products; the role of the FDA's Office of Combination Products (OCP); examples of expected, near-term regulatory developments in the US that may be of interest to combination product developers; international harmonization and coordination activities with foreign counterparts; and FDA resources for obtaining additional information.

22.2 What Products Are Considered Combination Products

In the United States, the term "combination product" refers to a product comprising any combination of a drug and a device; a device and a biological product; a biological product and a drug; or a drug, a device, and a biological product (21 CFR 3.2; see 21 USC 353(g)). Types of combination products include physically or chemically combined products (such as drug-eluting stents or syringes marketed prefilled with a drug or biological product); co-packaged products (such as an ampule of a drug packaged together with a delivery device, first aid kits that include bandages and drugs to treat wounds and other injuries, or surgical kits that include devices and drugs that might be used for a particular type of surgical procedure); and certain separately marketed but "cross-labeled" products (such as a laser and a light-activated drug that are marketed separately from one another but labeled specifically for use with one another). See 21 CFR 3.2(e).

22.3 The Standards for Determining If a Product Is a Combination Product

Because a combination product comprises two or more different types of medical products (constituent parts), a determination of whether a product is a combination product begins with determining the classification of the articles of which it is comprised. If the product includes at least two, distinguishable medical products that are classified differently from one another, it is a combination product. Generally, it may be fairly obvious whether a product is a combination product. A prefilled syringe, for example, clearly consists of a device (the syringe) and the drug or biological product contained in the syringe. In some cases, classification may be more difficult to determine. Regardless of how apparent the classifications may be, the answer depends on an assessment of which of the statutory definitions — that for biological product, device, or drug — best applies to each article of which a product is comprised.[1]

22.4 The Standards for Determining Which FDA Component has Primary Responsibility for Regulating a Combination Product

The FDA has three components, called "Centers," that regulate medical products for humans: the Center for Biologics Evaluation

---

[1]Section 201(g) of the Federal Food, Drug, and Cosmetic (FD&C) Act (21 USC 321(g)) provides that the term "drug" means:

(A) articles recognized in the official United States Pharmacopoeia, official Homoeopathic Pharmacopoeia of the United States, or official National Formulary, or any supplement to any of them; and (B) articles intended for use in the diagnosis, cure, mitigation, treatment, or prevention of disease in man or other animals; and (C) articles (other than food) intended to affect the structure or any function of the body of man or other animals; and (D) articles intended for use as a component of any articles specified in clause (A), (B), or (C)… .

Section 201(h) of the FD&C Act (21 USC 321(h)) provides that the term "device" means:

… an instrument, apparatus, implement, machine, contrivance, implant, *in vitro* reagent, or other similar or related article, including any component, part, or accessory, which is—

(1) recognized in the official National Formulary, or the United States Pharmacopeia, or any supplement to them,

(2) intended for use in the diagnosis of disease or other conditions, or in the cure, mitigation, treatment, or prevention of disease, in man or other animals, or

(3) intended to affect the structure or any function of the body of man or other animals, and which does not achieve its primary intended purposes through chemical action within or on the body of man or other animals and which is not dependent upon being metabolized for the achievement of its primary intended purposes.

Section 351(i) of the Public Health Services Act (42 USC 262(i)) provides that:

The term "biological product" means a virus, therapeutic serum, toxin, antitoxin, vaccine, blood, blood component or derivative, allergenic product, protein (except any chemically synthesized polypeptide), or analogous product, or arsphenamine or derivative of arsphenamine (or any other trivalent organic arsenic compound), applicable to the prevention, treatment, or cure of a disease or condition of human beings.

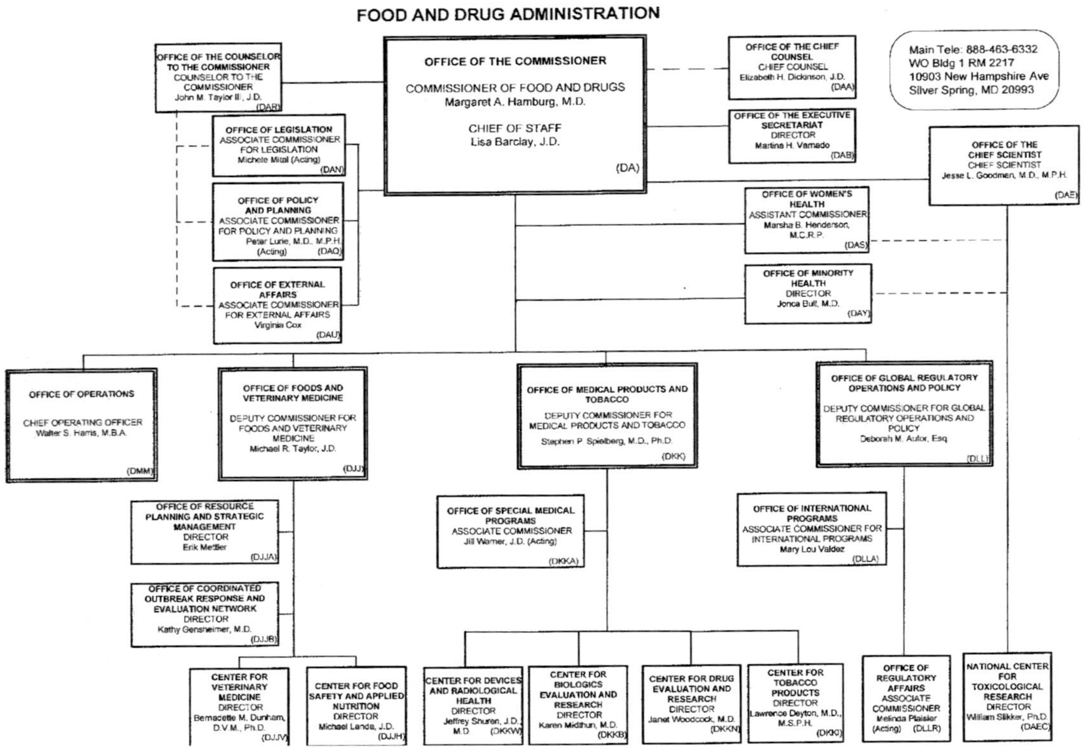

Figure 22.1 FDA chart.

and Research (CBER); the Center for Devices and Radiological Health (CDRH); and the Center for Drugs Evaluation and Research (CDER). Section 503 of the FD&C Act requires that the determination of which Center will have primary responsibility for the regulation of a combination product be based upon the "primary mode of action" (PMOA) of the combination product. See 21 USC 353(g). There are three modes of action for purposes of this analysis, that of a biological product, a device, or a drug. See 21 USC 353(g); 21 USC 3.2(k). If the PMOA is provided by a biological product constituent part, the combination product is typically assigned to CBER. If the PMOA is provided by a device constituent part, the combination product is typically assigned to CDRH, and if the PMOA is provided by the drug, the combination product is typically assigned to CDER. See 21 USC 353(g)(1); 21 CFR 3.4(a).

PMOA is defined as the mode of action that provides the greatest contribution to the overall therapeutic effect of the combination product. See 21 CFR 3.2(m). Like classification, the PMOA may be obvious in some cases. For example, the drug or biological product provides the PMOA for a prefilled syringe because the syringe serves merely to deliver the drug or biological product that then treats the disease or condition the combination product is intended to address. In other cases, PMOA may be more difficult to determine, for example, if more than one constituent part of the combination product directly contributes to the treatment effect. In such cases, data on the relative contribution of the different constituent parts may be needed to make the determination.

Further, in some cases, it may not be possible to determine PMOA directly. For example, a product may consist of two articles that address different diseases or conditions, so that there is no overall therapeutic effect to which either contributes more than the other. In such circumstances, PMOA is determined indirectly through the use of an algorithm. See 21 CFR 3.4(b). The first step of the algorithm asks whether one of the Centers already regulates a combination product that raises similar questions of safety and effectiveness to those raised by this combination product. If there is one such Center, the combination product will be assigned to that Center. If there is not such a Center, the second step of the algorithm applies. Under the second step, the combination product is assigned based on which Center has the most experience with the most significant safety and effectiveness issues presented by the combination product.

22.5 Requests for Designation

Section 563 of the FD&C Act provides that a request for designation (RFD) may be submitted to obtain a formal, binding determination from the FDA as to the classification or Center assignment for a product. 21 USC 360bbb-2. The FDA is required to respond to RFDs not later than sixty days after they are filed. See 21 USC 360bbb-2(b). If the agency does not respond within that time-frame, the classification or assignment recommended by the RFD submitter applies. See 21 USC 360bbb-2(c). A classification or assignment made through the RFD process can only be changed either with the consent of the RFD submitter or for public health reasons based on scientific evidence. See 21 USC 360bbb-2(b),(c); see 21 CFR 3.9.

RFDs are submitted to OCP, which is charged with determining whether products should be classified as biological products, devices, drugs, or combination products, and with assigning them to the appropriate Center. The FDA permits and encourages sponsors to seek guidance from OCP before submitting an RFD, to confirm whether one is needed and to help ensure that the RFD will be complete for filing. Among other requirements, an RFD must describe the product, its components and ingredients; state the product's intended use; provide the submitter's understanding of how the product works; and provide a justification for the product's PMOA if the product is a combination product. See 21 CFR 3.7. For further guidance see How to Write a Request for Designation (RFD), Guidance for Industry (http://www.fda.gov/RegulatoryInformation/Guidances/ucm126053.htm).

22.6 Premarket Review Considerations

There are no special premarket standards or requirements specifically for combination products. The basic concern for them, as for all medical products, is to ensure that they are safe and effective for their intended uses. While the lead Center for a combination product is determined based on the PMOA of the product as discussed above, other Centers may participate in the premarket review of combination products, bringing to bear their expertise and informing the review process. See, e.g., 21 USC 360bbb-2(g)(1), (4)(C).

A principal consideration for combination products is to ensure that product development and testing addresses all relevant considerations relating to each constituent part and their interactions. Accordingly, for example, in assessing whether a syringe is an appropriate delivery device for a particular drug, relevant considerations would include whether the syringe interacts with the drug, whether it will deliver the correct drug dosage, and whether the integrity of the syringe material can be maintained in accordance with the combination product's shelf-life. Similarly, in the case of a drug-eluting stent for example, considerations for the drug constituent part would include (in addition to its effectiveness to achieve its intended therapeutic purpose) such factors as whether the formulation of the drug is appropriate in light of the need to control the elution rate and resist flaking from the stent.

Strong, clear business arrangements between regulated entities can be important to obtaining marketing authorization. Access to third-party proprietary data submitted by one manufacturer, for example, can reduce data development demands and expedite product review and approval, including with respect to post-market changes. A related issue with regard to cross-labeled combination products in particular, is whether it makes better sense to seek a single marketing authorization for the combination product or to seek separate marketing authorizations for each of the separately marketed constituent parts of the combination product. Separate applications may facilitate further development of these constituent parts for independent uses not involving the other constituent part. However, reliance upon separate applications may also pose challenges, for example, with respect to coordination of post-market modifications to either constituent part, particularly if the applications are held by different sponsors. The FDA has the authority to require two applications in appropriate cases for combination products. See 21 CFR 3.5(c).

22.7 Post-Market Regulatory Considerations

In the context of two rulemakings, for postmarketing safety reporting (PSR) and for current good manufacturing practices (CGMPs) for combination products, among other contexts the FDA has stated that combination products are subject to the legal requirements applicable to their constituent parts, and that combination products comprise a distinct category of medical products that can be regulated in light of the distinct regulatory considerations they raise. See Current Good Manufacturing Practice Requirements for Combination Products (final rule), 78 FR 4307 (https://www.federalregister.gov/articles/2013/01/22/2013-01068/current-good-manufacturing-practice-requirements-for-combination-products); Postmarketing Safety Reporting for Combination Products (proposed rule), 74 FR 50,744 (http://edocket.access.gpo.gov/2009/pdf/E9-23519.pdf).

The FDA has taken a similar approach in both rulemakings for PSR and for CGMPs. Specifically, for each topic the agency reviewed the regulations applicable to biological products, drugs, and devices, and assessed in which ways those sets of regulations overlap and in which ways they may be distinct. Based on this review, the FDA developed approaches it states are intended to enable regulated entities to comply with the multiple sets of regulations applicable to their combination product without unnecessary redundancy of requirements or burden. In both cases, the FDA has pursued an approach under which some regulations applicable to constituent parts of the combination product must be implemented in their entirety while only specified provisions of other such regulations need to be met. These two rulemakings offer some insight as to the FDA's thinking regarding what requirements apply to combination products and how to clarify and streamline appropriate measures to comply with them. Further insight can be expected from the finalization of the PSR rule and other policy initiatives announced by the FDA such as those noted in the discussion of near-term developments below.

As in the premarket context, various staff from Centers other than the lead Center and from other FDA components may participate in post-market regulatory activities for combination products. Such coordination may be appropriate, for example, to ensure staff with appropriate expertise participate in site inspections and the review of post-market changes to products.

22.8 Role of Office of Combination Products

OCP is a statutorily mandated office whose responsibilities include ensuring the timely, effective premarket regulation of combination products and their consistent and appropriate post-market regulation. See 21 USC 353(g)(4). OCP undertakes a wide range of

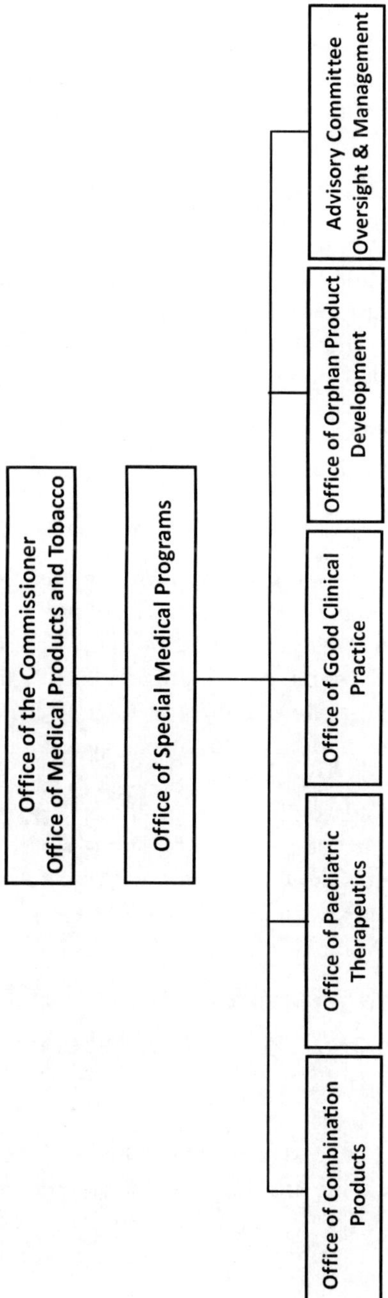

Figure 22.2 The OCP chart.

activities in accordance with this mandate, including: responding to RFDs as discussed above; facilitating the consultation process between Centers on combination product regulatory issues; offering input on product-specific regulatory issues; convening working groups and coordinating initiatives to develop policies; participating in agency working groups and initiatives that may affect regulation of combination products; and resolving disputes within the FDA and between FDA and regulated entities. In addition, OCP acts as a resource to combination product developers and manufacturers to answer regulatory questions and facilitate interactions with the agency, including Center review staff, field staff, and enforcement and inspectional personnel.

22.9 Near-Term Developments That May Arise in the US

OCP and other FDA components have announced various projects for combination products that may be of particular interest to combination product developers and manufacturers. These include: continued development of product-specific guidance for imaging products, injectors, and companion diagnostics. In addition, OCP has announced plans to develop further general guidance for combination products on post-marketing changes, registration and listing, and cross-labeled combination products. Also, the FDA is continuing efforts to finalize guidance on standards to determine whether medical products should be classified as biological products, devices, drugs, or combination products.

22.10 International Harmonization and Coordination Activities with Foreign Counterparts

The FDA has expressed interest in working with foreign counterpart agencies to promote harmonization and coordination of activities with respect to combination products. Some preliminary discussions have taken place with Australian, Canadian, European, and Japanese regulators regarding identification of topics of shared interest. In addition, OCP continues to work with and provide technical assistance to foreign counterparts throughout the world. A practical consideration is that harmonization and coordination with respect to combination products largely depends on related efforts with respect to biological products, devices, and drugs. Accordingly, progress on some topics may depend on preliminary work with respect to each of these types of products from which combination products are comprised.

22.11 FDA Resources for Obtaining Additional Information

For further information, OCP's Web page on the FDA Web site is an excellent resource: http://www.fda.gov/CombinationProducts/default.htm. In addition, as noted above OCP itself is an important resource to address questions and obtain assistance for engaging with the FDA on regulatory issues for combination products and medical product classification issues. Contact information for OCP is available on its Web page.

Chapter 23

Regulation of Combination Products in the European Union

Janine Jamieson and Elizabeth Baker

Licensing Division, Medicines and Healthcare Products Regulatory Agency, London SW1W 9SZ, UK

janine.jamieson@mhra.gsi.gov.uk, elizabeth.baker@mhra.gsi.gov.uk

23.1 Introduction: Legal Basis

In Europe, there are two regulatory routes for drug–device combination products, either as medical devices incorporating ancillary medicinal substances or as medicinal products utilizing a delivery device.

Following are the regulations covering these two options:

- Medical Devices Directive 93/42/EEC (MDD)/Active Implantable Medical Devices 90/385/EEC (AIMDD)
- Medicinal Products Directive 2001/83/EC (MPD)

As a general rule, a combination product is regulated **either** by the MDD/AIMDD for the conformity assessment procedure relevant to medical devices **or** by the MPD for the marketing authorization

Handbook of Medical Device Regulatory Affairs in Asia
Edited by Jack Wong and Raymond K. Y. Tong

ISBN 978-981-4411-21-9 (Hardcover), 978-981-4411-22-6 (eBook)
www.panstanford.com

procedure applicable to medicinal products. The procedures of both Directives do not apply cumulatively; however, some cross-references are made within one regime to specific requirements of the other regime.

The two procedures have different requirements and the correct classification is crucial for development and regulatory approval of a combination product in Europe.

The appropriate regulatory procedure depends upon the principal mode of action of the combination product.

- Drug-delivery products presented as an integral combination with a medicinal product are regulated as **medicinal products.**
  Example: pre-filled syringes
  See Section 1.2.
- Drug-delivery products presented separately from the medicinal product are regulated as **medical devices.**
  Example: drug delivery pump
  See Section 1.3.
- Medical devices incorporating, as an integral part, an ancillary medicinal substance are regulated as **medical devices but with additional requirements for the ancillary medicinal substance.**
  Example: drug-eluting stent
  See Sections 1.4, 1.5 and 1.6.

Guidance on which regulations are applicable, particularly in cases where the principal mode of action is not clear, can be found in the MEDDEV 2.1/3: EC Guidance document on "Borderline products, drug-delivery products and medical devices incorporating, as an integral part, an ancillary medicinal substance or an ancillary human blood derivative". See the European Commission website [1].

The information provided in the following sections is based, to a large extent, on the text of the MEDDEV 2.1/3 document. The reader is directed to this document for more detailed information and examples of drug–device combination products.

23.1.1 Definitions

23.1.1.1 Medical device

Article 1(2) (a) MDD defines a medical device as

Any instrument, apparatus, appliance, software, material or other article, whether used alone or in combination, including the software intended by its manufacturer to be used specifically for diagnostic and/or therapeutic purposes and necessary for its proper application, intended by the manufacturer to be used for human beings for the purpose of:

- diagnosis, prevention, monitoring, treatment or alleviation of disease,
- diagnosis, monitoring, treatment, alleviation of or compensation for an injury or handicap,
- investigation, replacement or modification of the anatomy or of a physiological process,
- control of conception,

and which does not achieve its principal intended action in or on the human body by pharmacological, immunological or metabolic means, but which may be assisted in its function by such means.

The medical device function is usually achieved by physical means (including mechanical action, physical barrier, replacement of or support to organs or body functions).

23.1.1.2 Medicinal product

Article 1(2) MPD defines a medicinal product as follows:

(a) Any substance or combination of substances presented as having properties for treating or preventing disease in human beings; or

(b) Any substance or combination of substances which may be used in or administered to human beings either with a view to restoring, correcting or modifying physiological functions by exerting a pharmacological, immunological or metabolic action, or to making a medical diagnosis.

This definition comprises two limbs, one relating to presentation and the other to function. A product constitutes a medicinal product if it is covered by one or other or both of those limbs.

The definition of a medicinal product is applied on a case by case basis and determination takes into account current European Case Law. The Medicinal Products Directive (MPD), Article 2(2), is clear that, in cases of doubt, taking into account all of a product's characteristics, if a product meets both the definition of a medical device and a medicinal product, then the MPD will apply.

23.1.1.3 Combination products: Principal mode of action

The principal intended action of a combination product is determined based on the mechanism of action of the device and medicinal substance aspects.

The manufacturer's labelling and claims are also taken into account, but they should be in line with, and not contradict, current scientific data. The product manufacturer should be able to justify scientifically their rationale for the design and classification of the combination product.

Useful definitions from MEDDEV 2.1/3

"**Pharmacological means**" is understood as an interaction between the molecules of the substance in question and a cellular constituent, usually referred to as a receptor, which either results in a direct response, or which blocks the response to another agent. Although not a completely reliable criterion, the presence of a dose-response correlation is indicative of a pharmacological effect.

"**Immunological means**" is understood as an action in or on the body by stimulation and/or mobilisation of cells and/or products involved in a specific immune reaction.

"**Metabolic means**" is understood as an action which involves an alteration, including stopping, starting or changing the speed of the normal chemical processes participating in, and available for, normal body function.

Medical devices may be assisted in their function by pharmacological, immunological or metabolic means, but as soon as these means are not ancillary with respect to the principal intended action of a product, the product no longer fulfils the definition of a medical device and the product will be regarded as a medicinal product.

Examples

Bone cements and gentamicin-loaded polymethylmethacrylate (PMMA) beads are useful examples of combination products for illustration of the classification rules:

- Plain bone cement without antibiotics is a medical device since it achieves its principal intended action (the fixation of prosthesis) by physical means.

- Bone cements containing antibiotics, where the principal intended action remains fixation of prosthesis, are also medical devices. In this case the action of the antibiotic, which is to reduce the possibility of infection being introduced during surgery, is clearly ancillary.
- If, however, the principal intended action of the combination product is to deliver the antibiotic (for example, gentamicin-loaded beads for insertion into and withdrawal from an infected bone cavity), this will be regarded as a medicinal product with the beads acting as a delivery device for local action of the gentamicin.

23.1.1.4 Borderline products: MEDDEV 2.1/3

The EC guidance document MEDDEV 2.1/3 is an extremely useful document which provides detailed information on the classification criteria between medical devices and medicinal products. In cases where it is not clear which regulatory regime applies, numerous examples and explanatory notes are provided to aid in the decision making process.

23.1.1.5 Borderline products: Manual of decisions

There have been a number of cases of disagreement about classification over the years, between manufacturers and notified bodies and also between different notified bodies and competent authorities (the EU national regulatory bodies for medicines). A Medical Device Expert Group (MDEG) on Borderline and Classification issues has been set up to discuss products where there is a divergence of opinion across Europe. The Expert Group meets regularly to help reach agreement on classification issues. The decisions of the MDEG on Borderline and Classification are published in the Manual of Decisions available on the European Commission website [2]. However, the manual is designed to aid case-by-case application of the legislation by the competent authorities and is not a legal document itself.

23.2 Combination Products Regulated as Medicinal Products

This classification refers to devices that are intended to administer a medicinal product in the case where the device and the medicinal product form a single integral product, which is intended exclusively for use in the given combination and which is not reusable.

According to the MDD, this single product is governed by the MPD but the relevant essential requirements of Annex I to the MDD apply as far as the safety and performance-related device features are concerned.

23.2.1 Examples of Combination Products Regulated as Medicinal Products

- Pre-filled syringes
- Aerosols containing a medicinal product
- Patches for transdermal drug delivery
- Implants containing medicinal products in a polymer matrix whose primary purpose is to release the medicinal product
- Intrauterine contraceptives whose primary purpose is to release progestogens
- Temporary root canal fillers incorporating medicinal products, whose primary purpose is to deliver the medicinal product

23.3 Combination Products Regulated as Medical Devices

This category refers to devices that are intended to administer a medicinal product, but are not combined with a specific medicinal product. They may be re-useable and may be used with different medicinal products.

In this case, that device is governed by the MDD or the AIMDD.

23.3.1 Examples of Combination Products Regulated as Drug-Delivery Devices

- Drug delivery pump
- Implantable infusion pump
- Iontophoresis device
- Nebulizer
- Syringe, jet injector
- Spacer devices for use with metered dose inhalers
- Port systems

23.4 Combination Products Regulated as Devices Incorporating, as an Integral Part, an Ancillary Medicinal Substance

These relate to a device that incorporates, as an integral part, a medicinal substance which, if used separately, may be considered to be a medicinal product and which is liable to act upon the body with action that is ancillary to that of the device.

In this case, the principal mode of action is attributable to the device element and the medicinal substance has a lesser, secondary effect.

The device is assessed and authorised in accordance with the MDD or the AIMDD, with additional requirements in line with MPD applied to the medicinal substance component.

According to the directives, the substance incorporated in the device must meet the three following conditions:

- The substance, if used separately, may be considered to be a medicinal product.
- The substance is liable to act upon the human body.
- The action of this substance is ancillary to that of the device.

In addition, a medical device incorporates a medicinal substance *as an integral part*, within the meaning of the directives only if the device and the substance are physically or chemically combined at the time of administration (i.e., use, implantation, application, etc.) to the patient.

23.4.1 Examples of Devices Incorporating an Ancillary Medicinal Substance

- Drug eluting stents
- Catheters coated with heparin or an antibiotic agent
- Bone cements containing antibiotic
- Root canal fillers which incorporate medicinal substances with ancillary action
- Bone void filler intended for the repair of bone defects where the primary action of the device is a physical means or matrix, which provides a volume and a scaffold for osteoconduction and where an additional medicinal substance is incorporated

to assist and complement the action of the matrix by enhancing the growth of bone cells
- Condoms coated with spermicides

23.4.2 Examples of Drug Substances Incorporated into Devices

- Antibiotics, e.g. gentamicin, vancomycin
- Other anti-microbials, e.g. silver, chlorhexidine, rifampin
- Anti-proliferatives, e.g. paclitaxel, sirolimus
- Heparin
- Dexamethasone
- Nonoxinol
- Benzocaine

23.4.3 Assessment of the Medicinal Substance Aspects of a Device Incorporating an Ancillary Medicinal Substance

For devices incorporating, as an integral part, an ancillary medicinal substance, the notified body should first of all verify the usefulness of the substance as part of the medical device themselves. They must then seek a scientific opinion from one of the EU competent authorities for medicines on the quality and safety of the substance including the clinical benefit/risk profile of the incorporation of the substance into the device.

The aspect of "usefulness" is interpreted as the rationale for using the medicinal substance in relation to the specific intended purpose of the device. It refers to the suitability of the medicinal substance to achieve its intended action, and whether the potential inherent risks (aspect of "safety") due to the medicinal substance are justified in relation to the benefit to be obtained within the intended purpose of the device.

23.5 The Consultation Process

The notified body and the manufacturer may choose the EU competent authority with whom they consult. However, the European Medicines Agency (EMA) must be consulted for all medical devices incorporating ancillary human blood derivatives, e.g. human albumin or medicinal products manufactured using biotechnological processes (i.e., those falling within the scope of Annex I to Regulation (EC) No. 726/2004 [1]).

In accordance with MEDDEV 2.1/3, Section C, the notified body should ensure that data supplied by the manufacturer in relation to the device and its intended use includes a specific segment regarding the medicinal substance being incorporated with ancillary purpose. Detailed submission guidance is available on the websites of EMA, MHRA and other competent authorities.

23.6 Information to Be Provided on the Ancillary Medicinal Substance

23.6.1 General

Information addressing the safety, quality and usefulness of the medicinal substance should be prepared by the manufacturer, submitted to the notified body, and then forwarded by the notified body to the competent authority (MHRA in UK). In addition, a report on the usefulness of the medicinal substance should be prepared by the notified body and included with the application form.

Because of the wide range of medical devices which incorporate, as an integral part, an ancillary medicinal substance, a flexible approach to the data requirements is necessary. However, the information should be based in principle and to the relevant extent on Annex 1 to Directive 2001/83/EC (MPD).

23.6.2 Quality, Safety, Usefulness (Clinical Benefit/Risk)

23.6.2.1 Quality

Relevant information should be provided on both

- the drug substance itself and
- the drug substance as incorporated into the medical device.

With regard to the drug substance, evidence should be provided that the drug substance is manufactured to a high, reproducible quality and is suitably controlled by an appropriate specification.

Where a European Pharmacopoeia (PhEur) monograph exists for a substance, the specification should be that of the PhEur as a minimum.

With regard to the combination product, information relevant to the medicinal substance should be provided, i.e. on the quantitative composition, details of manufacture, control of critical excipients, and control of intermediate and finished products. Validation data should be provided where appropriate, in particular for analytical methods. The data submitted should demonstrate that the amount of medicinal substance incorporated is based on safety and efficacy considerations, that it can be suitably controlled within specified limits, that it is evenly distributed within/across the device as necessary and maintains satisfactory performance over the shelf-life of the product.

23.6.2.2 Safety and usefulness (clinical benefit/risk)

There should be a clear rationale and safety consideration for including the ancillary medicinal substance at the proposed dose.

Where well-known medicinal substances for established purposes are involved, original data on all aspects of safety and usefulness may not be required and many of the headings of Annex 1 to Directive 2001/83/EC will be addressed by reference to literature sources, including standard textbooks, experience and other information generally available. However, all headings should be addressed, with either relevant data or justification for absence of data, based on the manufacturer's risk assessment.

For new active substances and for known medicinal substances for a non-established purpose, comprehensive data is required to address the requirements of Annex 1 to Directive 2001/83/EC. The evaluation of such active substances would be performed in accordance with the principles of evaluation of new active substances.

23.6.2.3 Guidance

MEDDEV 2.1/3, Section C, provides guidance on the consultation procedure for devices incorporating ancillary medicinal substances or ancillary human blood derivatives [1]. In addition, the EMA and national competent authorities publish guidance on procedures and documentation requirements for the consultation.

There are also a number of useful European guidelines relating to the quality, safety and efficacy of medicinal substances as used in medicinal products which can be found on the EMA website [3] and in these consultation guidance documents.

It is not intended that the guidelines should be strictly adhered to for ancillary medicinal substances used in devices, however, as for medicinal product evaluation, justification for the use of different approaches should be provided.

23.7 Other Combination Products

This chapter has focused on the combination of medical devices with chemical medicinal substances. There are also other combination products in the early developmental stage, e.g. gene therapy, cell therapy, tissue engineered products combined with medical devices such as scaffolds, implants, stents and extracorporeal circuits.

These combinations are regulated as advanced therapy medicinal products (ATMP) and are assessed centrally by the Committee for Advanced Therapies (CAT) at EMA.

In this case, consultation with a notified body is required on the device aspects in a similar manner to consultation with a competent authority on the medicinal substance aspects of devices incorporating an ancillary medicinal substance.

More information on ATMP products can be found on the EMA [3] and MHRA websites [4].

References

1. MEDDEV 2.1/3: "EC Guidance document on 'Borderline products, drug-delivery products and medical devices incorporating, as an integral part, an ancillary medicinal substance or an ancillary human blood derivative," retrieved (April 2012) from http://ec.europa.eu/health/medical-devices/documents/guidelines/index_en.htm.
2. Medical Devices Expert Group on Borderline and Classification: Manual of Decisions, retrieved (April 2012) from http://ec.europa.eu/health/medical-devices/documents/borderline/index_en.htm.
3. European Medicines Agency website: Ancillary medicinal substances: Regulatory and procedural guidance, retrieved (April 2012) from http://www.ema.europa.eu/ema/index.jsp?curl=pages/regulation/

document_listing/document_listing_000133.jsp&mid=WC0b01ac05800267b9&jsenabled=true; Advanced therapies, retrieved (April 2012) from http://www.ema.europa.eu/ema/index.jsp?curl=pages/regulation/general/general_content_000294.jsp&mid=WC0b01ac05800241e0.

4. MHRA website: Borderline with Medicines, retrieved (April 2012) from http://www.mhra.gov.uk/Howweregulate/Devices/MedicalDevicesDirective/Borderlinewithmedicines/index.htm; Consultation with MHRA on Devices incorporating an ancillary medicinal substance, retrieved (April 2012) from http://www.mhra.gov.uk/Howweregulate/Devices/MedicalDevicesDirective/Drug-deviceconsultations/index.htm; Regulation of Advanced Therapy Medicinal Products, retrieved (April 2012) from http://www.mhra.gov.uk/Howweregulate/Advancedtherapymedicinalproducts/Aboutadvancedtherapymedicinalproducts/index.htm.

Part 5

Medical Device Regulatory System in Asia-Pacific Region

Chapter 24

Australian Medical Device Regulations: An Overview

Petahn McKenna

ASEAN Regulatory Affairs Manager,
Johnson & Johnson Medical Singapore

PMCKENN1@its.jnj.com

24.1 Medical Device Market in Australia

One of the wealthiest healthcare markets in Asia-Pacific, Australia's spending on health is at par with European markets such as Finland, Norway, and the United Kingdom. Similar to many other developed countries in the world, increased life expectancy, income, and demands for a higher quality of life are driving an increase in health expenditure.

Healthcare provision in Australia is made up of public and private funding: Public expenditure is funded by the Commonwealth (central) Government under a health care system called Medicare: Australia's universal, tax-financed insurance scheme covering medical, pharmaceutical, and public hospital services. Private

Handbook of Medical Device Regulatory Affairs in Asia
Edited by Jack Wong and Raymond K. Y. Tong

ISBN 978-981-4411-21-9 (Hardcover), 978-981-4411-22-6 (eBook)
www.panstanford.com

expenditure is largely funded through insurance. However, Medicare also pays 75% of the schedule fee for services and procedures provided in private hospitals.

Australia's medical device manufacturing industry is also growing: There were 655 medical devices companies in Australia in 2007, 30 more than the previous year. In 2009, Australia had domestic medical device sales of AUD 6 billion and earned export revenue of AUD 1.7 billion, employing at least 17,500 people.

Table 24.1 Australian health demographics

Population (June, 2011) [1]	22,620,600	
Population Growth Rate (over previous year) [1]	1.4%	
Life Expectancy (years) [2]	82	
Economics		
GDP Per capita (USD) [3]	39,975	
GDP Growth Rate [2]	2.5%	
Healthcare statistics		
Total expenditure on health as percent of gross domestic product (2009) [3]	8.5% (2009)	8.4% (2009)
Per capita total expenditure on health (PPP int. $) [3]	3,382 (2009)	2,980 (2005)

24.2 Medical Device Regulations

24.2.1 Overview

In Australia, medical devices are regulated by the Therapeutic Goods Administration (TGA). The Australian medical device regulatory requirements, which were implemented in 2002, are largely based on the European Council Medical Device Directive (MDD) 93/42/EEC (1). Since July 2010, *In vitro* diagnostic devices (IVDs) have also been regulated as a subset of medical devices.

The TGA regulates medical devices via the following platforms:

(i) pre-market assessment
(ii) post-market monitoring and enforcement of standards
(iii) licensing of Australian manufacturers and verifying overseas manufacturers' compliance with the same standards as their Australian counterparts

The following text will concentrate on pre-market assessment and the requirements that must be fulfilled in order to place a medical device on the Australian market. Much of the information within this section has been extracted from the Australian Regulatory Guidelines for Medical Devices (ARGMD), accessible via the TGA website. Wherever any more detail or clarification is required, readers should always refer to the TGA website or contact the TGA directly.

For details of the Australian post-market vigilance and monitoring requirements, please refer to Section 22 of the ARGMD.

24.2.2 Regulating Authority

The body responsible for regulating medical devices in Australia is the Office of Devices Authorisation, within the Therapeutic Goods Administration (TGA). The TGA is a division of the Australian Government Department of Health and Ageing.

24.2.3 Legislation and Guidance

All regulatory decisions applicable to medical devices are made using legislation as set out in the Therapeutic Goods Act 1989, Therapeutic Goods Regulations 1990, and the Therapeutic Goods (Medical Devices) Regulations 2002.

The TGA, in collaboration with the medical devices industry sector, has developed a consolidated reference document detailing the Australian regulatory requirements for medical devices. This document is called the Australian Regulatory Guidelines for Medical Devices.

24.3 Definition of Medical Device

The Therapeutic Goods Act 1989 defines a medical device as

> any instrument, apparatus, appliance, material or other article (whether used alone or in combination, and including the software necessary for its proper application) intended by the person under whose name it is to be supplied, to be used for human beings for the purpose of one or more of the following:
>
> (i) Diagnosis, prevention, monitoring, treatment or alleviation of disease;

(ii) Diagnosis, monitoring, treatment, alleviation of or compensation for an injury or handicap;

(iii) Investigation, replacement or modification of the anatomy or of a physiological process; control of conception;

and that does not achieve its principal intended action in or on the human body by pharmacological, immunological or metabolic means, but which may be assisted in its function by such means*; or

(i) an accessory to such an instrument, apparatus, appliance, material or other article.

*There are therapeutic goods that have both a medicine and a medical device component, and it is the combination of the two components that deliver the desired therapeutic effect. In deciding how these products are regulated, the TGA considers

(i) the primary intended purpose

(ii) the mode of action of the product

as they relate to the definition of a medicine and a medical device.

Further guidance is provided in Section 14 of the ARGMD: Medical Devices Incorporating a Medicine.

The regulations define a medical device to be an IVD if it satisfies the following criteria:

(i) It is a reagent, calibrator, control material, kit, specimen receptacle, software, instrument, apparatus, equipment or system, whether used alone or in combination with another diagnostic product for *in vitro* use; and

(ii) It is intended by the manufacturer to be used *in vitro* for the examination of specimens derived from the human body, solely or principally for

   (a) giving information about a physiological or pathological state or a congenital abnormality; or

   (b) determining safety and compatibility with a potential recipient; or

   (c) monitoring therapeutic measures.

24.4 Classification of Medical Devices

Medical devices are classified on the basis of risk, through consideration of the manufacturer's intended use, degree of invasiveness in the human body, and duration of use. The classification follows the EU system except that the Australian system includes a separate class for active implantable medical devices. The classification levels are shown in Table 24.2.

Table 24.2 Classification of medical devices

Classification	Level of risk
Class I	Low
Class I—supplied sterile Class I—incorporating a measuring function Class IIa	Low–medium
Class IIb	Medium–high
Class III	High risk
Active implantable medical devices (AIMD)	High risk

Note: Differences between the Australian and European classification systems are detailed in Section 8 of the ARGMD.

The TGA has adopted a risk-based approach to regulation of medical devices, through consideration of the risk to the patient, versus potential benefit of the device. The level of TGA regulatory control increases with the level of risk of the medical device.

24.4.1 Classification of IVD Medical Devices

The Australian medical device regulatory framework has a separate classification system for IVD medical devices (IVDs). The manufacturer is responsible for determining the class of an IVD (as described in Table 24.3) using a set of classification rules with regard to

(i) the manufacturer's intended use of the device; and
(ii) the level of risk to the patient and the public (taking into account the likelihood of harm and the severity of that harm).

Table 24.3 Classification of IVD medical devices

Classification	Level of risk
Class 1 IVD	No public health risk or low personal risk
Class 2 IVD	Low public health risk or moderate personal risk
Class 3 IVD	Moderate public health risk or high personal risk
Class 4 IVD	High public health risk

Note: The same classification rules apply to both commercial IVDs and in-house IVDs.

24.5 Inclusion of Medical Devices on the ARTG

The majority of medical devices must be included in the Australian Register of Therapeutic Goods (ARTG) before being made available for supply in Australia. Exceptions to this requirement are devices that are supplied through one of the four mechanisms for supplying medical devices in Australia not included in the ARTG:

(i) clinical trials in Australia
(ii) authorised prescribers
(iii) Special Access Scheme
(iv) personal importation
(v) custom-made medical devices

For a medical device to be included in the ARTG, the TGA must be satisfied that available evidence demonstrates that the device is safe and effective and that an appropriate system is in place for monitoring the ongoing performance and safety of the device. As such, a sponsor can only apply to include a medical device in the ARTG if

(i) the device complies with the Essential Principles
(ii) appropriate conformity assessment procedures have been applied to the device

Applications for inclusion of a medical device in the ARTG are submitted through the TGA eBusiness (eBS) services, accessed via the TGA website, http://www.tga.gov.au.

There are different levels of access for registered users and the general public. Only an Australian sponsor can apply to include a medical device in the ARTG.

Following the inclusion of a medical device in the ARTG, the TGA issues a Certificate of Inclusion, which can be downloaded by the Sponsor from the eBS.

Class 1–3 in-house IVD medical devices are required to be entered on an in-house IVD database that is separate from the ARTG — For more information, please refer to Part 6A, Schedule 3, of the Regulations.

24.5.1 Process for Supplying a Medical Device in Australia

The following processes must be followed in order to include a medical device on the ARTG:

(i) process for all Class I non-sterile and non-measuring devices
(ii) process if the medical device is manufactured in Australia (other than Class 1)
(iii) process if the medical device is manufactured overseas (other than Class 1)
(iv) process if the device contains a medicine or materials of animal, microbial recombinant, or human origin

This chapter only outlines the latter two processes as these will be of most interest to the majority of readers. Please refer to the ARGMD on the TGA website for a detailed description of the up-to-date processes.

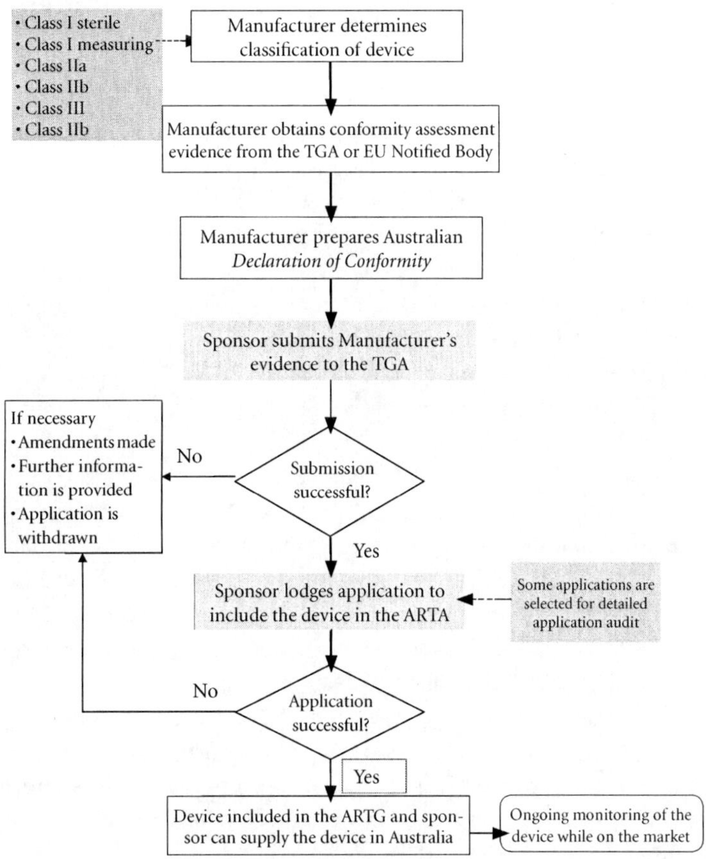

Figure 24.1 Process to supply a medical device in Australia if the medical device is manufactured overseas.

The following processes must be followed in order to include an IVD medical device on the ARTG:

(i) process for including Class 1 IVD medical devices (other than export only) in the ARTG

(ii) process for including IVD medical devices (other than Class 1) in the ARTG

For most Class I and II devices, successful electronic submission of the medical device application form is followed by inclusion of the device in the ARTG.

Applications for Class III, AIMD, and certain Class IIb devices (refer to Section 11, ARGMD) are subjected to a mandatory Level 2 application audit prior to inclusion in the ARTG whereby all supporting documentation will be submitted to the TGA for evaluation.

In addition, any application for a medical device of any Class may be randomly selected for a Level 1 Application Audit. In such cases, the sponsor is required to provide the requested documentation to the TGA within 20 working days.

Since the Australian regulatory system is closely aligned with the European system, evaluation requirements for all devices (other than those containing a medicine or material of animal, human or microbial origin) are significantly reduced for products which have already been approved for CE Marking by a European Notified Body. Products which have not been CE Marked must go though full Conformity Assessment evaluation by the TGA.

Additionally, an abbreviated approval route through the Aust-EC Mutual Recognition Agreement (MRA) is available for devices other than those containing a medicine or material of animal, human or microbial origin, which are substantially manufactured within the European Community (and have a EC legal manufacturer). Devices with MRA certificates issued by a European Notified Body may be approved by the TGA within 1 week.

Full TGA Conformity Assessment evaluation is required for devices that include human blood or plasma derivative, derivatives of animal or microbial origin, or incorporate a medicine. TGA approval for such products may involve a TGA audit of the manufacturing facility.

Once issued, TGA Conformity Assessment certificates are valid for 5 years.

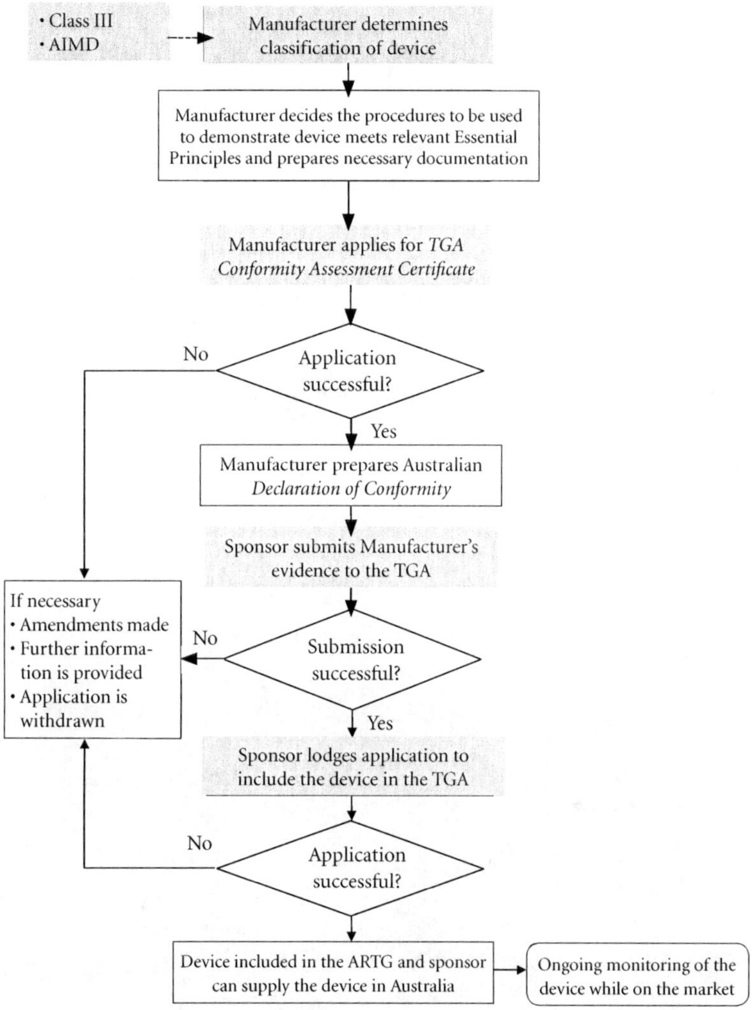

Figure 24.2 Process to supply a medical device in Australia if the device contains a medicine or materials of animal, microbial recombinant, or human origin.

24.5.2 Process for Including Class 1 IVD Medical Devices (Other Than Export Only) in the ARTG

The flowchart in Fig. 24.3 summarises the steps for including in the ARTG a Class 1 IVD that is to be supplied in Australia:

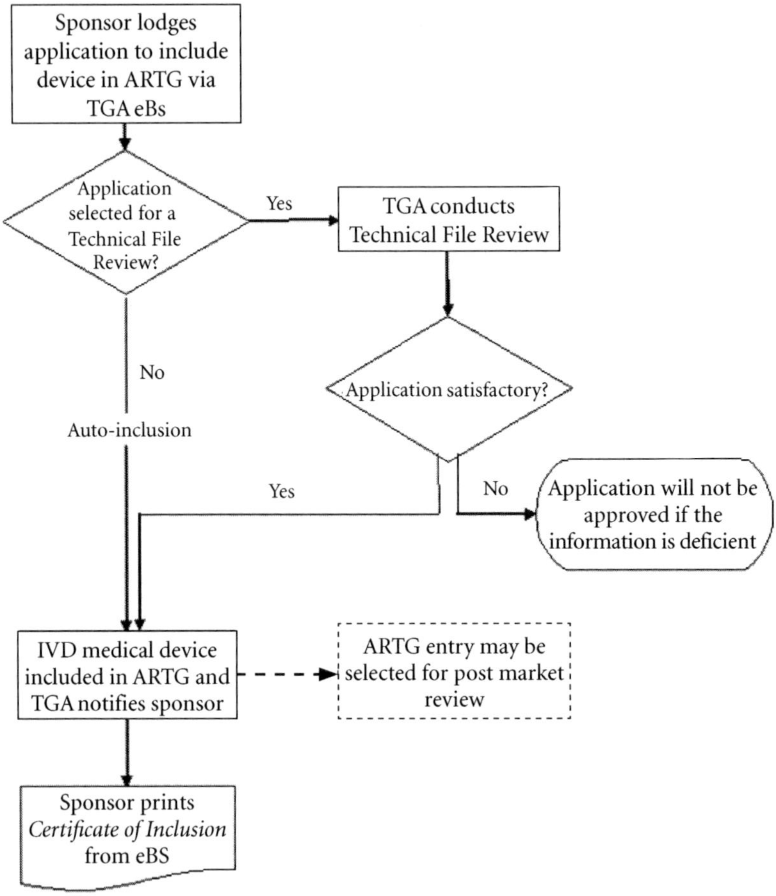

Figure 24.3 Steps for including in the ARTG a Class 1 IVD that is to be supplied in Australia.

24.5.3 Process for Including IVD Medical Devices (Other Than Class 1) in the ARTG

The flowchart in Fig. 24.4 summarises the steps for including in the ARTG an IVD that is to be supplied in Australia, other than a Class 1 IVD:

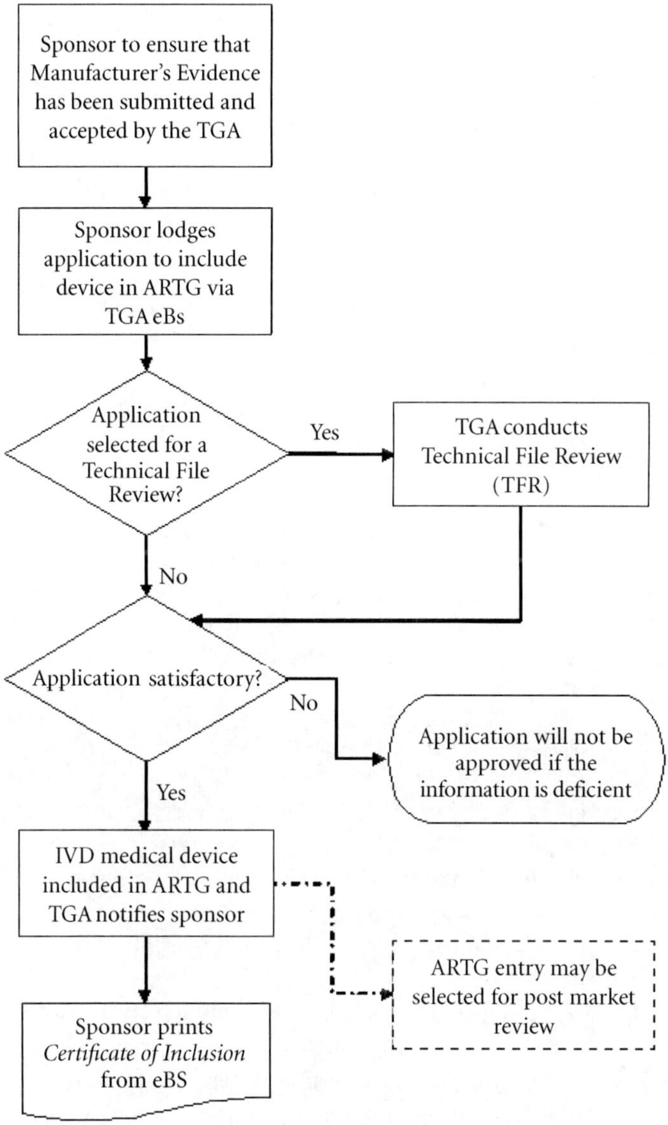

Figure 24.4 Steps for including in the ARTG an IVD that is to be supplied in Australia, other than a Class 1 IVD.

24.6 Same Kind of Medical Device (SKMD)

In the case of Class I, Class I sterile, Class I measuring, Class IIa, and Class IIb medical devices, and Class 1, Class 2, Class 3 IVDs and Class 4 immunohaematology reagents (IHRs), one medical device is considered to be of the "same kind" as another medical device, if both devices

(i) have the same manufacturer
(ii) have the same sponsor and
(iii) are the same classification
(iv) have the same GMDN code

Medical devices which are identical in respect to these criteria can be grouped under one ARTG inclusion. There is no record kept in the ARTG of the product family name, model numbers, or catalogue numbers for these classes of device.

For Class III and Class AIMD medical devices, and Class 4 IVDs (that are not IHRs) a further requirement is added to the definition of same kind of medical device — they must have the same Unique Product Identifier (UPI), described in the following section.

24.7 Unique Product Identifier

As specified in Regulation 1.6, of the Therapeutic Goods (Medical Devices) Regulations 2002, the unique product identifier (UPI) is the combination of words, numbers, symbols, or letters assigned by the manufacturer to uniquely identify the device and any of its variants. The UPI is distinct from the catalogue identifier assigned to the device.

The TGA recognizes that different manufacturers identify their product lines in different ways such as

(i) using family names to identify a range of similar devices
(ii) uniquely identifying each device with a model number
(iii) adopting a combination of both of these approaches

Figure 24.5 explains UPI showing the example of a family of prosthetic heart valves, as provided within the ARGMD. In this example, the family name does not uniquely identify all of the device models in the product range. Therefore, the term "Globus prosthetic heart valves" is not considered a UPI, because it does not distinguish between the different intended purposes of each model in the product range — atrial-versus mitral-valve replacement.

However, the model names

(i) Globus atrial prosthetic heart valve
(ii) Globus mitral prosthetic heart valve

are considered UPIs because the model/catalogue numbers are only variations of the diameter of the device that do not change its intended purpose.

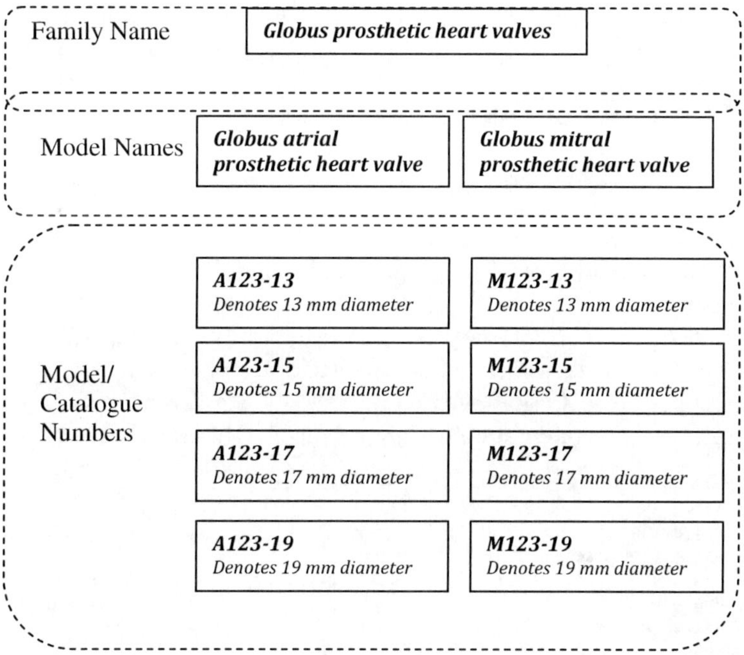

Figure 24.5 Example of a UPI provided within the ARGMD.

24.8 *In vitro* Diagnostic UPIs

The UPI for an IVD uniquely identifies an individual IVD, or a combination of IVDs which together constitute an IVD closed system (a combination of reagents, calibrators and quality control materials that share a common intended purpose; and are to be used only in combination with each other as components of a single assay).

24.9 Renewal

In Australia, the requirement for sponsors to renew or resubmit their regulatory approvals on a periodic basis is restricted to those supported by a TGA Conformity Assessment certificate, which requires renewal every 5 years.

Once a medical device is included in the ARTG, the sponsor is obligated to ensure the medical device remains in compliance with the Essential Principles and that changes are submitted to the TGA for evaluation as required.

Sponsors are required to pay an annual fee for each ARTG inclusion, equivalent to the original fee for inclusion on the ARTG.

24.10 Documentation Requirements

24.10.1 Conformity Assessment Applications

Manufacturers who apply for a TGA Conformity Assessment Certificate are required to prepare technical documentation to demonstrate that the medical device complies with the Essential Principles. This will vary on a case by case basis, depending on the, type of device, risk associated with its manufacture and use, and period that it has been on the market. However, the minimum technical documentation will always include the elements described in Fig. 24.6.

Documentation Required
Conformity Assessment
Copy of all current conformity assessment evidence for the medical device and/or manufacturer
Clinical evidence
Risk management records (ISO 14971)
Essential Principles compliance summary (e.g., Essential Principle checklist or similar)
Evidence to support compliance with any standards or test methods utilised for compliance (for example, test reports or assessment reports, labels and Instructions for Use)

Microbial, or recombinant origin; or medicinal substances
Evidence to support the quality and safety of animal derived material, in accordance with the TGA approach to minimising the risk of exposure to Transmissible Spongiform Encephalopathies (TSEs) through medicines and medical devices, available on the TGA website.
Drug Master File and GMP Clearance for medicine manufacturer.

Figure 24.6 Minimum documentation required, applications for Conformity Assessment Certificate.

The TGA refers sponsors to the GHTF Summary Technical Documentation for Demonstrating Conformity to the Essential Principles of Safety and Performance of Medical Devices (STED), for guidance on the technical documentation that should be assembled and submitted to demonstrate conformity to the Essential Principles.

Devices containing materials of human blood or plasma derivatives, animal, microbial or recombinant origin or medicinal substances are regulated more stringently by the TGA. As such, the TGA reserves the right to conduct an on-site audit of manufacturing facilities as part of the application process if they are not completely satisfied with the supporting documentation.

At a minimum, the TGA requires evidence to support the quality and safety of animal derived material, in accordance with the TGA approach to minimising the risk of exposure to Transmissible Spongiform Encephalopathies (TSEs) through medicines and medical devices, available on the TGA website.

24.11 Application Audits

The TGA will write to the sponsor requesting the information that is required to conduct the application audit. The TGA may ask for any documentation relating to the device and/or manufacturer (Fig. 24.7).

Level 1

- Original or correctly notarised copy of the manufacturer's Australian Declaration of Conformity
- Copy of the latest and current conformity assessment evidence for the medical device and/or manufacturer
- Information about the device, including copies of the
  - label
  - instructions for use
  - advertising material such as brochures, web pages, advertisements

Level 2

- All the documentation listed above for a Level 1 audit
- Risk management report
- Clinical evaluation report
- Efficacy and performance data for medical devices that disinfect including sterilisation of other medical devices

Figure 24.7 Minimum documentation requirements for each level of an application audit.

24.12 Access to Unapproved Medical Devices

There are four mechanisms for accessing unapproved medical devices in Australia which do not require inclusion in the ARTG prior to supply:

(i) clinical trials in Australia
(ii) authorised prescribers
(iii) the Special Access Scheme
(iv) personal importation

Importantly, these schemes cannot be used to facilitate the commercial supply of therapeutic goods.

Further information on these mechanisms is available on a web page titled "Accessing unapproved products", on the TGA website, http://www.tga.gov.au/hp/access.htm.

References

1. Australian Demographic Statistics (June 2011). *Australian Bureau of Statistics.* Retrieved (18 May 2012) from http://www.abs.gov.au/.
2. AusMedtech (28 Nov 2011). Retrieved (22 February 2012) from http://www.ausbiotech.org/ausmedtech/.
3. Department of the Treasury. *Australia to 2050: Future Challenges, January 2010 (Intergenerational Report 2010).*
4. TGA. Australian Regulatory Guidelines for Medical Devices (ARGMD) (May 2011). *Therapeutic Goods Administration* Version 1.1. Retrieved (25 January 2012) from www.tga.gov.au.
5. TGA. Accessing unapproved products. *Therapeutic Goods Administration.* Retrieved (25 January 2012) from http://www.tga.gov.au/hp/access.htm.
6. World Health Organisation. Global Health Observatory (GHO)(2011). *Country Statistics* 2011. Retrieved (18 January 2012) from http://www.who.int/gho/countries/en/.
7. Year Book Australia (2008). *Australian Bureau of Statistics.* Retrieved (22 January 2012) from http://www.abs.gov.au/ausstats/abs@.nsf/0/A50BD9743BF2733ACA2573D2001078D8?opendocument.

Chapter 25

China: Medical Device Regulatory System

Jack Wong

Asia Regulatory Professional Association (ARPA)

speedxquality@yahoo.com

Disclaimer

The regulatory information contained in this chapter is intended for market planning and is subject to change frequently. Translations of laws and regulations are unofficial.

25.1 Introduction

China's overall registration framework is under revision and amendment, and certain regulation outlined below may have been revised recently. Certain explanation of the regulation may also be updated accordingly. Please refer to the most updated regulation from the State Food and Drug Administration's (SFDA) official website or consult your local regulatory affairs staff/consultant for up-to-date explanation and practice.

Handbook of Medical Device Regulatory Affairs in Asia
Edited by Jack Wong and Raymond K. Y. Tong

ISBN 978-981-4411-21-9 (Hardcover), 978-981-4411-22-6 (eBook)
www.panstanford.com

25.2 Market Overview

China's medical device market is forecasted to have a value of US$23.2 billion in 2011 with strong growth in two-digit annual growth rate. China has the world's largest population.

In 2009, the Chinese government committed 850 billion yuan (US$124 billion) to develop/enhance the country healthcare system over a three-year period. The plan is to create a platform for universal healthcare access for all by 2020. The prospects for medical device spending are huge. The government has committed heavily in the construction of thousands of hospitals, healthcare centres and clinics, and this will inevitably lead to spending on capital goods, most notably medical devices.

25.3 Overview of Regulatory Environment and What Laws/Regulations Govern the Medical Devices

China's regulatory system for medical devices is still in its rapid development phase, which unavoidably leads to a certain degree of difficulty to catch up on the latest regulatory requirement. Language can also be a major problem for foreign manufacturers as most of regulation and product standards are in Chinese. Product registration submission files are also required to be in Chinese as well

There are three levels of legislation, all of which are considered mandatory and apply to both local and foreign manufacturers:

- Regulations for the Supervision and Administration of Medical Devices, which were promulgated by the State Council on 4 January 2000 and came into force on 1 April 2000;
- SFDA Orders, which provide the detail for implementing the Regulations
- Normative documents of the central or local FDAs, which are similar to standards

Regulations for the Supervision and Administration of Medical Device basic content include

- Chapter I: General Provisions

    - Scope: All units or individuals engaged in the research and development, production, distribution, use, supervision and administration of medical devices within the territory of P.R. China
    - Definition of medical device
    - Competent authority : SFDA
    - Classification: Class I, II and III
- Chapter II: The Administration of Medical Devices
    - Registration
    - Requirements of clinical trial
- Chapter III: Administration of Production, Distribution and Use of Medical Devices
- Chapter IV: Supervision of Medical Devices
- Chapter V: Penalties
- Chapter VI: Supplementary Provisions

The English version of the China regulations for the supervision and administration of medical devices can be found at the following link: http://eng.sfda.gov.cn/WS03/CL0767/61641.html.

25.3.1 Measuring Function

Medical devices produced and used for the purpose of providing concrete measuring values shall comply with the requirements of the metering law. The detailed product list shall be formulated and promulgated by the drug regulatory authority under the State Council, jointly with the metering authority.

25.3.2 Standards

China has National Standard for medical device. A medical device must follow China National Standard specification. More than 35% of all IEC and ISO standards have now been adopted by China, but many are not direct transpositions and contain China-specific requirements. Table 25.1 lists some of the main medical device-related international standards and their Chinese equivalents. The standards ISO 14155 and ISO 13485: 2003 have also recently been adopted.

Table 25.1 Primary medical device related international standards and their Chinese equivalents

International standard	Chinese equivalent
ISO 13485/13488	YY/T0287/0288
ISO 14971: 2000	YY/T0316 – 2003
IEC 60601-1: 1988	GB 9706.1 – 1995

National medical devices standards can be found at National Standardisation Technical Committee's website (www.sac.gov.cn). Industry standards can be found at the websites of the SFDA (www.sfda.gov.cn) and the Centre for Medical Device Evaluation (www.cmde.org.cn).

The SFDA recognizes products' country-of-origin approval to kick off imported product registration.

25.4 Regulatory Body

The SFDA is directly under the State Council, which is in charge of comprehensive supervision on the safety management of medical device, drug, food, health food and cosmetics and is the competent authority of drug regulation.

The drug regulatory authority under the State Council is responsible for supervision and administration of medical devices nationwide. The drug administration of the local government at county level and above is responsible for supervision and administration of medical devices in each administrative region. The drug regulatory authority under the State Council shall coordinate with other departments under the State Council, responsible for comprehensive economic administration, in the implementation of policies for the medical device industry

The detailed organization chart of the SFDA can be found at http://eng.sfda.gov.cn/WS03/CL0763/.

SFDA contact details

State Food and Drug Administration

26 Xuanwumen Xidajie, Beijing, 100053, P.R. China

Fax: +86-010-68310909

Email: inquires@sda.gov.cn

25.5 Regulatory Overview

25.5.1 Definition of Medical Device

The definition of a medical device that is used in China is very similar to the definition provided by the GHTF, although there are some differences in interpretation of the definition (e.g. spectacles are not medical devices in China). The definition given in the Regulations is any instrument, apparatus, appliance, material, or other article whether used alone or in combination, including the software necessary for its proper application. It does not achieve its principal action in or on the human body by means of pharmacology, immunology or metabolism, but which may be assisted in its function by such means; the use of which is to achieve the following intended objectives:

1. Diagnosis, prevention, monitoring, treatment or alleviation of disease;
2. Diagnosis, monitoring, treatment, alleviation of or compensation for an injury or handicap conditions;
3. Investigation, replacement or modification for anatomy or a physiological process;
4. Control of conception.

25.5.2 Classification of Medical Device

Medical devices are classified according to the risk level associated with their intended use. In general, the risk level depends on the design of a medical device as well as its intended use.

The State shall classify medical devices and administer them on the basis of the following classification:

- Class I medical devices are those for which safety and effectiveness can be ensured through routine administration.
- Class II medical devices are those for which further control is required to ensure their safety and effectiveness.
- Class III medical devices are those which are implanted into the human body or used for life support or sustenance or pose potential risk to the human body and thus must be strictly controlled in respect to safety and effectiveness.

The classification catalogue for medical devices shall be stipulated, adjusted and promulgated by the drug regulatory authority under the State Council, in accordance with classification principles after consulting with health authority under the State Council.

These class definitions are not the same as those used in the European Union or by the GHTF, and the Class III classification is much broader than many manufacturers may be used to. There are many reasons for these classification differences in China. The two key reasons are

1. Historical reason, i.e. some devices are classified as different classification or even as drug even before medical device regulation came into being and hence the device may follow the old classification
2. Social reason, i.e. the SFDA may consider some device to have higher risk in China, e.g. after some adverse events

For further information on the classification of devices, readers are referred to "The Provisions for Medical Device Classification (SFDA Order No 15)".

The handling of administration matters relating to medical devices is also determined by the device's classification. For locally produced devices

- Class I devices are administered by a city level regulatory authority.
- Class II devices are administered by a provincial/municipal regulatory authority.
- Class III devices are administered by the central SFDA.

All imported medical devices are administered by the central SFDA.

25.5.3 Registration Process

25.5.3.1 Medical devices registration certificate

Each medical device or medical device family should have a Medical Devices Registration Certificate before it can be placed on the market in China. The certificate is owned by the local manufacturer or the distributor and must be renewed every four years (the new regulation will suggest the expiry after a five-year term). The precise requirements for product registration vary depending on the device class but can include sample testing, clinical evaluation/investigation and site inspection.

A simplified flow chart depicting the process for product registration is shown in Fig. 25.1. For every imported medical device, before registration, the applicant should write a product standard which follows China National Standard as the first step. The manufacturer can use an ISO/IEC standard as product standard, but the standard should be translated into Chinese. The applicant should arrange product testing by the national Testing Centre to ensure that the product passes the test as per the China National Standard. Once the SFDA Application Receiving Office has all the required information, the application is passed to the Medical Devices Evaluation Centre, then to the Department of Medical Devices Registration at the SFDA, then to the Director of the Medical Devices Department, and then to the Director General of the SFDA for final approval. Finally, the result of the application and certificate of approval is sent back to the Application Receiving Office for collection by the applicant.

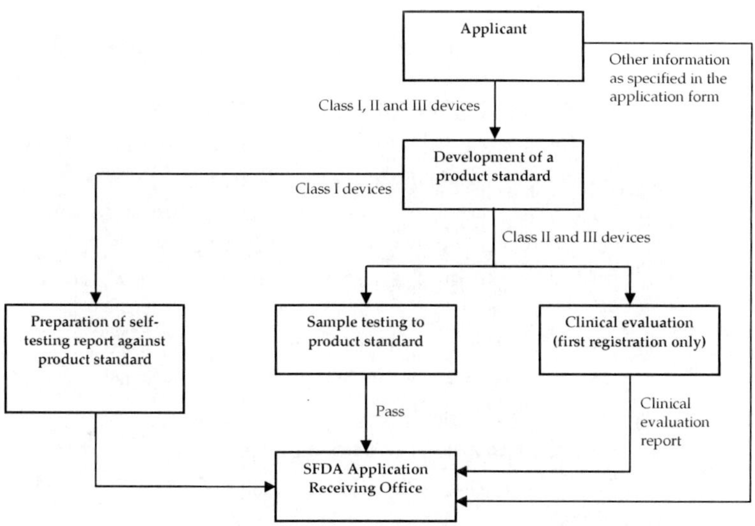

Figure 25.1 Procedure for obtaining a Medical Devices Registration Certificate.

25.4.5.2 Product testing

Testing is performed by a local testing centre.

No product testing is required for the following types of devices:

(1) Among the laboratory equipment, the electrophoresis apparatus "centrifuge" ultra low temperature refrigerator,

paraffin slicing machine, paraffin embedding machine, cell centrifuge smearing machine, and full automatic dying machine no clinical trial reports and Product Type Test Reports issued by the medical devices quality test agency and recognized by the State Drug Administration are required to be provided .

(2) The products of Class I in accordance with catalogue of classification of the medical device products of China.

(3) As for the medical devices in conformance with both of the following conditions, the application for exemption from test may be made if

(a) The domestic enterprise has received the authentication certificate of GB/T19001+YY/T0287 or GB/T19002+YY/T0288 issued by the quality system authentication agency recognized by the State Drug Administration, and the quality system concerned has covered the products for application.

(b) The product abroad has received the authorization of launching from the competent department of the country of origin, and the certificate is still valid, and the enterprise has been authenticated in accordance with the ISO 9000 Serial Standards (or equivalent).

(c) The difference between the structure and performance of the products for application and those of the registered products of a kind is insignificant in terms of safety and effectiveness.

(d) The products for application are not implantable devices.

(e) No radioactive sources exist in the products for application.

(f) In case of any malfunction, no grave injury accidents such as death of and body injury of the user or operator will be caused.

25.5.3.3 Clinical trials

In application for medical device registration, Class III medical devices are subject to clinical trials, Class II medical devices are generally subject to clinical trials, and Class I medical devices are exempt from clinical trials.

This is very significant for Class III medical device manufacturers that are looking to register their products in China.

Currently, the only Class III devices that absolutely require clinical trials are long-term implantable devices. This language implies that clinical trials will be required for all Class III devices. While the final regulations have yet to be released, this change could greatly affect the time to entry for foreign Class III products.

25.5.3.4 Exemption of clinical trial data for Class II devices

In November 2011, the SFDA issued Decree 475, exempting several types of domestically produced Chinese products from clinical trial requirements. These clearances are very similar to the exemptions listed in Section 510(k) of the US Food, Drug, and Cosmetic Act.

During the application process, a manufacturer may request exemption from clinical trial data requirements by demonstrating the similarity of their device with an approved product already on the market. The list of products that qualify for this exemption is currently limited to 21 device groups, including medical surgery tools, syringes, thermometers, ECG machines, ophthalmic equipment, nebulisers, electrodes, sterilisers, protective clothing, dentures, cryogenic tools and single-use urology equipment.

While at first glance this exemption seems like a big advantage for domestic companies, most foreign firms that register Class II devices are already exempt from clinical trials as they can provide safety data from their home countries. In addition, once a company has an approved product on the market, it is typically exempt from clinical trial requirements for similar future products. In the short term, these exemptions will likely be most advantageous for start-up Chinese companies that wish to quickly bring new devices to the market; in the long term, however, these regulations may facilitate the *de novo* development, manufacture and distribution of medical devices in China by foreign companies.

25.5.3.5 Enforcing GMPs

With Decree 54, the SFDA officially implemented the new medical device GMP regulations.

The GMPs are divided into 13 chapters covering general risk management procedures, management responsibilities, resource management, documentation, procurement and other sections equivalent to international GMP requirements.

The most detailed sections of the new regulations cover production management. The production management guidelines require manufacturers to devise, implement and document production processes at all steps under their control and formulate guidelines for each device they manufacture. Each product must be marked and monitored during the entire production process to identify and prevent improper use of the device prior to or after official release.

To enforce the new GMPs, the SFDA is using a risk-based approach similar to that used by its US counterpart. This means that high-risk devices such as Class III and sterile Class II devices are being prioritised for SFDA review during the initial inspection and review process. After the SFDA has expanded its inspection teams and processed the backlog of high-risk inspections required during the first phase of this endeavour, other manufacturers can expect to be visited.

25.5.3.6 Timeframes

Table 25.2 lists the timeframes involved in each activity for obtaining registration of a product and its distributor.

Table 25.2 Timeframes

		Class II and III	
Process	**Class I**	**First registration**	**Re-registration**
Dossier compilation by the manufacturer and his distributor	2–3 months	2–3 months	2–3 months
Translation into Chinese, product standard compilation, modification of the Instructions for Use (manufacturer and distributor)	1–2 months	1–2 months	1–2 months
Sample tested by national Testing Centre*	n/a	3 months	3 months
Clinical trial or clinical data evaluation*†	n/a	To be determined	n/a
On-site inspection at overseas manufacturing site (Class III only)*	n/a	To be determined	To be determined

Registration dossier submission to, and approval by, the SFDA plus review and approval of the Instructions for Use by the SFDA	5 months	8 months	8 months
Total	~9 months	12–14 months	12–14 months

* These stages may be performed in parallel.
† May not be needed for some Class II devices (e.g. if equivalent to an approved, marketed product).

More registration guidelines can be found at http://eng.sfda.gov.cn/WS03/CL0770/61661.html.

25.5.3.7 The CCC mark

The CCC mark is an additional product testing mark for some medical devices. Products that do not bear the CCC mark may be held at customs; the mark applies to the following eight categories of medical devices:

- rubber condoms (under latex products)
- medical diagnostic x-ray equipment
- haemodialysis equipment
- hollow fibre dialysers
- extra-corporeal blood circuit for blood purification equipment;
- electrocardiographs
- implantable cardiac pacemakers
- artificial heart-lung machines

The CCC mark is issued by the China Quality Certification Centre (CQC), a parallel department to the SFDA.

CCC testing for medical devices is usually based on national standards such as GB 9706 (the Chinese equivalent of IEC 60601). The testing is usually performed at the same testing centre and at the same time as the testing for a Medical Devices Registration Certificate. Two separate test reports are issued (one is sent to the SFDA and one to the CQC) and the fees are charged separately.

There has been a concern about and opposition to this duplicative testing and certification of medical devices. Despite a formal announcement by the SFDA and the General Administration of Quality Supervision, Inspection and Quarantine (AQSIQ) that duplicative testing is no longer allowed, in reality this has yet to be implemented.

25.6 Monitoring Adverse Events

Tracking adverse events and reporting them in a timely manner has been the driving force behind the issuance of Decree 425 from the SFDA. The 45-page guidance document issued in 2011 details requirements for personnel, documentation, reporting times and annual reports. All medical devices that are registered for sale in China will have to comply with these new requirements. Foreign firms that do not have a China office and are working through local third-party agents and distributors should ensure that their local representatives are aware of, and can comply with, these new regulations.

Each company must have designated staff for reporting adverse events in at least a part-time capacity and a system to properly track, collect and analyse the root cause of an adverse event. Depending on the severity of the incident, and prior to a cause being discovered, the sale of the device may be suspended and could require co-ordination with hospitals and clinics that dispense the device.

For Class III devices, a system must be in place to collect global adverse event data from wherever the device is sold. Severe adverse events must be reported to the SFDA within 15 days irrespective of its location in the world.

The SFDA sets forth detailed requirements for all stakeholders, from device manufacturer personnel to distributors and patients.

Any company whose medical devices are sold in China should carefully review the guidance to ensure that they are in compliance with the guidelines; otherwise, they risk running foul of the SFDA and possible blockage of their product's sale due to improper adverse event monitoring, reporting or response.

25.7 Managing Recalls

If an adverse event investigation warrants the recall of a medical device, then the company should follow the Medical Device Recall

Management Guidelines laid out in SFDA Decree 82. The decree contains 38 articles laying out the requirements that should be followed in case of a recall.

A recall notice should have

- name, batch and other basic information
- reasons for the recall
- recall requirements, such as an immediate moratorium on the sale and use of the product

Everyone in the process, from the manufacturer to the distributor, shares the liability for medical device problems. Foreign companies that are working through local Chinese distributors and agents, therefore, must also ensure that all regulations are being followed properly.

There are three levels of recalls as determined by the SFDA:

- Recalls are classified as Class I if use of the medical device has caused, or may cause, serious health hazards that are of a permanent nature.
- Recalls are classified as Class II if a medical device may cause a health issue of a temporary nature.
- Class III recalls are the least stringent and are used for devices that are not likely to cause harm but are still defective.

These recalls can be of a voluntary nature or ordered by the SFDA.

In carrying out a medical device investigation and evaluating its defects, an analysis should be done to determine

- whether the use of the medical device caused the adverse event
- whether there is relevant scientific literature, research, testing or validation to explain the causes of injury
- the geographical area effected by the damaged device and its population characteristics
- the extent of the damage to human health
- the probability of injury
- the short-term and long-term consequences of the injury
- other potential harm to human health

References

1. SFDA website: http://www.sfda.gov.cn.
2. S. Goldenberg, E. Zhao (13 April 2012), *The Implications of Medical Device Regulatory Change in China*, RAJ Pharma.

Chapter 26

Hong Kong: Medical Device Regulatory System

Jack Wong
Asia Regulatory Professional Association (ARPA)
speedxquality@yahoo.com

Disclaimer

The regulatory information contained in this chapter is intended for market planning and is subject to change frequently. Translations of laws and regulations are unofficial.

26.1 Market Overview

26.1.1 Market Environment

(i) Hong Kong is a prosperous economy and acts as a hub for trade throughout Asia.
(ii) The population is about 7 million and very receptive to use of advanced medical products. All medical and healthcare

Handbook of Medical Device Regulatory Affairs in Asia
Edited by Jack Wong and Raymond K. Y. Tong

ISBN 978-981-4411-21-9 (Hardcover), 978-981-4411-22-6 (eBook)
www.panstanford.com

products, subject to the China and Hong Kong Closer Economic Partnership Arrangement's (CEPA) rules of origin, are able to enjoy duty-free access to the China mainland.

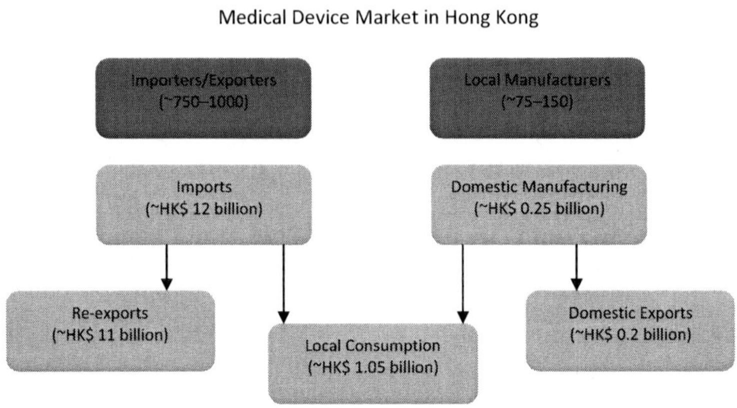

Figure 26.1 Medical device market in Hong Kong.

26.2 Overview of Regulatory Environment and What Laws/Regulations Govern Medical Devices

Medical device regulation is developing in Hong Kong. The new regulatory system will largely be based on the recommendation of the Global Harmonization Task Force (GHTF). The GHTF is a voluntary consortium with representatives from the trade and regulatory authorities from the United States, Canada, Australia, Japan, and the European Union formed in 1992 to harmonize the standards and principles of regulating medical devices

Currently, the import or sale of medical devices in Hong Kong except those containing pharmaceutical products or emitting ionizing radiation does not require registration.

An "irradiating apparatus" is defined by the Radiation Health Unit as one intended to produce or emit ionizing radiation, or capable of producing or emitting ionizing radiation at a dose rate exceeding 5 microsievert per hour at a distance of 5 cm from any accessible point of the surface of the apparatus. The Radiation Health Unit's Irradiating Apparatus Licence Section processes applications for and handles renewal of licences required to import, sell, manufacture, produce, deal in/with, possess and/or use irradiating medical equipment.

The Consumer Goods Safety Ordinance (Cap.456) provides protection against the supply, manufacture or import of unsafe products, including some medical devices that can be regarded as consumer goods, unless otherwise specified in the Schedule. The Electrical Products (Safety) Regulation (Cap.406G) provides protection against the supply of unsafe electrical products including medical devices designed for household use except those products specified otherwise. Details are available at: http://www.justice.gov.hk/home.htm.

The statutory regulation of certain health care professionals, whereby the practitioners are required to ensure the safe and appropriate treatment for patients, also provides incidental control on the use of medical devices.

The Undesirable Medical Advertisements Ordinance (Cap.231) prohibits advertisements related to the curative or preventive effects of products on diseases listed in the Ordinance. Details are available at: http://www.justice.gov.hk/home.htm.

To raise public awareness on the safe use of medical devices and enable traders to familiarize themselves with the future mandatory requirements, the Medical Device Control Office (MDCO) was established in July 2004. Its mission is to set up a risk-based and cost-effective regulation on the supply and use of medical devices with reference to harmonized standards and procedures recommended by the GHTF. The government launched a Medical Device Administrative Control System (MDACS) on 26 November 2004. The first phase of MDACS starts with voluntary listing of Class IV (High Risk) Medical Devices. The second phase of MDACS, which includes voluntary listing of Class II and Class III (medium risk) medical devices, was launched on 14 November 2005.

26.3 Regulatory Body

The MDCO is the regulatory body in Hong Kong.

Contact information for medical devices
Medical Device Control Office,
Department of Health,

The Government of Hong Kong SAR,
31/F, Hopewell Centre,
183 Queen's Road East,
Wan Chai, Hong Kong
Website: http://www.mdco.gov.hk/

Contact information for irradiating apparatus
Electrical & Mechanical Services Department (EMSD),
Health Sector Division,
16/F Multi-Centre Block A,
Pamela Younde Nethersole Eastern Hospital,
Chai Wan, Hong Kong
Website: http://www.info.gov.hk/emsd/english/about/organisation/index.html

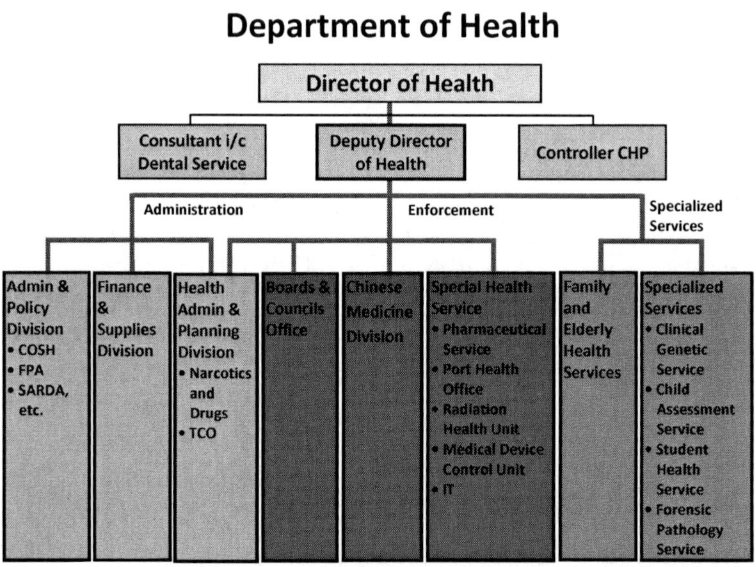

Figure 26.2 Organizational Chart of Medical Device Control Office (MDCO) in the Department of Health.

26.4 Regulatory Overview

26.4.1 Definition of Medical Device (It Follows GHTF)

Medical devices range from sophisticated equipment such as cardiac pacemakers used by health care professionals to simple products such as bandages and thermometers bought over the counter.

In essence, a medical device refers to any instrument, apparatus, appliance, material or other article, excluding drugs, used for human beings for diagnosis, prevention, treatment and monitoring of diseases or injuries; for rehabilitation purposes; or for the investigation, replacement or modification of body structure or function. In addition, it includes devices used for examination of human specimens.

An accessory to a medical device is subject to the same regulations that apply to the medical device itself. However, devices designed for the treatment or diagnosis of diseases and injuries in animals are outside the scope of the proposed regulatory framework.

An "irradiating apparatus" is defined by the Radiation Health Unit as one intended to produce or emit ionizing radiation, or capable of producing or emitting ionizing radiation at a dose rate exceeding 5 microsievert per hour at a distance of 5 cm from any accessible point of the surface of the apparatus. The Radiation Health Unit's Irradiating Apparatus Licence Section processes applications for and handles renewal of licences required to import, sell, manufacture, produce, deal in/with, possess and/or use irradiating medical equipment.

26.4.2 The Classification of Medical Devices

The Principle

Medical devices are classified according to the risk level associated with their intended use. In general, the risk level depends on the design of a medical device as well as its intended use. The actual classification of each device also depends on several factors, such as the duration of device in contact with the body, the degree of invasiveness, whether the device delivers medicines or energy to the patient, whether they are intended to have a biological effect on the patient and local versus systematic effects (e.g. conventional versus absorbable sutures). These factors may, alone or in combination, affect device classification. For details, please refer to rules of classification in the MDCO's guidance document called GN-01 (Overview of the Medical Device Administrative Control System).

Details are available at http://www.mdco.gov.hk/english/mdacs/mdacs_gn/files/gn_01.pdf.

(*Note*: The "Classification Rules for Medical Devices" given in Appendix 1 of this guidance document may be updated from time to time. You may wish to refer to the most updated version included in the Technical Reference [TR-003] Classification Rules for Medical Devices published by Department of Health.)

Table 26.1 Classification of medical devices according to the risk level associated with their intended use.

Classification	Risk level	Examples of medical devices
I	Low	Tongue depressor, bandage, dressing
II	Medium–low	Suction pump, gastroscope, transdermal stimulator
III	Medium–high	Lung ventilator, orthopaedic implant, X-ray machine, medical laser
IV	High	Prosthetic heart valve, implantable cardiac pacemaker, heparin-coated catheter

Note: 1. The classification is in accordance with the Principles of Medical Devices Classification proposed by the GHTF.

2. Class IV medical devices bear the highest risk, whereas Class I medical devices bear the lowest risk.

Similar to Europe, it is the manufacturer's responsibility to assign the classification of their medical devices.

26.4.3 Role of Distributors or Local Subsidiaries

The local responsible person (LRP) is the one who applies for the inclusion of a medical device into the List of Medical Devices under the MDACS. They have the following roles related to the device in the list:

(i) effective communication with the manufacturer, importers, users, the public and the Department of Health
(ii) keeping of distribution records
(iii) arrangement of maintenance and services
(iv) tracking of specific medical devices
(v) management of alerts and recalls

The reporting of adverse incidents follows MDCO guidance document [GN-03] *Guidance Notes for Adverse Incident Reporting by Local Responsible Persons.*

It is the manufacturer's responsibility to assign the classification of their medical device. The LRP should understand the classification rationale. More than one LRP for the same product is allowed in Hong Kong, but the manufacturer needs to have a proper recall system to identify which LRP should recall which batch of the same product. Details on the LRP's roles can be found in the MDCO's Code of Practice Document — [COP-01] Code of Practice for Local Responsible Persons.

26.4.4 Product Registration or Conformity Assessment Route and Time Required

The MDACS is basically divided into three parts: Pre-market Approval, Post-market Surveillance and Recognition of Conformity Assessment Bodies.

Pre-market Approval is in the form of voluntary listing of medical devices, importers and local manufacturers complying with specific requirements. They will be listed in one of the following lists:

- The List of Devices, including Class IV, Class III and Class II
- The List of Importers
- The List of Local Manufacturers

Post-market Surveillance is the review of the experience of using those devices that have been placed on the market. The surveillance system would monitor and co-ordinate the management of adverse incidents, safety alerts and recalls related to the use of medical devices.

Recognition of Conformity Assessment Bodies (CAB) is the acceptance of a list of agencies from which manufacturers could ask them to assess their medical devices for compliance with the requirements related to safety and performance. BSI Product Service is the first CAB approved in Hong Kong on 13 April 2007. TUV SUD and SGS were also approved as CAB afterwards.

Table 26.2 Summary of the requirement for product registration

	Class I	Class II	Class III	Class IV
Product registration	Not required	Required	Required	Required
Registration of local manufacturers	Required	Required	Required	Required
Registration of overseas manufacturer or its local representative	Not required	Required	Required	Required
Registration of importer	Required	Required	Required	Required
Registration of retailer	Not required	Not required	Not required	Not required

26.4.4.1 Suggested registration routes/steps

(i) The manufacturer understands the essential principles and gets quality system certification, e.g. ISO 13485.
(ii) The manufacturer appoints an LRP.
(iii) The LRP submits product registration to the MDCO or the CAB.
(iv) A review is conducted by the MDCO or the CAB.
(v) The documentation receives acknowledgement, and the application number is given two weeks after submission.
(vi) The MDCO takes about 12 weeks for review after getting all required documentation.

26.4.4.2 Technical material requirement

For Classes II to IV, please follow [GN-02] *Guidance Notes for Listing Class II, III and IV Medical Devices* (July 2011 Edition).

26.4.4.3 The labelling requirement of medical device

Please follow Technical Reference document on the MDCO website: [TR-005] *Additional Medical Device Labelling Requirements.*

26.4.4.4 Post-marketing surveillance requirement

Please follow the MDCO's guidance document [GN-03] *Guidance Notes for Adverse Incident Reporting by Local Responsible Persons.*

26.4.4.5 Manufacturing-related regulation: Do manufacturers need registration/authorization?

Voluntary listing is recommended. For details, please see [GN-08] *Guidance Notes for Listing of Local Manufacturers.*

26.4.4.6 Clinical trial-related regulation: Are medical device clinical trials regulated?

No, medical device clinical trials are not regulated at the moment, but a consultation document had been released in the past. The process is very similar to pharmaceuticals. Details are available at http://www.mdco.gov.hk/english/mdacs_gn/files/dgn_eng.pdf.

26.4.4.7 Is there a procedure for mutual recognition of foreign marketing approval or international standards?

Yes, Hong Kong recognizes ISO standards. Product registration approvals in GHTF countries will simplify the registration process.

26.5 Commercial Aspect

Currently, there is not any control over the price of a medical device.

Are parallel imports allowed?

As the MDACS is only a voluntary system, there is no regulatory requirement on parallel imports. However, only those products supplied through (or with consent of) the LRP can use the assigned listing number, as it is impractical, if not impossible, to verify whether a parallel-imported product is of the same quality and performance as those listed products supplied through the LRP. In this way, the LRP can effectively control and recall the product when required.

Is there any regulation regarding the advertisement of a medical device?

The Undesirable Medical Advertisements Ordinance (Cap.231) prohibits advertisements related to the curative or preventive effects of products on diseases listed in the Ordinance. Details are available at http://www.justice.gov.hk/home.htm.

26.6 Next Steps

The government launched the MDACS on 26 November 2004. The MDACS has been implemented in different phases as follows: The first phase started with the voluntary listing of Class IV (high risk) medical devices. The second phase, launched on 14 November 2005, continued with the voluntary listing of Class II and Class III (medium risk) medical devices. Phase III, which commenced on 13 October 2006, involved the recognition of designated Conformity Assessment Bodies (CAB), in which BSI was the first designated HK CAB. In phase IV, which began on 23 March 2007, local (Hong Kong) manufacturers were listed, and phase V, which began on 17 July 2007, listed importers of medical devices (except Class I devices). Since 2009, Class D *in vitro* diagnostic medical devices have been listed.

We expect the listing of medical device distributors and Class 1 medical device products in the future.

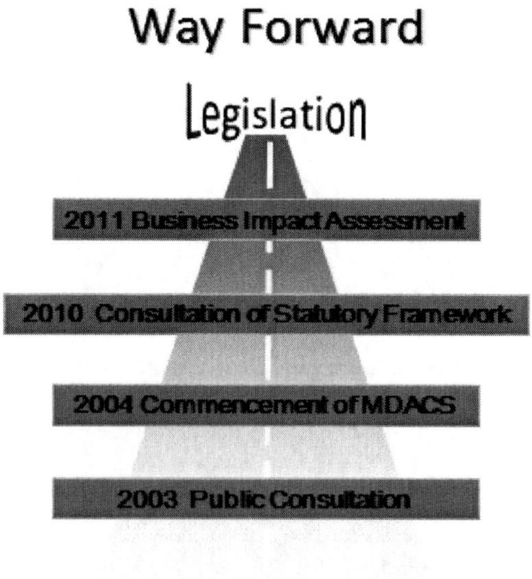
Way Forward
Legislation
2011 Business Impact Assessment
2010 Consultation of Statutory Framework
2004 Commencement of MDACS
2003 Public Consultation

Chapter 27

India: Medical Device Regulatory System

Kulwant S. Saini

Johnson & Johnson Medical, India,
A division of Johnson & Johnson Ltd,
9/43, Kirti Nagar, New Delhi 110015, India

ksaini@its.jnj.com, kulwantsaini@hotmail.com

Disclaimer

The regulatory information contained in this report is intended for market planning and is subject to change frequently. Translations of laws and regulations are unofficial.

27.1 Market Overview

27.1.1 Market Environment

- India, a parliamentary democracy and an emerging market in Asia Pacific, is the most populous (1.24 billion) democracy in the world.

Handbook of Medical Device Regulatory Affairs in Asia
Edited by Jack Wong and Raymond K. Y. Tong

ISBN 978-981-4411-21-9 (Hardcover), 978-981-4411-22-6 (eBook)
www.panstanford.com

- India's next five-year plan is poised to increase the healthcare expenditure to 3% of GDP and to 5% by 2020. Nearly 60 million middle-class households get added every 10 years, and this increased affordability and access would drive the 75% of the growth in healthcare. Healthcare remains in the top three categories in terms of consumption growth. India has the potential to show the fastest growth over the next 30–50 years and slated to be third largest economy by 2030.
- The total healthcare expenditure per capita has grown from US$ 28 in 2000 to US$ 43 in 2010 at a compound annual growth rate of 4.4% pa. The medical device industry is estimated to be approximately US$ 3.0 billion and the medical equipment industry is around half a billion. The medical device industry is growing at a rate of over 15%. India has been recognized for its quality pharmaceuticals and is largely self-sufficient, but for medical devices it is mostly dependent on imports (65–75%). There are a lot of local manufacturers that are also exporting their products worldwide, but barring a few simpler medical devices, most of the advanced medical devices and implants are being imported into India.
- Healthcare spending trends
  - Self-pay will continue to be major part of healthcare spend (currently at 58% going down to ~50% by 2017).
  - Increased penetration of insurance (no. of insured [private] to grow at 15% over the next seven years).

27.1.2 Overview of Regulatory Environment and What Laws/Regulations Govern Medical Devices

Currently, there are no separate medical device (MD) regulations in India, and there is a serious mix up of drug and device regulations. The MD regulations are evolving and the direction is that the MD regulations would shape up in line with Global Harmonization Task Force (GHTF) guidelines.

The Drugs and Cosmetics Act 1940 (Act) and the Drugs and Cosmetics Rules 1945 are currently applicable to drugs as well as medical devices. In addition to the aforementioned act, following other acts and rules also are applicable to regulate the drugs.

- Pharmacy Act, 1948
- Drugs and Magic Remedies (Objectionable Advertisements) Act, 1954
- Narcotic Drugs and Psychotropic Substances Act 1985
- Medicinal and Toilet Preparations (Excise Duties Act, 1955
- Drugs (Price Control) Order, 1995 (under the Essential Commodities Act)

Following are the other laws that have a bearing on the manufacture, distribution and sale of drugs and cosmetics:

- Industries (Development and Regulation) Act, 1951
- Trade and Merchandise Marks Act, 1958
- Indian Patents and Design Act, 1970
- Factories Act, 1948.
- Legal Metrology Act 2009 (in force from 1.4.2011),
- Draft Legal Metrology Packaged Commodities Rules 2011

The **Drugs and Cosmetics Act 1940** regulates the import, manufacture, distribution and sale of drugs and cosmetics (and medical devices). It is a comprehensive act for the requirements applicable for the drugs and cosmetics but not yet for the medical devices (except for Schedule M III, provisions applicable to hypodermic needles and syringes) which have been mentioned in some sections (drug definition, labelling, standards for MDs) under drugs.

When we talk of MD regulations in India, we talk of two different periods, one before October 2005 and the other after October 2005, when 10 categories of medical devices were notified by the Government of India (MOH) through Gazette notification SO No. 1468(E) and GSR 627(E).

Before 2005, the following medical devices were regulated as drugs as these fall under either the definition of the drug or were part of the monograph of a Pharmacopoeia or were of a biological origin (Schedules C and C1):

- Blood grouping sera
- Ligature, surgical sutures (and staplers)
- Intra uterine devices
- Condoms
- Tubal rings

- Surgical dressings
- Umbilical tapes
- Blood/blood component bags
- Disposable hypodermic syringes and needles, disposable perfusion sets (GSR 365(E), dated March 17, 1989)
- *In vitro* diagnostic devices for HIV, HBsAg and HCV

The first major notification on medical devices was released in October 2005 post court intervention in one of the case (filed by the Maharashtra FDA), involving a Mumbai hospital using unapproved drug-eluting stents (classification issue, drug or device) which were not approved in country of the origin. The court directed the Drugs Controller General of India (DCGI) to regulate these critical medical devices. The following list of categories of sterile products, intended for internal or external purpose, was notified:

- Cardiac stents
- Drug-eluting stents
- Catheters
- Intra ocular lenses
- IV cannulae
- Bone cements
- Heart valves
- Scalp vein sets
- Orthopaedic implants
- Internal prosthetic replacements

Later, in August 2006, a clarification was issued that the devices which are imported non-sterile and sterilized by the hospitals before use would also fall under the ambit of the October 2005 notification (SO No 1468(E)).

Each brand under the aforementioned categories of notified medical device needs to be registered with the regulators before these can be imported into India.

Post October 2005 notification, other lists of products and accessories were put on the Central Drugs Standard Control Organization (CDSCO) website (September 2007) but were never implemented or notified through a gazette notification, as the act states under the definition of drug. Hence, those were still being freely imported. On 5 March 2012, the DCGI sent a circular to State Drug Controllers and CDSCO branch offices categorizing

11 products from the aforementioned list into various notified categories of the main gazette notification of products notified in October 2005. This correlation of additional products to notified categories eliminates the need for a tedious gazette notification process. Table 27.1 shows a list of these products:

Table 27.1 Additional medical devices classified under categories notified in October 2005

Name of devices	Class of notified devices
Spinal needle	Disposable hypodermic needle
Insulin syringes	Disposable hypodermic syringes
Three-way stop cock as an accessory of IV cannula/catheter/perfusion set	Disposable perfusion set
Introducer sheath	IV cannula
Cochlear implant	Internal prosthetic replacement
Close wound drainage set	Catheter
AV fistula needle	Disposable hypodermic needle
Extension line as an accessory of infusion set	Disposable perfusion set
ANGO kit/PTCA/cath lab kit	IV cannula/disposable perfusion set
Measure volume set	Disposable perfusion set
Flow regulator as an accessory of infusion set	Disposable perfusion set

Another requirement for drug-eluting stents was put in September 2007, which stated that before approval/registration, a manufacturer needed to perform a clinical trial in India on 100 patients for six months (products already in use and approved by USFDA or CE marked) or 12 months (new products and not yet approved elsewhere). Through this clarification, peripheral stents were also brought under the list of regulated products.

Radiation-emitting devices need to be approved by the Bhabha Atomic Research Centre for the radiation safety.

Operationally, the regulatory mechanism in India consists of a two-tier system, one in the centre, the DCGI, and one each in the states (total 28) and in the union territories (total 7). These two regulators operate independently, and the DCGI reports to the central government and the state regulators (the Food and Drug

Administration or the Drugs Control Department) report to their ministry of health. Both the central regulator and the state regulator are responsible for the implementation of the Drugs and Cosmetics Act provisions. Their major responsibilities are listed in the following subsections.

Under the Drug and Cosmetics Act, the regulation of the manufacture, sale and distribution of drugs is primarily the concern of the state authorities, while the central authorities are responsible for approval of new drugs, clinical trials in the country, laying down the standards for drugs, control over the quality of imported drugs, coordination of the activities of state drug control organizations and providing expert advice with a view to bringing about uniformity in the enforcement of the Drugs and Cosmetics Act.

27.1.3 Functions Undertaken by DCGI and Central Government

27.1.3.1 Statutory functions

- laying down standards of drugs, cosmetics, diagnosis and devices
- laying down regulatory measures, amendments to acts and rules
- regulating market authorization of new drugs
- regulating clinical research in India
- approving licenses to manufacture certain categories of drugs as the Central License Approving Authority, i.e. for blood banks, large-volume parenterals and vaccines and sera.
- regulating the standards of imported drugs
- carrying out tasks relating to the Drugs Technical Advisory Board (DTAB) and Drugs Consultative Committee (DCC)
- overseeing testing of drugs by central drugs laboratories
- overseeing publication of Indian Pharmacopoeia

27.1.3.2 Other functions

- coordinating the activities of the State Drugs Control Organization to achieve uniform administration of the act; policy guidance
- providing guidance on technical matters
- participating in the WHO GMP certification scheme
- monitoring adverse drug reaction (ADR)

- conducting training programs for regulatory officials and Government Analysts
- looking after the distribution of quotas of narcotic drugs for use in medicinal formulations
- screening drug formulations available in the Indian market
- evaluating/screening applications for granting no-objection certificates for the export of unapproved/banned drugs

27.1.4 Functions Undertaken by the FDA and State Governments

27.1.4.1 Statutory functions

- licensing of drug manufacturing and sales establishments
- licensing of drug testing laboratories
- approval of drug formulations for manufacture
- monitoring of quality of Drugs and Cosmetics, manufactured by respective State units and those marketed in the State
- investigation and prosecution in respect of contravention of legal provisions
- administrative actions
- pre- and post-licensing inspection

Importers and manufacturers face difficulties in compliance and registration of their products as there had been no separate regulations written and implemented for MDs. For the registration of MDs, the drug registration/approval process has been followed since 2006 although a brief list of contents of the technical dossier was published in 2006, which was modified later and published (last quarter of 2010) on the website (http://cdsco.nic.in/).

To streamline the work for designing proper MD regulations, a core group of industry members and regulators was constituted. Various industry agencies (Federation of Indian Chambers of Commerce and Industry [FICCI], Confederation of Indian Industry [CII], American Chamber of Commerce in India [AMCHAM], Advanced Medical Technology Association [ADVAMED]) were also involved into the process through their MD regulatory subgroups. The efforts of this core group during 2009 and 2010 culminated into the compilation of a base document (Schedule M III) which was based on the European Medical Device Directive and the GHTF guidelines. This comprehensive document was submitted to the

DCGI office at the end of 2010 and the highlights of this document are as follows:

1. includes the GHTF definition of a medical device
2. based on the risk-based (GHTF) classification of medical devices
3. includes the QMS certification (ISO 13485) and Conformity Assessment Procedures (MDD and GHTF) involving notified bodies and the regulators (for Class C and D products)
4. post marketing surveillance (PMS)

Schedule M III document need to be wetted by the legal ministry and has to be linked with various sections of Drugs and Cosmetics Act in such a way that it becomes a standalone guideline for MDs within the act. Currently there is no proper definition of the MD in the Drugs and Cosmetics Act, which is the main hindrance in the inclusion of the MD guidelines/regulations in the act. A Drugs and Cosmetics (Amendment) Bill was introduced in the Parliament in 2007. This bill has been modified in the last four years to amend the act with respect to the provisions for the drugs as well medical devices. It includes a proper definition for the MD and separate provisions for MDs in the act. It even recommends the change of the name of the Act to "Drugs, Cosmetics and Medical Devices Act" so as to provide proper recognition to MDs. This bill, which is now pending approval by the Parliament, would enable the government to make rules for MDs and inclusion of the Schedule M III into the act.

As the passing of the aforementioned bill by the Parliament is a time-consuming exercise, as it is busy with other priorities, in the meantime the DCGI office has come out with guidelines to streamline the process of registration, manufacture, PMS and clinical trials. These guidelines have been published on the CDSCO website. A dialogue is going on between the DCGI and industry members to further refine these interim guidelines.

27.1.5 Guidance Documents

- Guidance Document on Common Submission Format for **Registration of Medical Devices** in India (4 August 2010)
- Guidance Document on Common Submission Format for **Import License in Form 10** of Medical Devices in India (25 August 2010)
- Requirements for **Conducting Clinical Trial(s)** of Medical Devices in India (4 August 2010)

- Guidance document on application for grant of **License in Form-28** for manufacture of Medical Devices in India under Central Licensing Authority Scheme (12 August 2010)
- Guidance on clinical trial inspection (1 November 2010)
- Guidance Document on Common Submission Format for Registration of Notified Diagnostics Kits in India (5 January 2011)
- Guidance Document on Common Submission Format for Import License of Notified diagnostics kits in India (5 January 2011)
- Guidance Document on Common Submission Format for Import License of Non-Notified diagnostic kits in India (5 January 2011)

27.1.6 Indian Pharmacopoeial Commission

The Indian Pharmacopoeial Commission (IPC) is an autonomous institution under the Ministry of Health and Family Welfare, Government of India, dedicated to laying down standards for drugs, pharmaceuticals and healthcare devices/technologies besides providing reference substances and training.

27.1.7 Detail of Key Regulator(s)

The CDSCO headquarters are located in New Delhi, and it functions under the Directorate General of Health Services (see Figs. 27.1–27.3 for details).

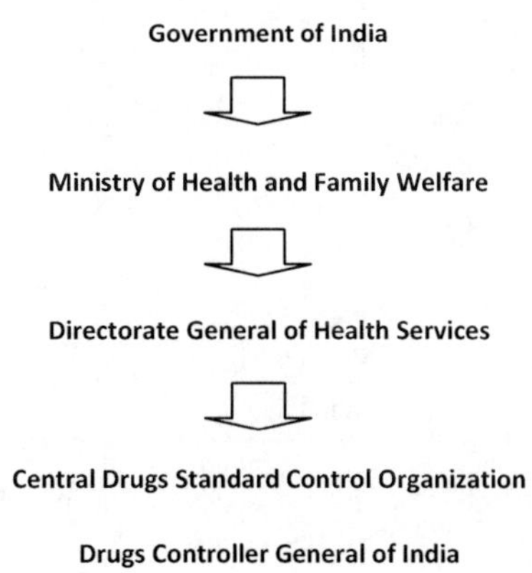

Figure 27.1 The Central Drugs Standard Control Organization: The central agency.

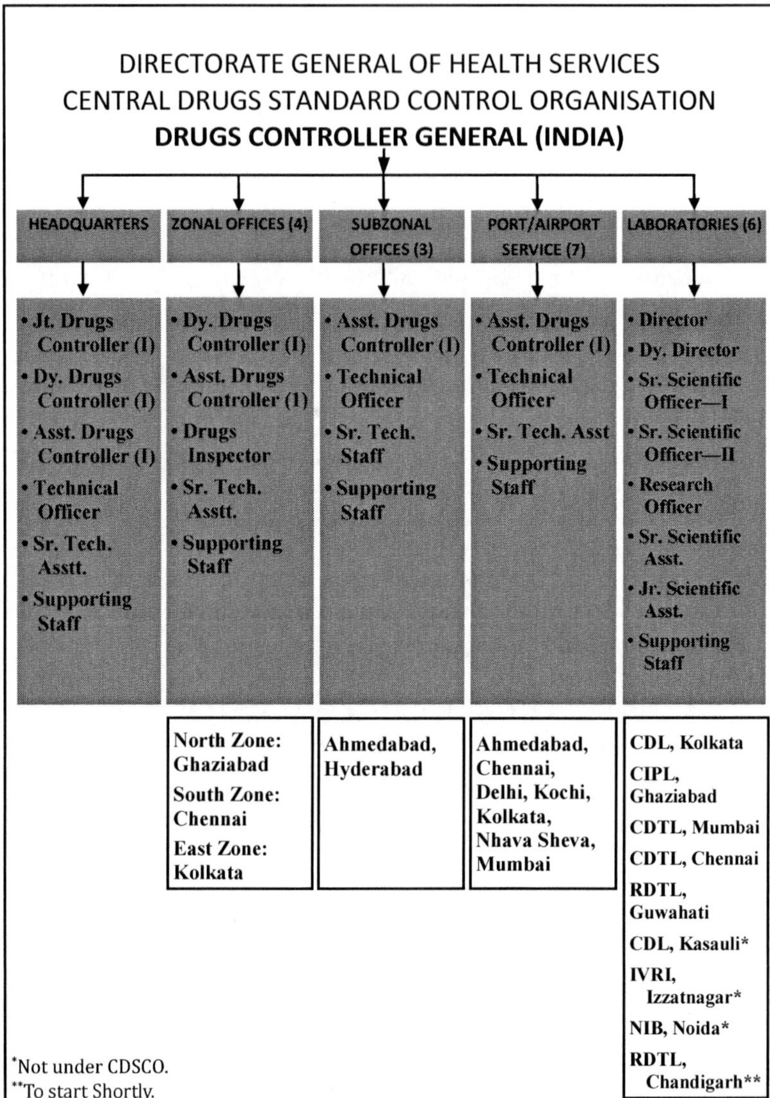

Figure 27.2 Organization Chart — CDSCO.

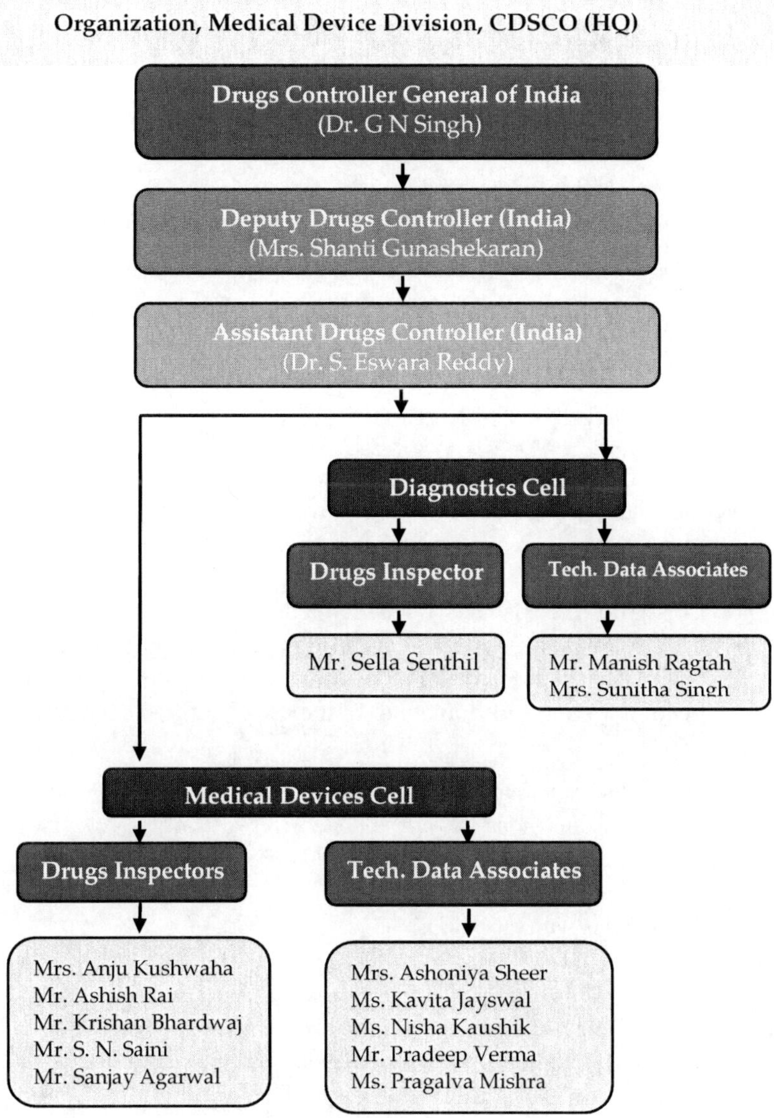

Figure 27.3 Organization chart: CDSCO — Medical Devices Division.

Contact Information

Drugs Controller General of India
Dr. G. N. SINGH
FDA Bhawan, Kotla Road, New Delhi 110002
Phones: +91 11 23236965 (D)
Fax: +91 11 23236973.
Email: dci@nb.nic.in
CDSCO website: http://cdsco.nic.in/
Medical Device Division website: http://cdsco.nic.in/Medical_div/medical_device_division.htm

27.2 Regulatory Overview

27.2.1 Definition of Medical Device

Medical devices are partially regulated in India and some (as listed Section 27.1.2) of the critical devices have been notified as drugs and regulated as drugs. Rest of the devices are still being freely imported into India.

Currently, the MD has been defined under the definition of the drug in Section 3(b)(iv) of the Drugs and Cosmetics Act. This definition is not close to GHTF definition and requires a gazette notification for any addition of MD to the list of notified devices:

> 3 (b) (iv)
>
> ... such devices intended for internal or external use in the diagnosis, treatment, mitigation or prevention of disease or disorder in human beings or animals, as may be specified from time to time by the Central Government by notification in the Official Gazette, after consultation with the board.

In view of the partial and incomplete MD regulations, currently, there is no definition of the accessory in the Drugs and Cosmetics act.

The proposed definition of the MD in the Drugs and Cosmetics Amendment bill is based on the GHTF definition of the MD. This bill still awaits the approval by the Parliament before these new provisions can be made part of the Act. Similarly, the Schedule M III (document compiled for base regulations for MDs) now available with the regulator also has a GHTF definition of MD. The contents of the bill and the base regulations would become part of the act in due course after review and approval by the Parliament and other ministries involved in the process. This complete definition would eliminate the need for the involvement and review by the advisory board in future.

27.2.2 Classification of Medical Device

In absence of the base medical device regulations, currently, there is no system for the risk-based classification of MDs. Medical devices have been notified from time to time as per the recommendation of the Advisory Board although the last notification contained mostly the critical and implantable MDs.

The proposed base MD regulations in the comprehensive Schedule M III document are in line with the GHTF and the European MD Directives. A comprehensive risk-based classification on the lines of GHTF (Class A, B, C, D) requirements has been included in this document. This considers various factors such as the duration of contact, degree of invasiveness, biological origin and combination with drugs. Once implemented, this document also proposes a phased implementation of regulations starting with Class D devices.

27.2.3 Role of Distributors or Local Subsidiaries (LRP)

A notified MD can be sold in India by a local manufacturer (having a manufacturing license) or the foreign manufacturer or importer (licensee), after registration of the manufacturing site and obtaining an import license for the products manufactured at that particular site, either by the manufacturer himself or by an affiliate of the manufacturer having an office in India or by an agent/importer/distributor. This person is responsible for the compliance to the provisions (also the GMPs) of the Drugs and Cosmetics Act in India on behalf of the manufacturer (if situated outside India):

- An authorization from the manufacturer to be its agent in India in the form of a Power of Attorney.
- Need to have a valid wholesale license for sale and distribution of products in any state of India, issued by the state's FDA/DCA.
- Make sure the premises where the imported products are to be stocked are equipped with proper storage accommodation and equipment (temperature/humidity).

- The importer is a link between the regulators and the source company for compliance:
  - Customer complaints management in coordination with manufacturer and adverse incident reporting; also responsible for the reporting of the MDR to the regulator in India
  - Management of the field actions as communicated by the manufacturer
- The manufacturer shall at all times observe the undertaking given by them or on their behalf in Form 9.
- The licensee shall allow any inspector authorized by the licensing authority to enter with or without notice any premises where the imported products are stocked, to inspect and to take samples, if required, for testing.
- If the licensing authority directs, the licensee shall not sell or offer for sale any batch of the products.
- For traceability, the licensee shall maintain a record of all sales showing particulars of the products and of the person to whom products have been sold.

27.2.4 Product Registration or Conformity Assessment Route and Time Required

The pre-market product and site registration process currently followed in India is based on the drug regulations. Figure 27.4 illustrates the process of the registration of the site and product (mandatory for Notified MDs). The evaluation process as defined for MDs in 2006 for expedited review is based on the prior approval (USFDA, CE Mark or Conformity Assessment Procedure, approval in any of the GHTF countries) of the products. A new product not approved previously in any of the countries may be asked to go for the clinical trials for the generation of evidence for any of the new indication and then would go for an additional complete evaluation (for Form 45 new product approval). Almost all of the MDs approved by DCGI office since year 2006 have gone through the "Me Too" route, which involves two steps:

- Application in Form 40 and DCGI approval in Form 41 (Registration Certificate)
- Application in Form 8 and DCGI approval in Form 10 (Import License)

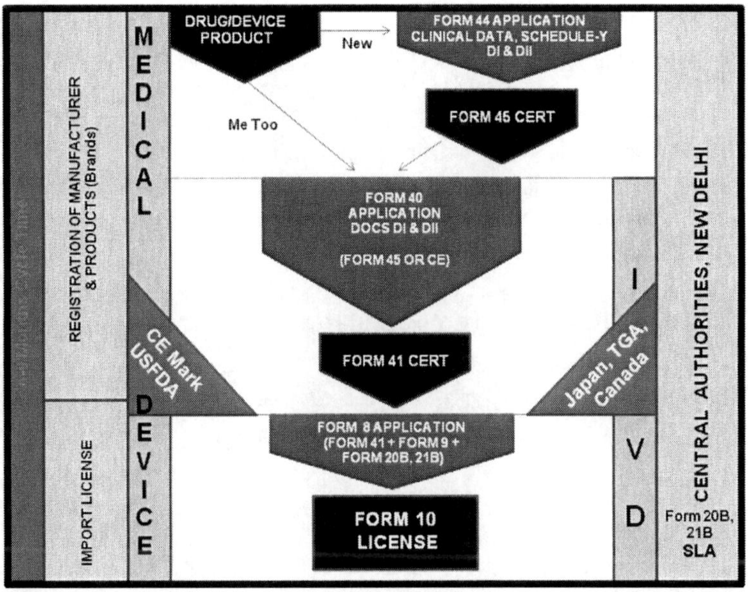

Figure 27.4 Manufacturing site and product registration: process flow chart.

This evaluation for the indigenous manufacturers involves DCGI as well as the state FDAs. For foreign manufacturers, it involves only the DCGI office. The process also involves a site inspection by the joint team of CDSCO and FDA for indigenous manufacturers. If required (as per conditions of the license), a site inspection may be performed for a foreign manufacturer, although such inspection has not been performed since 2006. Generally, the Conformity Assessments Procedures performed by the NBs are acceptable for this purpose.

For *in vitro* diagnostics (IVDs) (non-critical), only the second step is required and no site registration is needed. A registration certificate (RC) for a particular site is generally valid for three years and then re-registration is required. The import license is valid till the registration certificate is valid. During the currency of the Registration Certificate, additional products from the same site can be endorsed on the RC. The import license in this case would be valid for the remaining period of the RC. The manufacturing license issued to an Indian manufacturer is valid for five years.

The dossier format (various forms), contents and submission process is defined in the guidance documents listed in

Section 27.2.8 and also available on the CDSCO site and the Drugs and Cosmetics Act. In case of "Me Too" products, the DCGI office evaluation process/documentation review takes about 6–9 months to issue the RC and the import license. In case of a new product/new indication, performing a clinical trial and the issue of Form 45 may need additional cycle time. In such cases, the technical dossier may also be additionally referred to an expert committee for review/comments.

27.2.5 Quality System Regulation

Currently as MDs are notified as drugs, it is expected that the local manufacturer will comply with Schedule M GMPs (Drugs and Cosmetics Act). Source companies situated outside India, generally, comply with ISO 13485, or USFDA QSRs or the QMS requirements in the country of origin. These are also acceptable, currently, as part of the submission for the registration certificate to be issued by the Indian regulators. The Plant Master file required in India is generally replaced by the Quality Manual of the source company for the submission.

Future proposed regulations in the Schedule M III draft would be based on ISO 13485 requirements as per GHTF.

27.2.6 Product Registration and Quality System Regulation for Combined Device–Drug Product

As mentioned above, there are no base MD regulations yet in place in India. MDs are notified and regulated as drugs. Hence, there is no definition of combination product and no specific requirements laid down for the combination products.

Proposed Schedule M III has provisions similar to GHTF and would require such combination products to be evaluated by drug as well as device section of the CDSCO depending on the status of approval of drug in India. Combination product definition is proposed to be similar to GHTF and the product as such would be treated as MD.

27.2.7 Registration Fee

Table 27.2 shows the fees that are applicable for the various activities/submissions/functions carried out by the CDSCO, state FDA and test laboratories.

Table 27.2 Fees applicable for various activities/submissions/functions carried out by CDSCO, state FDA and test laboratories

Type of license	Form name as per D&C Act	Type of registration/ activity	Fee
Registration and re-registration	Form 40	Mfg. site registration	US$ 1,500
		Product registration (per product)	US$ 1,000
Import license	Forms 8 and 9	With one product	INR 1,000
		Subsequent additional Product	INR 100
Foreign manufacturer site inspection with respect to site registration	As per conditions of license	GMP inspection (if required)	US$ 5,000
Clinical trials	Form 122A		INR 50,000
Manufacturing licenses	Form 27 (Sterile)	Site fees	INR 6,000
		Product fees (per product)	INR 1,250
	Form 24 (non-sterile)	Site fees	INR 3,750
		Product fees (per product)	INR 750
Renewal of plant layout			INR 5,000
Test license	Form 12	1st product	INR 100
		Subsequent product	INR 50
Government lab testing fees	Rule 7, 48 and 168-F	Product testing	Refer to Schedule B, B-1 of Act

Abbreviation: INR, Indian rupee.

27.2.8 Technical Material Requirement

The dossier submissions for the site and medical device product registration follow the guidance document available on the CDSCO website under the MD section (Guidance Document on Common Submission Format for Registration of Medical Devices in India (4 August 2010), Guidance Document on Common Submission Format for Import License in Form 10 of Medical Devices in India (25 August 2010)). These are also listed in section 27.1.5 for MDs and IVDs.

27.2.9 The Labelling Requirement of Medical Device

The labelling requirements for drugs (and MDs) are defined under Rule 96 (Manner of Labelling) of the Act. Additional labelling requirements for the Non-Sterile Surgical Ligatures and Sutures are provided under Rule 102. For special products, the labelling requirements are provided under Rule 109-A, wherein it is stated that the labelling of MDs shall conform to "Indian Standard Specifications" laid down from time to time by the "Bureau of Indian Standards" in addition to other requirements.

Generally, for imported medical devices, ISO or GHTF guidelines are considered sufficient, but they are occasionally superseded by Indian regulations.

According to the Drugs and Cosmetics Act, it is a mandatory requirement that the product should have 60% residual shelf-life period as on the date of import.

Additionally, as per "Legal Metrology Act, 2009" (Declaration on Pre-packaged Commodities), all products sold in retail must carry the following information prior to commercial access:

(a) name and address of the importer
(b) generic or common name of the product
(c) net quantity in terms of standard units of weights and measures
(d) month and year of packing in which the product is manufactured or packed or imported
(e) maximum retail sale price (inclusive of all taxes) at which the product in packaged form may be sold to the ultimate consumer
(f) the approval number (import license number) for the notified devices category
(g) customer contact number

This labelling is generally done (if not labelled by the manufacturer) in warehouses in India by the importers before the product can be sold in the market.

Recent requirements by the Ministry of Health specify the inclusion of the GS1 bar code and serialization on products supplied to the MOH. The Director General of Health Services also specified the products to be exported from India for the purpose of tracking products and to identify counterfeits.

27.2.10 Post-Marketing Surveillance Requirement

The Drugs and Cosmetics Act specifies the reporting requirements for the Complaints and Adverse Reactions for drugs under Schedule M (GMPs) and additionally, under the Schedule Y for the new drug clinical trials. There are currently no specific requirements for MDs.

The proposed Schedule M III has a separate section on PMS and is based on the GHTF guidelines.

27.2.11 Manufacturing-Related Regulation

The manufacturing site and the product (if notified) need to be registered in India with the regulators. Licenses to manufacture medical devices in India can usually be obtained from the state FDA/DCA, after joint inspection from State FDA and CDSCO. However, for recently notified devices (see the list of 10 categories of MDs, Section 27.1.2), DCGI approval is needed. The required information for a device manufacturing license includes the implementation of Good Manufacturing Practices (GMP), as well as some other requirements. Licensing usually involves an inspection by the CDSCO and the state FDA. The license is valid for five years and is renewable.

GMPs are provided under Schedule M of the act. As with the product registration process, much of its requirements were prepared with drugs in mind. Its provisions include the adequacy of the manufacturing site, production area, quality control process, record keeping, testing and adverse event and recall handling system. Schedule M also calls for the maintenance of a Site Master File, as well as a self-inspection to be conducted before the official inspection. For the companies having CE-marked products, the QMS as per ISO 13485 is considered. Schedule L-1 lays down the "Good Laboratory Practices and Requirements of Premises and Equipment".

Future proposed regulations (Schedule M III) are based on the Conformity Assessment Procedures (GHTF) involving notified bodies and the CDSCO (Class C and D MDs).

Finally, if a product such as a drug-eluting stent contains a patented or proprietary drug, a good deal of information on the drug being manufactured must be submitted with a manufacturing license application.

After the DCGI office formulated guidelines for the import and manufacture of medical devices in the country, it also specified that all importers, stockists and retailers of medical devices will have to obtain sales licenses from the state FDAs within three months.

27.2.12 Clinical Trial-Related Regulation

The requirements for the new drugs and clinical Trials are provided under Part X-A of the act (Import or Manufacture of New Drug for Clinical Trials or Marketing). Rule 122 and its various subparts specify the process of Application for Permission to Import New Drug (and device) and to obtain permission for conducting the clinical trials. The details of requirements for the clinical trials are provided in Schedule Y of the act. These requirements are written basically for drugs/pharmaceuticals.

Following are the clinical trial draft guidelines specific to MDs, available on the CDSCO website under MDs section:

Requirements for Conducting Clinical Trial(s) of Medical Devices in India (4 August 2010)
Guidance on clinical trial inspection (1 November 2010)

Following additional clarification was issued on 5 September 2007 pertaining to the clinical trial requirements for drug-eluting stents:

- In case of manufacturers whose stents are already in use abroad and they wish to introduce the same in India, a six-month clinical trial has to be carried out on 100 patients.
- In case of stents which are new in nature and have not been used anywhere, a 12-month clinical trial has to be carried out on 100 patients.
- Global clinical trials: Whenever a firm applies only for a global clinical trial to be carried out in the country, this can be permitted as per the present norms followed in case of drugs. However, if the same company wishes to also market the product in India, it has to comply with the aforementioned norms.

- It is clarified that "All Peripheral Stents" are covered under the provisions of the Drugs and Cosmetics Rules and, hence, need to be registered for import and licenses approved by Central License Approving Authority (CLAA) for indigenous manufacture.

27.2.13 Is There a Procedure for Mutual Recognition of Foreign Marketing Approval or International Standards?

There are no mutual recognitions currently in place with any countries, but India recognizes ISO standards. Product registration approvals by the USFDA or in GHTF countries and the CE mark are recognized, and these have formed the basis for the site and product registrations since 2006. The proposed Schedule M III regulations are based on the GHTF guidelines and European regulations.

27.3 Commercial Aspect

27.3.1 Any Price Control of Medical Device

MDs are notified and regulated as drugs in India. For drugs, there are price control requirements (Drugs (Prices Control) Order 1995) in India. The National Pharmaceutical Pricing Authority (Department of Pharmaceuticals, under the Ministry of Chemicals and Fertilizers) is an organization responsible for the price controls (to fix/revise) and availability of medicines in India. In the last three years, there have been some attempts by the authority to bring MDs under the price control, due to high visibility of the prices of stents and orthopaedic implants. There have been many interactions and representation on this subject from the industry to dissuade the agency from implementing the manufacturing cost-based price controls on MDs.

In the mean time, the Ministry of Health and Family Welfare has put certain ceiling limits for reimbursement of stents (drug-eluting stents, bare-metal stents and non-coronary stents) for its Central Government Health Scheme beneficiaries. These are based on the type of approval the product has in India (approved by DCGI) or in the country of origin (USFDA approved or CE marked). There has been strong representation from importers as well as local manufacturers on this *ad-hoc* approach to pricing.

27.3.2 Are Parallel Imports Allowed?

For importing the notified MDs, one needs to have an import license from the DCGI. This is issued on the basis of the Registration Certificate for a manufacturing site of a foreign company. These licenses can be used by the authorized agent to whom these have been issued. An importer may authorize another importer to use its Registration Certificate and allow the issue of another import license to the latter by the DCGI. Both of these need to maintain the distribution records as per the requirements of the act.

27.3.3 Any Advertisement Regulation of Medical Device?

MDs are regulated as drugs in India. Rule 106 A states,

> No drug (or MD) may purport or claim to prevent or cure or may convey to the intending user thereof any idea that it may prevent or cure, one or more of the diseases or ailments specified in Schedule J.

The Drugs and Magic Remedies (Objectionable Advertisement) Rules, 1955: This Act is meant to control the advertisements related to drugs (or MD).

27.4 Upcoming Regulation Changes

Since the notification (October 2005) of 10 categories of MDs, the registration and product approval process followed by the DCGI office has been the same as followed for drugs. This has led to a mix-up of the drug and device regulations. The industry and the regulators in India have realized this, and some attempts have been made by them collectively to resolve this in the near future. Some of the things are listed below:

- Currently there is no proper definition of a medical device in the act. A complete definition of the MD (in line with GHTF) has been proposed in the Drugs and Cosmetics amendment Bill.

This bill was reviewed by Parliament Standing Committee in 2009–2010, and the bill after modification was re-submitted to the Parliament again in October 2010. This bill is now pending the Parliament approval. The Parliament's approval of this bill will lead to the inclusion of the definition of a medical device and related regulations/guidelines in the Drugs and Cosmetics Act. Following are the features of the bill:

  - The bill proposes a proper definition of a medical device and a clinical trial and also proposes separate chapter II A in the Act for the provisions related to MDs.
  - The preamble changes in the act have been proposed, and the proposed name would be "Drugs, Cosmetics and Medical Devices Act".
  - The bill proposes the Powers of Central Government to make rules regarding classification, pre-market evaluation, standards, conformity assessment procedures, labelling and registration of MDs, etc.

- A core industry–regulator group has compiled (during 2008–2010) a comprehensive document Schedule M III containing MD regulations. These can form part of the Drugs and Cosmetics Act once the MD definition becomes part of the act through the passage of the aforementioned bill by Parliament. Schedule MII is based on the following:
  - the GHTF guidelines and the European Medical Device Directive
  - risk-based classification of MDs as per GHTF guidelines
  - the conformity assessment procedures involving the notified bodies
  - the adverse event reporting in line with GHTF guidelines
  - requirements for the clinical trials
- As the aforementioned bill approval by Parliament and finalization of the Schedule M III is a time-consuming process, the DCGI office has come out with MD-specific interim guidelines. These guidelines cover the registration of the site/product and import license submission requirements (common submission dossier) and approval process for MDs and *in vitro* devices, clinical trials, etc. These are available on the CDSCO website under the MDs section.

27.5 Related Agencies/Departments and Ministries

- Ministry of Health (MoH)
  - Directorate General of Health Services (DGHS)
  - Central Drugs Standards Control Organization (CDSCO)
- Ministry of Chemicals and Fertilizers
  - Department of Pharmaceuticals (DoP)
  - National Pharmaceutical Pricing Authority (NPPA)
- Department of Science and Technology (DST)
- Federation of Indian Chambers of Commerce and industry (FICCI)
- Confederation of Indian Industries (CII)

Chapter 28

Indonesia: Medical Device Regulatory System

Mita Rosalina

PT. Johnson & Johnson Indonesia

mrosalin@its.jnj.com

Disclaimer

The regulatory information contained in this chapter is intended for market planning and is subject to change frequently. Translations of laws and regulations are unofficial.

28.1 Introduction

Indonesia, with a population of more than 220 million, is a medical device market that has a large potential. However, foreign manufacturers of medical devices have always been faced with numerous obstacles and challenges in entering this market. This is despite the fact that Indonesia relies mainly on imported medical devices due to the lack of any established local manufacturer.[4]

Handbook of Medical Device Regulatory Affairs in Asia
Edited by Jack Wong and Raymond K. Y. Tong

ISBN 978-981-4411-21-9 (Hardcover), 978-981-4411-22-6 (eBook)
www.panstanford.com

Penetrating this huge market of medical devices is difficult due to the wide and extensive geographical boundaries in the country. Also, highly bureaucratic medical device import and trading regulations have made it more difficult for foreign manufacturers to enter the market. Indonesia also imposes tariffs of up to 30% on imported medical devices depending on the type, use, and value of these devices.[4]

Indonesia has a centralized healthcare system, headed by the Ministry of Health (Kementerian Kesehatan R.I.). The Ministry of Health purchases most of the medical disposables and hospital equipment for the 900 public hospitals around the country. Due to the highly rigid nature, there is limited budget for most of the hospitals in the country. Recent changes, however, have been encouraging in de-centralizing healthcare services in the country. This will spur the growth of the medical devices market in the country as individual regions collect and plan the healthcare budget individually themselves.[4]

There is a market disparity in the standard of healthcare between rural and urban areas. The capital city, Jakarta, enjoys relatively good levels of primary care as well as a range of modern private specialist facilities, while healthcare coverage in remote regions tends to be insufficient.

The majority of the Indonesian medical device market is supplied by imports, which dipped by 1.5% over the previous year to US$ 348.4 million in 2009. Imports have grown at a CAGR of 35.2% in 2005–2009.[5] During the 24th ASEAN Consultative Committee on Standards and Quality Meeting on August 3–4, 2004, the formation of a Product Working Group on Medical Device (ACCSQ-MDPWG) was proposed to implement specific measures on medical device under the road map for healthcare integration. This is to be in line with the ASEAN leaders' decision on the establishment of the ASEAN Economic Community (AEC) by 2020 and fast-track integration of the 11 priority sectors, including the healthcare sector. Therefore, as one of ASEAN member country, Indonesia is committed to the implementation of ASEAN Harmonization in 2014.

To welcome it, at this time, Indonesia has some regulations relating to medical devices:

- Ministerial Regulation of Health Republic Indonesia No. 1189/ MENKES/Per/VIII/2010. *Production of Medical Devices and Household Device.* Issued on August 23rd, 2010.
- Ministerial Regulation of Health Republic Indonesia No. 1190/ MENKES/Per/VIII/2010. *Marketing Authorization Medical Devices and Household Device.* Issued on August 23rd, 2010.
- Ministerial Regulation of Health Republic Indonesia No. 1191/MENKES/Per/VIII/2010. *Distribution Medical Devices and Household Device.* Issued on August 23rd, 2010.

28.2 Regulating Authority

Medical devices in Indonesia are regulated by the Ministry of Health of the Republic Indonesia; Directorate of General Pharmaceutical Service and Medical Device; and Directorate of Medical Device Production and Distribution Development with the following address of office:

Kementrian Kesehatan RI
Jl. H.R. Rasuna Said Blok X-5
Kav No. 4–9; Jakarta 12950
Indonesia
Web site: www.binfar.depkes.go.id

28.3 Definition of Medical Device

A medical device means any instrument, apparatus, implement, machine, appliance, implant, *in vitro* reagent, software, material, or other similar or related article

(a) intended by the manufacturer to be used, alone or in combination, for human beings for one or more of the specific purpose of
- diagnosis, prevention, monitoring, treatment, or alleviation of disease
- diagnosis, monitoring, treatment, or alleviation of or compensation for an injury
- investigation, replacement, modification, or support of the anatomy or of a physiological process

- supporting or sustaining life
- control of conception
- disinfection of medical device
- providing information for medical or diagnostic purposes by means of *in vitro* examination of specimens derived from the human body

(b) that does not achieve its primary intended action in or on the human body by pharmacological, immunological or metabolic means, but may be assisted in its intended function by such means.

28.4 Classification of Medical Devices

Medical devices are classified into three classes based on risk[2]:

- **Class I**: In case of malfunction or misuse, these low-risk devices would not cause serious harm. The evaluation of these health instruments shall focus on the quality and the product.
- **Class IIa**: In case of failure or misuse, these medical devices can result in a significant impact on the health of patients, but not a serious accident. Before distribution, such health instruments will have to comply with a sufficient requirement for evaluation, but they do not require a clinical test.
- **Class IIb**: In case of failure or misuse, these medical devices can have significant effect on the health of patients, but not a serious accident. Before distribution, these health instruments shall have to comply with a complete requirement for evaluation, including a risk analysis and security facts for the evaluation, but they do not require a clinical test.
- **Class III**: The failure or misuse of these medical devices can result in serious implications for patients or nurses/operators. Before distribution, these health instruments shall have to comply with a complete requirement for evaluation, including a risk analysis and security facts for the evaluation, and they also require a clinical test.

Currently Indonesia does not have any guidelines on combination products. Therefore, it is strongly recommended that prior to the registration process, the product specification, intended use, and product claims be discussed with the Ministry of Health staff to ensure the classification of the product. Attached classification of product from legal manufacturer on application is recommended as reference.

28.5 Registration of Medical Devices

All medical devices (for all classes) with each code should be registered with the Ministry of Health before they can be freely imported, distributed, and sold in the market. Unit package that needs to be registered depends on unit sales.

Safety, quality, and efficacy of the product will be considered during evaluation to grant marketing authorization.

Abridged evaluation is not recognized by Indonesia authority. A full assessment is required for all classes of product. Approval status from others countries serves only as reference for the Ministry of Health staff in the reviewing process.

28.5.1 Process

The application must have distribution license "IPAK" from the Ministry of Health and the company that as applicant officially appointed by the source company or the legal manufacturer as the sole agent. This letter of appointment from source/legal manufacturer explains that the representative company in Indonesia has authorization to register, import, and distribute the product in Indonesia. The minimum appointment granted by the source company is two years, and this document needs to be legalized by the Indonesian embassy. It should be noted that the company that has the right to import the product is the same company that is the license holder for the products.

Currently, application is done by submitting the hard copy of registration documents and follow-ups directly to the Ministry of Health. English and Indonesian are the acceptable languages for the documents.

All classes of medical devices follow the registration process as shown in Fig. 28.1.

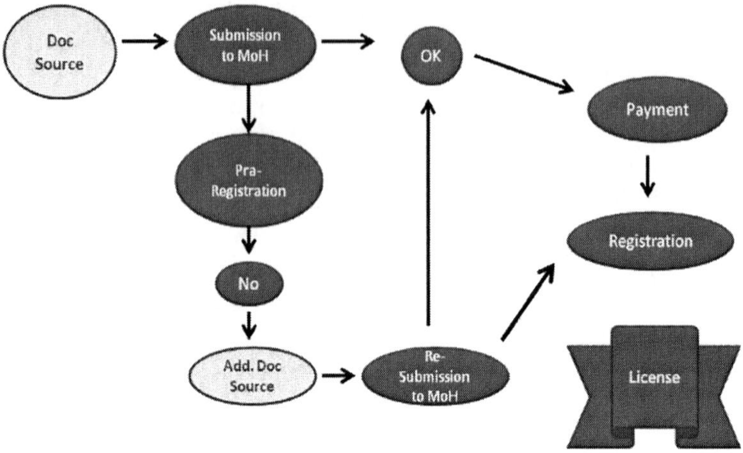

Figure 28.1 Medical device registration process followed by the Ministry of Health.

28.5.2 Documents Required

Please refer to Appendix 1.

28.5.3 Official Registration Fee

Type of medical device	New registration (mio rp)	Re-registration/variation/ renewal (mio rp)
Class III	5	1
Class II	3	1
Class I	1.5	0.5
	Explanation letter: 0.5 Mio Rp	

28.5.4 Time Line

The time frame needed to get approval is as follows:

- Class I: 30 working days after pre-registration
- Class II : 60 working days after pre-registration
- Class III: 90 working days after pre-registration

In general, it takes around six to nine months from the date of submission to get approval. This applies for new registration, re-registration, variation, and renewal.

28.5.5 Validity of Product License

The product license issued by the Ministry of Health will be effective for five years or in accordance with the term of validity of the letter of appointment. The certificate of license needs to be renewed three months before the expiry date.

28.5.6 Indonesian Labeling Requirement

Refer to Ministerial Regulation of Health Republic Indonesia No. 1190/MENKES/Per/VIII/2010: Marketing Authorization Medical Devices and Household Device; article 26.

Following is the minimum information that needs to be stated on the labeling:

- trade name/brand name/product name
- name and address of legal and physical manufacturer
- name and address of importer
- product component, formula (household device)
- active ingredient with percentage (household device)
- intended use and direction for use (must be in Indonesian)
- warning, precaution, and adverse effect (must be in Indonesian)
- expiry date
- batch number/production code/serial number, registration number, and net quantity of the product

28.5.7 Regulatory Action for Changes and Device Modifications

This is not specified in the regulations. Changes can be registered via a data amendment process, variation, or re-registration, and the requirements are judged on a case-by-case basis.

Any changes that have an impact on the following should be considered:

(1) size
(2) packaging specification
(3) LABELING
(4) tax payer number (NPWP)

28.6 Post Market Surveillance System

There can be severe consequences of faulty or substandard medical devices for public health and safety. Regulatory bodies all over the world are thus striving to achieve an optimal system of medical device controls that accommodates a device in all its permutations and combinations, balancing quality and safety with faster access to the market.

Regulatory systems need to be in place to manage the potential residual risks posed to the intended user. Because of this, the Indonesia authority is developing a post market surveillance process for medical devices. Post market surveillance mechanisms are required to monitor the medical devices already in the market. This is essential for such devices. In the event of any complications, the authorities are able to direct swift corrective actions.

In Indonesia, post market surveillance is still voluntary. However, it has been recommended by the authority for cases that have adverse health consequences for the patient or cause death. In such cases, it is mandatory for the company to report to the authority in 24 hours with details of the corrective action.

References

1. Ministerial Regulation of Health Republic Indonesia No. 1189/ MENKES/Per/VIII/2010. *Production of Medical Devices and Household Device.* Jakarta, August 23, 2010.
2. Ministerial Regulation of Health Republic Indonesia No. 1190/ MENKES/Per/VIII/2010. *Marketing Authorization Medical Devices and Household Device.* Jakarta, August 23, 2010.
3. Ministerial Regulation of Health Republic Indonesia No. 1191/ MENKES/Per/VIII/2010. *Distribution Medical Devices and Household Device.* Jakarta, August 23, 2010.
4. Wee, A. (2006). *Medical Device Distribution in Indonesia-Partnering Established Companies for Optimum Penetration.* Retrieved March 7, 2012, from http://www.frost.com/prod/servlet/market-insight-top.pag?docid=72640483.
5. Espicom (2012). *The Medical Device Market: Indonesia.* Retrieved March 7, 2012, from http://www.espicom.com/prodcat2.nsf/Product_ID_Lookup/00000554?OpenDocument.

Appendix 1

Indonesia CSDT Format

Attachment A: Administrative Documents

Sections	Documents required	Details	Class I	Class II a	Class II b	Class III
Administrative Documents	**1. Copy of Local Company Licence as Medical Devices Distributor**	- No need to do addendum process to add new principle in distribution license as long its products category already available in the list - If product category has not yet in the list, addendum process will be needed - JJMI will provide this himself.	*	*	*	*
	2. Power of Attorney	POA (Power of Attorney) from the legal manufacturer to local company as sole agent or sole distributor in Indonesia — Need ID embassy legalization from the country of legal manufacturer	*	*	*	*
	3. Certificate of Free Sale	No need ID embassy legalization Endorsed by regulatory body in country of physical manufacturer or country of legal manufacturer, including the following information: product name, product code, description and the manufacturing site	*	*	*	*

(Continued)

Attachment A (*Continued*)

Sections	Documents required	Details	Class I	Class II a	Class II b	Class III
4. Executive Summary	**A. Overview**	*Brief description of device	*	*	*	*
		*Intended uses and indications for use				
		*Any novel features				
	B. Commercial Marketing History	*Date of first introduction and use	*	*	*	*
		*List of countries where it is marketed				
	C. Intended Use and Indications	*Instructions for Use (IFU)	*	*	*	*
	D. List of regulatory approval or marketing clearance obtained and status of any pending request for market clearance	*Registration status in reference agencies	*	*	*	*
		*Copies of certificates or approval letters from the reference agencies (approval certificates from the 5 benchmark countries)				
		*Declaration on labeling, packaging and instructions for use (IFU)				
	E. Important safety/ performance related information	*Summary of adverse events and recalls	*	*	*	*
		*Description of the following (if the medical device contains these items):				
		1. Drugs (description about safety and efficacy drugs usage, doses, adverse effect, pharmacology, etc.) If applicable				
		2. Animal or human cells, tissues and/or derivatives thereof, rendered non-viable (e.g. porcine heart valves, catgut sutures, etc.); If applicable				

Sections	Documents required	Details	Class I	Class II a	Class II b	Class III
		3. Cells, tissues and/or derivatives of microbial or recombinant origin (e.g. dermal fillers based on hyaluronic acid derived from bacterial fermentation processes); If applicable 4. Irradiating components, ionizing (e.g. x-ray) or non-ionizing (e.g. lasers, ultrasound, etc.). If applicable				
5. Essential Principles	**Essential principles conformity checklist**	*Essential Principles of Conformity Checklist for the device. This checklist should contain all of the essential principles described in the Guidance on Essential Principles for Safety and Performance of Medical Devices	*	*	*	*
6. Evidence conformity with the standard	**Evidence conformity with the standard**	*Certificate of Analysis (COA) of products. COA should be matched with product specification. The template should mention about parameter, limitation and nominal result of test. COA should mention name of product that we register, batch/lot no. *ISO 13485 from Physical manufacture and legal manufacture *IEC 60-601 for electrical safety – if applicable *Declaration of conformity	*	*	*	*

Attachment B: Information of Device

Sections	Documents required	Details	Class I	Class II a	Class II b	Class III
Device Description	**1. Description ABCD**	Description about: – Direction for use – Indication – Brochure – Raw material specification – Expiry date (only for sterile products) – JJMI will provide this himself.	*	*	*	*
	2. Device Description and Features	*Description and principles of operation *Risk Class and applicable classification rules *Description of accessories and other devices to be used with the medical device *Description of key function elements of the medical device *Labeled pictorial representation (product drawing, picture, photo) *Explanation of any novel features	* (If Applicable)	* (If Applicable)	* (If Applicable)	* (If Applicable)
	3. Intended use, 4. Indications, 5. Instructions of Use, 6. Contraindications, 7. Warnings, 8. Precautions and 9. Potential Adverse Effects	*Information typically found in the Instructions for Use (IFU); for electromedic--> Manual book should be provided. These information should be provided in Indonesia language as well.	*	*	*	*

Sections	Documents required	Details	Class I	Class II a	Class II b	Class III
	10. Alternative Therapy	*Description of any alternative practices or procedures for diagnosing, treating, curing or mitigating the disease or condition for which the device is intended	*	*	*	*
	11. Materials	*List of materials of the medical device making direct contact (e.g. with the mucous membrane) or indirect contact (e.g. during extracorporeal circulation of body fluids) with a human body.		*	*	*
		* Include information regarding chemical material, biological and physical characterization of the medical devices		*	*	*
		*For medical devices intended to emit ionizing radiation, information on radiation source (e.g. radioisotopes) and the material used for shielding of unintended, stray or scattered radiation – if applicable		*	*	*
	12. Other Descriptive Information-manufacturer information	*Description of any other important characteristics of the medical device that is not addressed in the preceding sections. *Finished product specification test (protocol and result) – example PPQ protocol and result	*	*	*	*

(*Continued*)

Attachment B (*Continued*)

Sections	Documents required	Details	Class I	Class II a	Class II b	Class III
	13. Manufacturing Process	Must-cover method of manufacturing process, condition, environment, facilities and controls used for process, packaging, labeling and storage devices. This process can be represent by flow chart of manufacturing process. Include a summary of methods and sterilization processes (for sterile products) *Identify all sites (name and full address) for design and manufacturing activities (including contract manufacturers and contract sterilizers) 1. Identify the activities conducted at different manufacturing sites 2. Provide Quality Management System (QMS) certificates for all design and manufacturing sites (including contract manufacturers and contract sterilizers)	*	*	*	*
	13a. Sterilization validation (for sterile products)	*Information on the sterilization validation method used, sterility assurance level (SAL) attained; standards applied, sterilization protocol, summary of validation results	*	*	*	*

Sections	Documents required	Details	Class I	Class II a	Class II b	Class III
		*Initial sterilization validation including bioburden testing, pyrogen testing, testing for sterilant residues (if applicable) and packaging validation. If initial sterilization validation is not performed, adequate justification must be provided	*	*	*	*
		*Evidence of the ongoing revalidation of the process (e.g. evidence of revalidation of the packaging and sterilization processes)	*	*	*	*
		*Post-sterilization functional test on the medical device	*	*	*	*
		*If the sterilant is toxic or produces toxic residuals, test data and methods that demonstrates the post-process sterilant and/or residuals are within acceptable limits	*	*	*	*
	13b. Stability Studies (for devices with a shelf life)	*Data demonstrating that the relevant performances and characteristics of the medical device are maintained throughout the claimed shelf life which the "expiry" date reflects, including:	*	*	*	*
		1. Prospective studies using accelerated ageing, validated with real time degradation correlation; or	*	*	*	*

(*Continued*)

Attachment B (*Continued*)

Sections	Documents required	Details	Class I	Class II a	Class II b	Class III
		2. Retrospective studies using real time experience, involving e.g. testing of stored samples; review of the complaint history or published literature etc.; or	*	*	*	*
		3. A combination of (1) and (2).	*(If applicable)	*(If applicable)	*(If applicable)	*(If applicable)
		*Summary of stability studies conducted, stability protocols used, results of studies. This summary should include conclusions with respect to storage conditions and shelf life, and, if applicable, in-use storage conditions and shelf life.	*	*	*	*
	13c. Projected Useful Life (for devices without expiry dates)	* For devices that do not have expiry dates (e.g. infusion pump, digital thermometer), the projected useful life of the medical device must be provided. Manufacturers may refer to TS/ISO 14969 (Medical devices – Quality management systems – Guidance on the application of ISO 13485:2003) for information on how to determine the projected useful life	*	*	*	*

Attachment C: Specification and Quality Assurance Device

Sections	Documents required	Details	Class I	Class II a	Class II b	Class III
Specification and Quality Assurance Device	**1. Specification**	Finished product specification: functional characteristics and technical performance specifications for the device including, as relevant, accuracy, sensitivity, specificity of measuring and diagnostic devices, reliability and other factors; and other specifications including chemical, physical, electrical, mechanical, biological, software, sterility, stability, storage and transport, and packaging to the extent necessary to demonstrate conformity with the relevant Essential Principles.	*	*	*	*
	2. Other Relevant Specifications	List of features, dimensions and performance attributes of the medical device, its variants and accessories that would typically appear in the product specification made available to the end user, e.g. in brochures and catalogues		*	*	*
	3. Summary or reference or design verification and design validation	This section should summarize or reference or contain design verification and design validation data to the extent appropriate to the complexity and risk class of the device: Such documentation should typically include: declarations/certificates of conformity to the "recognized" standards listed as applied by the manufacturer; and/or		*	*	*

(*Continued*)

Attachment C (*Continued*)

Sections	Documents required	Details	Class I	Class II a	Class II b	Class III
		– summaries or reports of tests and evaluations based on other standards, manufacturer methods and tests, or alternative ways of demonstrating compliance. The data summaries or tests reports and evaluations would typically cover, as appropriate to the complexity and risk class of the device: a listing of and conclusions drawn from published reports that concern the safety and performance of aspects of the device with reference to the Essential Principles; • engineering tests; • laboratory tests; • biocompatibility tests; • animal tests; • simulated use; • software validation				
Clinical Study	**4. Pre-clinical Studies**	*Biocompatibility Testing (Protocol and result)			*	*
		*Physical Testing (Protocol and result)				
		*Animal Testing (Protocol and result)				
		*Software validation Studies (Protocol and result)				
	5. Devices containing Biological material (if applicable)	* results of studies in relation to the risks associated with transmissible agents. Statement letter for disease and virus free	* (If Applicable)	* (If Applicable)	* (If Applicable)	* (If Applicable)

Sections	Documents required	Details	Class I	Class II a	Class II b	Class III
	6. Software verification and validation studies (if applicable)	*Manufacturer should give design validation and software development. The manufacturer and/or device sponsor must provide evidence that validates the software design and development process. This information should include the results of all verification, validation and testing performed in-house and in a user's environment prior to final release, for all of the different hardware configurations identified in the labeling, as well as representative data generated from both testing environments.			*	*
	7. Clinical Evidence	*Clinical evaluation report of the device			*	*
		*Full reports of all studies referenced in clinical evaluation report *Note*: The documented evidence submitted should include the objectives, methodology and results presented in context, clearly and meaningfully. The conclusions on the outcome of the clinical studies should be preceded by a discussion in context with the published literature. Clinical evidence of effectiveness may comprise device-related investigations conducted domestically or other countries. It may be derived from relevant publications in a peer-reviewed scientific literature			*	*

(*Continued*)

Attachment C (*Continued*)

Sections	Documents required	Details	Class I	Class II a	Class II b	Class III
		Use of Existing Bibliography Copies is required of all literature studies, or existing bibliography, that the manufacturer is using to support safety and effectiveness. These will be a subset of the bibliography of references. General bibliographic references should be device-specific as supplied in chronological order. Care should be taken to ensure that the references are timely and relevant to the current application				
		Clinical evidence can be obtained from publications relating scientific literature which has been discussed with the experts.				
Risk Management	**8. Risk Management Documents**	*Risk Management report for the design of the device and its manufacturing process			*	*
		*Accompanying documents referenced in the report, including the risk management plan, results of risk assessment and risk control				
Raw material specification	**raw material specification**	Specification of raw material or components of product.			*	*
Packaging Material Specification (for diagnostic product)	**Packaging Material Specification (for diagnostic product)**	Packaging Material Specification (for diagnostic product),			*	*
Analysis Test Report	**Analysis Test Report**	Analysis Test Report and or clinical study for reagent/*in vitro* diagnostic product			*	*

Attachment D: Labeling and Intended of Use

Sections	Documents required	Details	Class I	Class II a	Class II b	Class III
Device Labeling ****Labels are required for each and every product codes which are to be registered.***	**1. Device Labeling**	*Copies (in original color) of:				
		1. Labels on the device and its packaging (primary and secondary levels)	*	*	*	*
		2. Instructions for use/IFU (including operating manual and user manual) -> Should be Indonesian language		*	*	*
		3. Patient information leaflet (where applicable)		*	*	*
		4. Product picture with address of manufacture for Electromedic device	*	*	*	*
		*Promotional material (including brochures and catalogues) *Note*: These following information must be available: – Name and address physical manufacturer medical devices and/or Household Medical Supply – IFU need to be translated in Indonesian language, at least with below information: – Indication and Direction of use must be in the Indonesian language – Adverse effect-warning signs must be in the Indonesian language – Importer-name and address as well as marketing authorization number				
Lot Numbering system		Lot numbering system or explanation letter regarding the lot system	*	*	*	*

Attachment E : Post Market Evaluation

Sections	Documents required	Details	Class I	Class II a	Class II b	Class III
Post Market Evaluation	1. SOP about handling product complaint, recall and stop shipment	This SOP should come from the legal manufacturer/source and local as applicant			*	*

Chapter 29

Japan: Medical Device Regulatory System

Atsushi Tamura

Pharmaceuticals & Medical Devices Agency,
Shin-Kasumigaseki Bldg., 3-3-2 Kasumigaseki, Chiyoda-ku Tokyo, JAPAN

tamura-atsushi@pmda.go.jp

Disclaimer

The regulatory information contained in this chapter is intended for market planning and is subject to change frequently. Translations of laws and regulations are unofficial.

29.1 Introduction

Japan is an island nation in East Asia, located in the Pacific Ocean, with a population of over 127 million. Regarding the international harmonization of medical device, Japan has been a founding member of the Global Harmonization Task Force and currently is a member of the International Medical Device Regulators Forum. Production, import and export values of medical devices have been 1713 (1576), 1055 (1074) and 453 (475) billion yen, respectively, in FY2010 (FY2009).[1]

Handbook of Medical Device Regulatory Affairs in Asia
Edited by Jack Wong and Raymond K. Y. Tong

ISBN 978-981-4411-21-9 (Hardcover), 978-981-4411-22-6 (eBook)
www.panstanford.com

29.2 Regulatory Agency in Japan

29.2.1 The Ministry of Health, Labour and Welfare

The Ministry of Health, Labour and Welfare (MHLW) designs and implements social systems and structures that are closely related to people's lives throughout their lifetime and entire life cycle. The MHLW covers a wide range of areas from medical care to employment and childcare support and each department of the ministry serves "for people, for life, and for the future" on a daily basis.[2] Figure 29.1 shows the key organization chart of the MHLW.

The Pharmaceutical and Food Safety Bureau

The Pharmaceutical and Food Safety Bureau sets consistent regulations from production to sales and post-marketing safety measures based on the Pharmaceutical Affairs Act, in order to ensure the efficacy and safety of drugs, medical devices, etc. The Bureau is also working on various issues that are directly linked to people's lives and health, including blood projects such as blood donation, and measures against drug abuse.

29.2.2 Pharmaceuticals and Medical Devices Agency

The Pharmaceuticals and Medical Devices Agency (PMDA) is the Japanese regulatory agency, working together with MHLW. The PMDA's obligation is to protect the public health by assuring safety, efficacy and quality of pharmaceuticals and medical devices. The PMDA conducts scientific reviews of marketing authorization application of pharmaceuticals and medical devices, monitoring of their post-marketing safety. The PMDA is also responsible for providing relief compensation for sufferers from adverse drug reaction and infections by pharmaceuticals or biological products.[3] The organization chart of the PMDA is shown in Fig. 29.2.

29.2.3 Shared Responsibility of MHLW and PMDA on Medical Device Regulation

The MHLW has ultimate responsibilities in policies and administrative measures, for example, the final judgment on approval, product withdrawal from market, and so on. On the other hand, the PMDA plays the role of a technical arm of the MHLW, through an actual review, examination, data analysis, etc., to assist the MHLW's

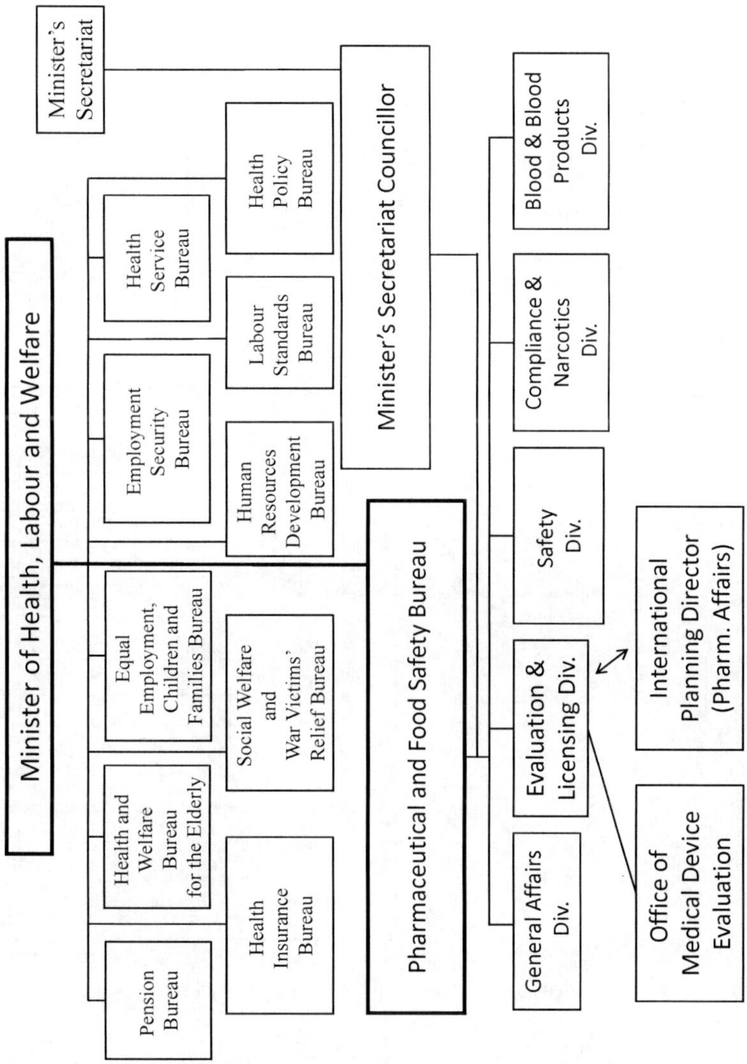

Figure 29.1 Organization Chart of MHLW.

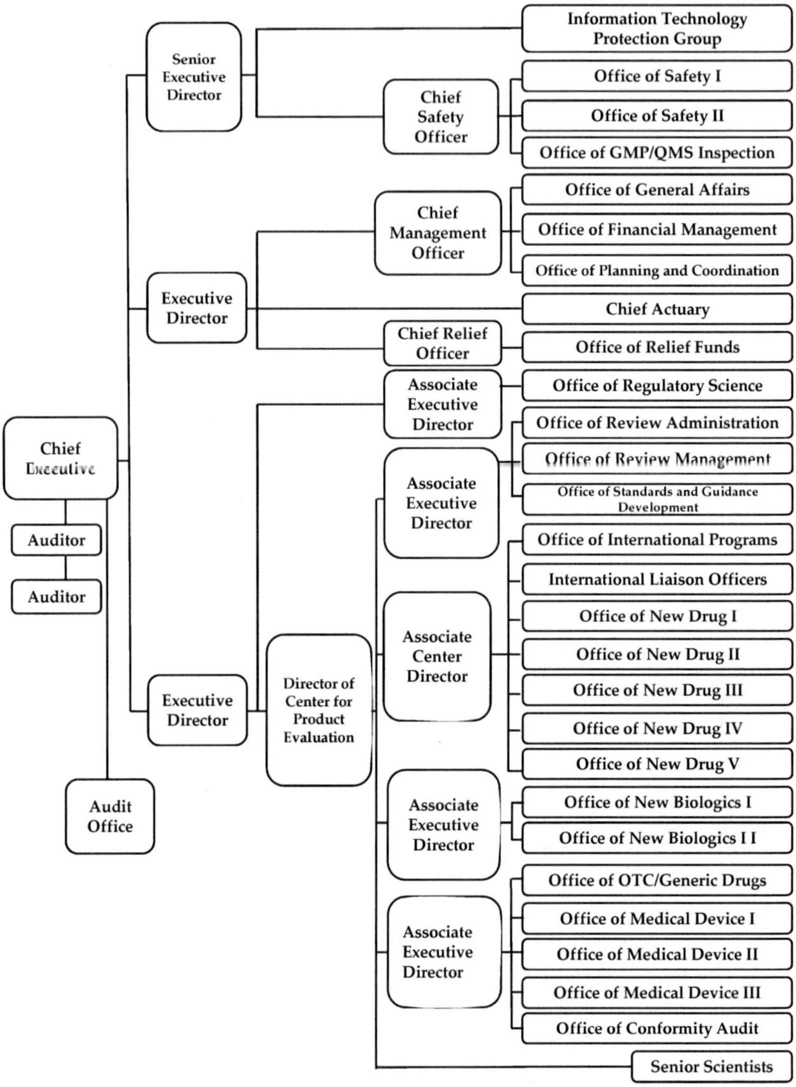

Figure 29.2 Organization chart of PMDA (as of 1 November 2011).

measures, for instance, approval review of medical devices, quality management system (QMS)/good laboratory practice/good clinical practice inspection, and collection and analysis of adverse event (AE) reports.

29.3 Legislation of Medical Devices

Medical device administration in Japan is maintained in accordance with a number of laws concerned as shown in Fig. 29.3 and Table 29.1. Among them, the Pharma-ceutical Affairs Law (PAL) is the supreme law. Some related cabinet ordinance, ministerial ordinance and ministerial notification are issued for enforcement of the PAL. Furthermore, notifications by the director general of bureau and/or notifications by director of division/office are also published as guidance documents for smooth enforcement of the PAL.

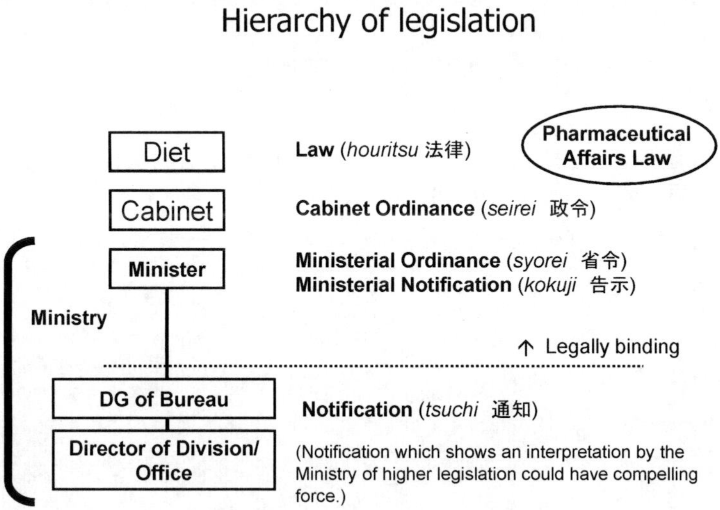

Figure 29.3 Hierarchy of legislation.

Table 29.1 Key pharmaceutical legislation

Law (*houritsu*)	Pharmaceutical Affairs Law (PAL, 1960)
Cabinet Ordinance (*seirei*)	Cabinet Ordinance on PAL, 1961 Cabinet Ordinance on PAFSC, 2000
Ministerial Ordinance (*shorei*)	Ministerial Ordinance on PAL, 1961 GCP for pharmaceuticals, 1997, for MD, 2005 Good Vigilance Practice (GVP), 2004 Good Quality Practice (GQP), 2004, etc.
Ministerial Notification (*kokuji*)	Essential Principles Certification standards for class II devices Classification of medical devices List of orphan designation, etc.
Notification (*tsuchi*) by Director General of Bureau or Director of Division/Office	Information on application procedures Guidelines for clinical evaluation, etc.

Medical devices are defined under Article 2, Paragraph 4, of the PAL, as follows:

> The term "medical device" in this Law refers to instruments and apparatus intended for use in diagnosis, cure or prevention of diseases in human or other animals; intended to affect the structure or functions of the body of man or other animals, as designated by cabinet ordinance, The Pharmaceutical Affairs Law, Enforcement Ordinance.

All medical devices have a generic name, which is called the Japanese Medical Device Nomenclature (JMDN). In JMDN, not only single product but also some grouping products such as surgical kit and ablation system are defined. At this moment, there is no clear definition of a product comprising two or more regulated components, a so-called combination product.

In order to bring medical devices into the Japanese market, under the PAL a legal procedure is required for products, companies and manufacturing sites, as shown in Table 29.2.

Table 29.2 Prerequisites to bring MDs into the Japanese market

Product	Minister's Approval (*shonin*) (Art. 14) or 3rd party Certification (*ninsho*) (Art. 23-2) or Marketing Notification (*todokede*) (Art. 14-9)
Company	License for Marketing Authorization Holder (*Seizohanbai-gyo-kyoka*) (Art. 12)
Manufacturing Site/ Manufacturer	License for Manufacturer (*seizo-gyo-kyoka*) (Art. 13) or Status as Recognized Foreign Manufacturer (*gaikoku seizo-gyosya nintei*) (Art. 13-3)

For medical devices, at least the following should be indicated on the device itself, wrappers or containers clearly in Japanese: name and address of the market authorization holder, brand name, generic name, serial number or manufacture sign, and device category. Since there are the other labelling requirements depending upon the type of the devices, the use of the specific materials and so on, it is necessary to check carefully the PAL and related regulations.

29.3.1 Classification of Medical Devices

The classification identifies the level of regulatory control that is necessary to assure the safety and effectiveness of a medical device. In Japan, medical devices are classified mainly into four classes, on the basis of risk-based system following the Global Harmonization Task Force (GHTF) rule as shown in Table 29.3.[4]

Table 29.3 Overview of classification and pre-market regulation for medical devices

Category		Risk-based classification	Technical stds. for certification	Type of regulation	Reviewed by	QMS
General MDs		Class I Extremely Low Risk	NA	Self-declaration	MAH (report to PMDA)	* Some exception
Cont-rolled MDs	Designated Controlled Medical Devices	Class II Low Risk	YES	3rd Party Certification	Registered Certification Body	Applied
	Others than above		NO	Minister's Approval	PMDA and MHLW	
Specially Controlled MDs		Class III Medium Risk	NA			
		Class IV High Risk				

29.3.2 Type of Product's Registration

29.3.2.1 Notification

Class I medical devices are categorized as "General Medical Devices" by PAL. A marketing authorization holder (MAH) who intends to market a "general medical device" is not required to obtain the minister's approval and is allowed to launch a medical device onto the Japanese market by submitting the marketing notification for the medical device to the PMDA.

29.3.2.2 Pre-market certification (third-party certification)

Class II medical devices are called "Controlled Medical Devices" in PAL. Among the controlled medical devices, medical devices to which there is the certification standard applicable are recognized as "Designated Controlled Medical Devices". To register and market a designated controlled medical device, the MAH needs to file pre-market certification application with a registered certification body (third-party certification body) and obtain their certification.

Application dossiers for pre-market certification have to be written in Japanese and the technical data and supporting information have to be submitted following the summary technical documentation (STED) format.

29.3.2.3 Pre-market approval

Class III and IV medical devices are defined as "Highly Controlled Medical Device" in PAL. When an MAH intends to launch a "specially controlled medical device" onto the Japanese market, the minister's approval to market the medical device is required. The minister's approval is granted on the basis of the scientific review at the PMDA.

Class II devices other than Specified Controlled Medical Devices are also subject to pre-market approval. In the case that no applicable certification standard has been established or that the product is deemed as a new medical device, the MAH is required to submit an application to the PMDA to obtain the minister's approval for the product.

Application dossiers for pre-market approval have also to be written in Japanese and the technical data and supporting information have to be submitted following the STED format, as shown in Fig. 29.4.

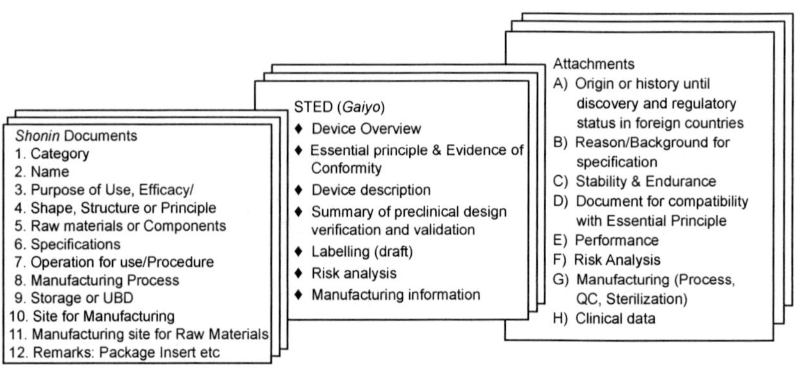

Figure 29.4 Application documents set for high-risk device.

29.3.3 Marketing Authorization Holder

To market, lease and/ or grant the products (which are manufactured or imported), it is necessary to have the appropriate class of MAH license, as shown in Table 29.4. Additionally, to obtain approval (certification) for a medical device, the appropriate class of MAH license is also needed (PAL Article 12, 14).

- MAH has to be responsible for the product distribution.
- MAH is required to be responsible for the quality of the product and manufacturing.
- MAH has to have an MAH general manager, a quality assurance manager and a post-marketing safety manager.

Table 29.4 Type of License for MAH (Art. 12)

Classification of medical device	Type of license needed
Highly controlled medical device	Type 1 MAH License
Controlled medical device	Type 2 MAH License
General medical device	Type 3 MAH License

29.3.4 Manufacturer License (Art. 13)/Accreditation of Foreign Manufacturer (Art. 13-3)

It is required by PAL that any person who intended to manufacture medical devices by professional shall obtain a license for each manufacturing facility from the heads of prefectures and the heads of regional bureau of health and welfares (RBHW) (Art. 81 and 81-4). Licenses are valid for five years and are renewable. If the manufacturing facilities are located outside of Japan, these foreign manufacturing facilities are required to obtain the Foreign Manufacturer Accreditation instead of a Manufacturer License.[5] Four categories of the accreditation, same as the License for Manufacturers, are valid for five years and are renewable. Application for the accreditation should be submitted to the PMDA, as shown in Table 29.5.

Table 29.5 Types of licenses for the manufacturer

Category	Operation	Authority
Biological	(1) All/Part of processes of manufacturing and quality management for MDs designated by the Minister (e.g. biological product)	Head of Prefecture (except for manufacturers of Specific Biological Products etc. Their licenses are issued by Head of RBHW)
Sterilization	(2) Sterilizing process (other than 1)	

(*Continued*)

Table 29.5 (*Continued*)

Category	Operation	Authority
General	(3) All/Part of processes of manufacturing and quality management for general MDs (other than 1 and 2)	
Packaging, etc.	(4) Only packaging, labelling and storage	

29.4 Related Requirements

29.4.1 Quality Management System

In Japan, manufactures for Class II–IV medical devices and Class I devices which are designated by the MHLW must demonstrate QMS compliance. Ministerial Ordinance 169 was issued in December 2004 and is the standard of manufacturing control and quality control for both medical devices and *in vitro* diagnostic reagents, known as the QMS Ordinance. This ordinance is the main regulation specifically listing QMS requirements. Japanese QMS fundamentally refers to ISO 13485, but there are some differences. These differences are including document control, record control, responsible engineering manager, infrastructure, etc. For example, there may be different requirements for the length of time required to keep copies of documents.

29.4.1.1 QMS conformity as an essential requirement

QMS conformity is an essential requirement for product approval/certification and for retention of approval/certification under the PAL. As requirements for product approval/certification, during the examination of application documents for approval/certification, a QMS conformity inspection is performed by the relevant review body. Approval/certification is granted only after conformity is established. As requirements for retention of approval/certification, approval/certification holders are obliged to undergo a QMS inspection every five years. If the approval/certification holder does not fulfil this obligation or does not follow improvement instructions resulting from the QMS inspection, approval/certification may be withdrawn by the relevant authorities.

29.4.1.2 QMS inspections

QMS inspections are conducted for medical device manufacturing facilities in Japan and in other countries based on the requirements set by the QMS Ordinance. The on-site and document-based inspections of manufacturing sites are performed by the PMDA, applicable prefecture or the RCB (registered certification body), according to its application category or other issues.

29.4.2 Good Quality Practices

The Good Quality Practices (GQP) specified in MHLW Ministerial Ordinance No. 136, 2004, are requirements for the MAH located in Japan. The MAH has to comply with the GQP, which is the standard of quality control of a medical device. GQP requires shipping control supervision of manufacturer handling of defective products etc.

The assessment of compliance to the GQP, for each MAH, is conducted by the prefectural government where the MAH has their registered place of business. Every manufacturer should familiarize themselves with the requirements of this ordinance, because of the specific requirements stipulating the cooperation between the MAH and the medical device manufacturer.

29.5 MAH'S Obligations during Post-Market Phase

Requirements for MAH (Art. 12-2)

The MAH has also to comply with the Good Vigilance Practice (GVP), which is the standard of post-marketing safety management of a medical device (issued as MHLW ordinance No. 135 dated 22 September 2004). In GVP requirements, the MAH must continue controlling risks by conducting investigation/consideration of information related to post-marketing safety management, planning/implementation of safety measure, and provision of information appropriately and smoothly. GVP includes standards concerning organization and staff engaged in post-market surveillance measurement, collection of safety information, internal audit and so on. Figure 29.5 shows the typical flow of an adverse event report.

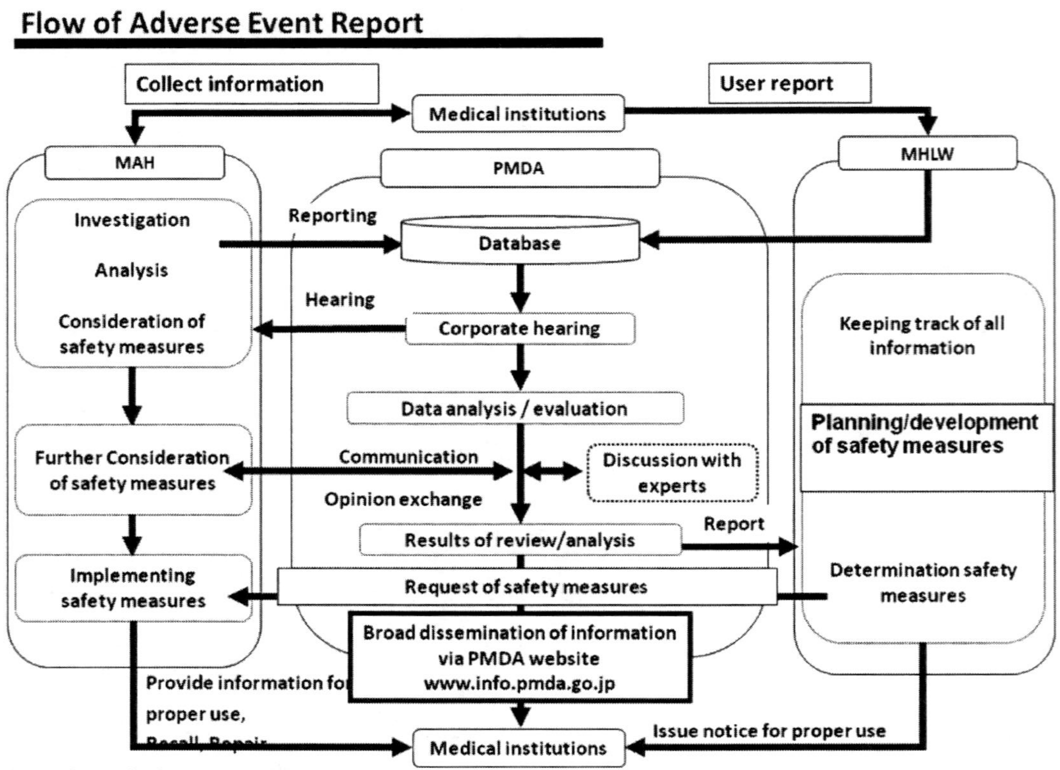

Figure 29.5 Flow of adverse event report.

29.5.1 Collection, Analysis and Reporting of Safety Information

When the MAH learns of adverse events, etc., suspected to be related to the efficacy and safety of medical devices, they must report the information to the PMDA within a certain period of time stipulated in MHLW ordinance (Tables 29.6 and 29.7).

Table 29.6 Report due date: malfunction, failure, breakage, leak, fault, etc. (in case it may cause health damage)

	Description to package inserts (IFU)	Report's due date
Serious	Unknown (unanticipated)	30 days
	Known (anticipated)	15 days (when the incidence rate of AE understood beforehand increase)
		30 days (except reports shown above)
Non-Serious	Unknown	Annual reports
	Known	—

Table 29.7 Report due date: health DAMAGE (death, injury, etc.)

		Description to package inserts (IFU)	Report's due date
Serious	Death	Known/unknown	15 days
	Except death	Unknown	15 days
		Known	15 days (When the incidence rate of AE understood beforehand increase)
			30 days (except reports shown above)
Non-serious		Unknown	Annual report
		Known	—

29.5.2 Recall

When the MAH undertakes recalls (including repairs) of medical devices, they must report to the governor of the prefecture where the company is located.

29.5.3 Post-Marketing Safety Management

The MAH must continue controlling risks by conducting investigation/consideration of information related to post-marketing safety management, planning/implementation of safety measure, and provision of information appropriately and smoothly.

The MAH must make efforts to collect information related to the efficacy and safety of medical devices and provide it to healthcare professionals (user).

When the MAH learns that the use of medical devices may cause the onset or spread of hazards, the necessary measures for safety should be taken, including recall, repair, discontinued distribution and provision of information to prevent such hazards.

The MAH must employ a person ("general marketing compliance officer") to undertake quality control and post-marketing safety control of medical devices.

The general marketing compliance officer must conduct the work concerning quality control and safety management impartially and appropriately.

When it is confirmed to be necessary for impartial and appropriate conduct of the work, the general marketing compliance officer must present to the MAH (head of the company) opinions in writing.

29.6 PMDA's Obligations during Post-Market Phase

The PMDA collects safety information promptly and efficiently; safety staff receive reports from companies when cases of adverse events and infections caused by drugs as well as malfunctions of medical devices are detected during the development and post-marketing periods.

The PMDA also consolidates all essential safety information reported by healthcare professionals, information from international sources, and conference papers and research reports. The collected information is then promptly compiled into a database and shared with the MHLW.

29.6.1 New Challenge

To improve and enhance safety measures, the PMDA takes various approaches such as the introduction of data mining methods (which allow statistical analyses of information on adverse drug reactions as reported by companies or medical institutions and the detection of cases to be investigated), promotion of the application of electronic medical records to safety measures in order to establish evaluation methods of safety (known as the MIHARI Project), building of a system for evaluating medical device malfunctions, and building of a system for gathering and evaluating data from medical devices subject to tracking.

29.6.2 Information Services

The PMDA makes available a wide range of information on the quality, efficacy, and safety of drugs and medical devices, such as the package inserts for drug products and medical devices, recalls, and urgent safety information ("Dear Healthcare Professional" Letters), on the Medical Product Information page on its website (http://www.info.pmda.go.jp). All cases of adverse drug reactions and malfunctions reported by companies on or after 1 April 2004 (the date the PMDA was established) are posted on the same Web page.

The PMDA provides information not only to healthcare professionals but also to the general public, such as the *Drug Guide for Patients*, which is an easy-to-understand explanation for patients to teach them about prescription drugs with warnings labels, and the *Manuals for Management of Individual Serious Adverse Drug Reactions* (for the general public), which outline individual ADRs, initial symptoms and key points for early detection and treatment in an easy-to-understand manner.

In addition, the agency offers a free email information service called "PMDA medi-navi" (available in Japanese only), through which important safety information is distributed to healthcare professionals who subscribe to the service.

References

1. *Yearbook of Statistics of Production by Pharmaceutical Industry* (in Japanese), retrieved (15 March 2012) from http://www.mhlw.go.jp/topics/yakuji/2010/nenpo/index.html.
2. *Organization of the Ministry of Health, Labour and Welfare*, retrieved: (9 March 2012) from http://www.mhlw.go.jp/english/org/detail/index.html.
3. *Organization of the Pharmaceuticals and Medical Devices Agency*, retrieved (9 March 2012) from: http://www.pmda.go.jp/english/about/organization.html.
4. *Summary Technical Documentation for Demonstrating Conformity to the Essential Principles of Safety and Performance of Medical Devices* (STED), retrieved (9 March 2012) from http:// http://www.ghtf.org/sg1/sg1-final.html.
5. *Application for Accreditation of Foreign Manufacturers*, retrieved (9 March 2012) from http://www.pmda.go.jp/english/service/pdf/application.pdf.

Chapter 30

Jordan: Medical Device Regulatory System

Anan Abu Hassan

Medical Devices and Cosmetics Section,
Jordan Food and Drug Administration
anan.abu_hassan@jfda.jo

Disclaimer

The regulatory information contained in this chapter is intended for market planning and is subject to change frequently. Translations of laws and regulations are unofficial.

30.1 Jordan Food and Drug Administration: Introduction

30.1.1 Vision

- To be the leading regulatory institution for the safety and quality of food and drugs at national and regional levels and well recognized at the international level.
- To gain the trust and confidence of citizens and institutions of Jordan through the exercise of efficient and effective

Handbook of Medical Device Regulatory Affairs in Asia
Edited by Jack Wong and Raymond K. Y. Tong

ISBN 978-981-4411-21-9 (Hardcover), 978-981-4411-22-6 (eBook)
www.panstanford.com

scientifically based decisions that ensure public health safety and welfare.

30.1.2 Mission

The Jordan Food and Drug Administration (JFDA) is an independent public sector regulatory institution whose main objectives are to ensure the safety and efficiency of drugs and food and the safety of products, including infant milk formula and its special formula, supplementary food, medicinal plants, natural products, disinfectants and antiseptics, medical equipment and supplies, pharmaceutical preparations containing vitamins and minerals, cosmetic preparations and any other substances related to treatment of diseases in human beings.

30.1.3 Overview of Structure of Jordan Food and Drug Administration

Medical devices sector in Jordan: The directorate of controlled MDs and Cosmetics controls medical devices, including antiseptics and disinfectants (see Fig. 30.1). In the past, the JFDA used to depend only on catalogues, free sale certificate (FSC), and some internal instructions to custom release for medical devices.

30.2 Medical Device Market in Jordan

The medical device market in Jordan comprises imported products and also products from local sources, including dental products, haemodialysis solutions, antiseptics, disinfectants, infusion set, plasters and surgical sutures. Local manufacturers should submit their site master file to the JFDA in order to be studied and to get an approval for manufacturing products.

30.3 Overview of Regulatory Environment and What Laws/Regulations Govern the Medical Devices

- Medical Device Importation Directives, Including antiseptics and disinfectants.

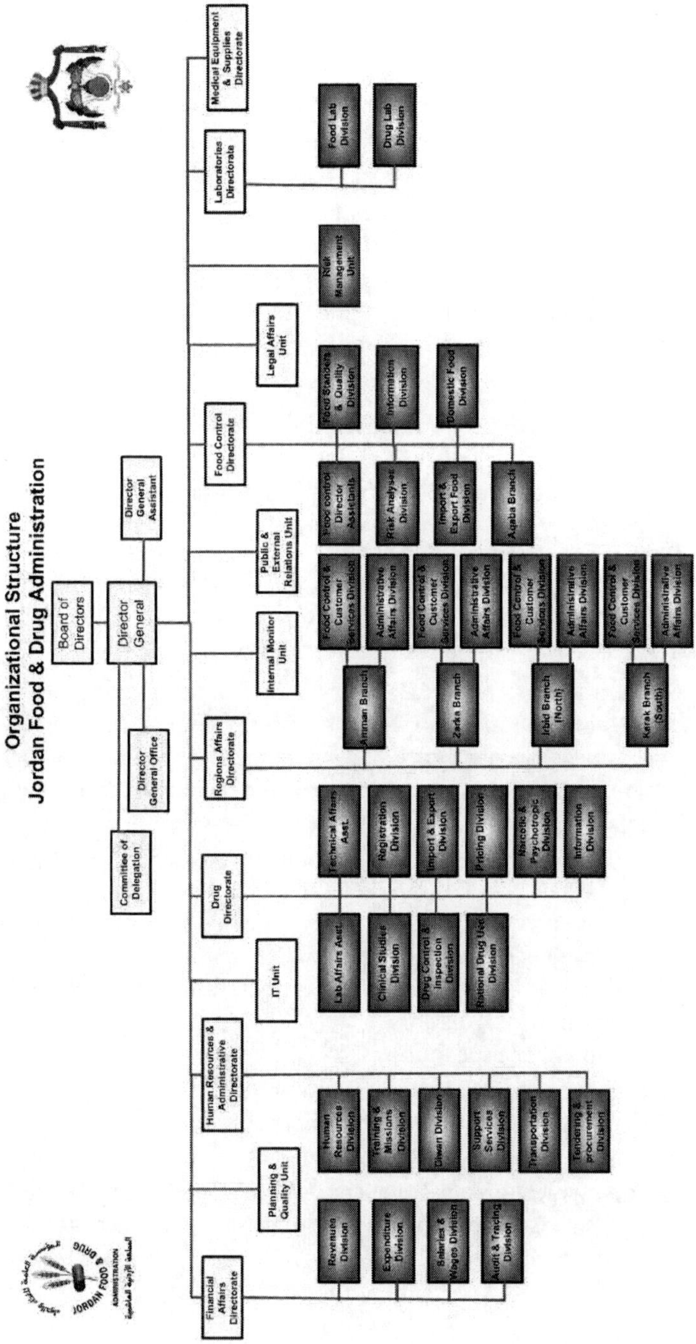

Figure 30.1 Organizational structure of JFDA.

- Issued in accordance with Article No. (5) of the Drug & Pharmacy Law No. 88
- Law No. 80 for the year 2001 & its relevant amendment law No. 30 for the year 2003
- Article 1: These Directives are called Medical Devices Directives including antiseptics and disinfectants. Effective Date was its publication date in the official Gazette
- Article 2: For the purpose of implementing these Directives, the terminology is set as mentioned in accordance with Article No. 2 of the law in addition to certain explanations for certain terminology such as

Article 1

These directives are called Medical Devices Directives, including antiseptics and disinfectants. The date from which they have been effective is the date of its publication in the official gazette.

Article 2

For the purpose of implementing these directives, the terminology is set in accordance with Article 2 of the law in addition to certain explanations for certain terminologies such as

1. **Definition of a medical device:** It is each device of substance, whether used alone or associated with others, including the software necessary for its use, prepared by the manufacturer to be used for a person in order to achieve any of the following goals:
   - diagnosis, prevention, monitoring, treatment, alleviation of disease
   - diagnosis, monitoring, treatment, alleviation and/or compensation for any injury or disability.
   - disclosure, compensation, or amendment from/to the anatomical situation.
   - control of conception
2. **Accessories:** Devices/tools prepared by the manufacturers for use with medical devices in particular class/category
3. **Medical device classification:** Following are the groups under which medical devices are classified with regard to safety/invasiveness, and these are classified in accordance to what is mentioned in the "Medical Devices Directives 93/42/EEC:
   - Class I
   - Class IIA

- Class IIB
- Class III
- Active Implants Class
- Active Implantable MDD 90/385/EEC.

4. **Laboratory:** FDA Drug Laboratory Control Department
5. **Committee:** The Medical Device Committee, covers both antiseptics and disinfectants

Article 3

A. It is allowed to import and freely use medical devices with the exception of what is stated in (B) after obtaining the approval of the Director General or its appointed personnel in accordance with Addendum Nos. 1, 3 and 4.
B. It is allowed to import and freely use the medical devices in the pharmaceutical forms and those whose components may be considered pharmaceutical/drug after obtaining the prior approval of the Medical Device Committee according to the items referred to in Addendum Nos 1, 3 and 4.
C. It is allowed to import antiseptics and disinfectants in accordance with the contents of Addendum Nos 2, 3 and 4
D. It is **prohibited** to import used or refurbished medical devices for all the health sectors in HKJ.

Article 4

The Medical Device Committee evaluates the importation requests for the items referred to in Items B and C pertaining to Article No. 3 and decisions regarding the same should be taken within a period of 30 working days from the date of the applicant initial importation request .

A. The applicant has the full right to submit an objection to the Medical Device Committee within a period of 30 working days from being officially notified in written.
B. The Medical Device Committee re-studies and re-evaluates the submitted objections, and decisions should be taken regarding the same within a period of 30 working days from date of submission to the Jordan Food and Drug Administration.

Article 5

The Director General of Jordan Food & Drug Administration has the full right to prohibit (based on the decision and recommendation of the Medical Device Committee) importation or marketing or to cancel previous approvals or call for recalls of medical devices, including antiseptics and disinfectants.

Article 6

It is obligatory to obtain the approval of the Medical Device Committee regarding any changes/updates to medical devices, antiseptics and disinfectants prior to implementation.

Article 7

The Director General of Jordan Food and Drug Administration issues Special Inspection Instructions for manufacturers/importers and distributors of medical devices, antiseptics and disinfectants and places/institutes where medical devices, antiseptics and disinfectants are being used, such as hospitals.

Article 8

The Director General submits all debatable issues which may rise in favour of the implementation of such importation directives to the Medical Devices Committee and take the necessary decisions and actions.

Article 9

Customs Authorities Employees are not allowed to clear any consignments of medical devices/antiseptics and disinfectants or any of their raw materials for the local manufacturers unless they obtain the prior approval of the Director General.

Article 10

It is prohibited to advertise any medical devices or antiseptics or disinfectants through any advertisement tools (audio/video advertisement) unless they have been officially approved by the Director General in accordance with the Medical Device Committee Recommendation.

The only exception to this is publication in specialized medical magazines.

Article 11

Post–Marketing surveillance requirement: All hospitals/clinics/ medical institutes centres should report to the JFDA any damage (whether serious/fatal incurred from the use of the medical devices/ antiseptics/disinfectants).

30.4 Data about Jordan

Table 30.1 MD&D market information

Year	Number of imported invoices/year	Number of registered medical devices/year
2006	12,000	104
2007	15,500	111
2008	17,900	285
2009	13,462	262
2010	18,91	390

Table 30.2 Clinical trials

Type of medical device	Clinical trial's name
Drug-eluting stents	1. Patient-related outcomes with endeavour vs. Cypher stenting trial Prospective, multi-centre, randomized, two-arm, open-label trial Clinical Investigation Plan 2. A post-market registry of the BioMatrix® drug-eluting stent. Prospective, multi-centre registry to be conducted at 40 European interventional cardiology centres

30.5 Price Control of Medical Device

At the moment, there is no control over the prices of medical devices by the JFDA in Jordan.

30.6 Priorities

Following is a brief summary of key priorities and focus of the JFDA for MDD in Jordan:

- Supplying the local market with safe, effective and qualified medical devices.
- To expand the scope of current regulation to cover other categories, including IVDs.
- Increasing public and private sectors', consumers' and manufacturers' awareness of the JFDA's role in medical devices regulations and defining the role of the JFDA in health technology assessments.
- Collaboration of JFDA with all involved sectors (customs, royal medical services, Ministry of Health, private hospitals)
- Allocating financial and human resources at the national level in order to support proper implementation of plans

Appendix 1

Importation/Registration Requirements for Medical Devices

General Conditions for the Importation of Medical Devices/ First Time

- The applicant should submit all of the following documents to the JFDA:

1. The Applicant Commercial Registry Certificate issued by the Ministry of Industry & Trade.
2. The original copy of any of the following certificates or a freshly signed notarized valid copy of the certificate (Notary Public Stamp on each page if more than one page) (the aforementioned certificate should be valid at the time of shipping):

   2.1 FDA Certificate (Certificate to Foreign Government) issued by the USA Dept. of Health and Human Services

   2.2 A Notarized CE Certificate issued by any authorized accredited EU notified body in accordance with the
   - Medical Devices Directives 93/42/EEC.
   - Active Implantable MDD 90/385/EEC and their amendments.

   2.3 A Free Sale Certificate issued by the health authorities in the country of origin in addition to a Free Sale Certificate from any of the following countries approved by the JFDA: Switzerland, Australia, Japan, Canada, and Norway. In case the origin of the medical device origin is none of these countries, following conditions should be met:

   2:3:1 To indicate that the medical equipment is allowed to be freely sold in the country of origin, any of the following statements can be applied:
   - freely marketed
   - freely sold
   - may be sold
   - may be marketed
   - allowed to be sold
   - authorized to sell

- no legal objection against the sale
- any other statement accredited by the Medical Device Committee

2:3:2 The certificate should state a validity period. A validity period of five years is considered valid from its initial date of issuance.

2:3:3 The name and the address of the manufacturer or the marketing authorization holder should be mentioned.

3. If the medical device is in the form of a pharmaceutical dosage or if it contains drugs, the following documents must be submitted:

3.1 Original catalogue containing the full information about the medical device composition, indication/contraindication/warnings, etc.

3.2 Commitment from the manufacturer clarifying the validity period of the medical device and its storage conditions and a stability statement guarantee regarding these conditions.

3.3 Outer pack and inner pack and insert leaflet (if available).

3.4 Finished product specifications and method of analysis of the medical device (with the exception of the medical device which contains drugs in its ingredients where Article No. 5/Addendum 4 should be applied.

3.5 For all medical devices which contain ingredients of animal origin, the TSE/BSE (transmissible spongiform encephalopathy)/(bovine spongiform encephalopathy) Certificate should be submitted.

Appendix 2

General Conditions for the Importation of Antiseptics and Disinfectants

The applicant should submit the following:

1. Applicant/Importer Registry Certificate, issued by the ministry of industry and trade.
2. The original free sale certificate issued by the health authorities in the country of origin, which should include the name of the product, composition, number and date of the certificate, name and address of the manufacturer and a statement showing that the product is freely sold in the country of origin according to the statement mentioned in Appendix 1, point 2.3.1, and the said certificate should have a validity period of five years. A validity period of five years is considered valid from its initial date of issuance.
3. Declaration from the manufacturer clarifying the validity period of the antiseptic and disinfectant and its storage conditions and a stability statement guarantee regarding these conditions.
4. Finished sample and insert leaflet (if available).
5. Finished product specifications.
6. Method of analysis.
7. For all antiseptics and disinfectants which contain ingredients of animal origin, the TSE/BSE Certificate should be submitted.

Appendix 3

Labelling Requirements for Medical Devices

1. Single-use medical device outer packs should clearly show
   (a) Batch or lot number
   (b) Expiry date
   (c) Name of the manufacturer or the Marketing Authorization Holder
   (d) Country of origin
   (e) Storage conditions
   (f) Sterilization method (in case the product is sterile); otherwise the applicant should show a certificate from the manufacturer showing the *sterilization* method used, with the exception of antiseptics and disinfectants.
2. If the medical device is CE marked, the CE mark should be present as a part of the label and it should be
   - clear
   - readable
   - irremovable
3. The medical device should pass the analysis test performed at the JFDA Lab if available in a pharmaceutical dosage form. This incudes the following products categories:
   - antiseptics, contact lenses solutions, haemostatic, vaginal douches, lubricants, IUDs.
   - mouth washes, infusion sets, bone cement, syringes, surgical gloves, condoms, surgical sutures (surgical sutures of bovine origin are prohibited)
   - dressings, cotton, plaster, hyaluronic acid, solutions that are used to keep/preserve Human body parts

Other categories of products will be refered to the Medical Device committee to decide whether analysis would be required.

Appendix 4

Importation Requirements for Medical Devices, Antiseptics and Disinfectants

1. Two copies of the invoice showing the following:
   - 1:1 Name of the manufacturer or the Marketing Authorization Holder
   - 1:2 The country of origin
   - 1:3 Names of the medical devices requested for importation, their models and catalogue numbers
   - 1:4 Names of antiseptics and disinfectants
   - 1:5 Batch number and expiry date for each item requested to pass the JFDA/Lab/Dept. analysis as per Addendum No. 3

2. Any of the accredited certificates by JFDA which compile with the specific class/category of the imported medical devices according to the following conditions:
   - 2:1 Medical Device Class I
     - 2:1:1 If it is sterile or calibrated for measuring: a general certificate issued in the name of the whole group/class.
     - 2:1:2 If differs from the above, then a declaration from the manufacturer stating that it is manufactured in accordance to worldwide specifications.
   - 2:2 Medical Devices Class IIA

     General certificate in the name of the group class/category should be submitted.
   - 2:3 Medical Device Class IIA

     General certificate in the name of the group with the exception of implants, where a separate certificate should be submitted.
   - 2:4 Medical Devices Class III

     A comprehensive/detailed certificate showing the trade name and models should be submitted.
   - 2:5 Medical Devices (Active Implants)

     A separate comprehensive detailed certificate showing the trade name and models should be submitted.

2:6 Free Sale Certificate showing the name of the anti-septic/disinfectant

1. Catalogue or brochure from the manufacture showing the name of each imported antiseptic/disinfectant.
2. Certificate of analysis for each imported batch of the (IVF media) materials used in the dentistry, such as filling, sticklers or others.
3. Quality Control Release certificate for each imported lot of the medical device which contains drugs in any of its ingredients.
4. Medical device containing human albumin requires certificate according to the current regulations. For imported batches, lot numbers should be submitted.
5. For devices which contain ingredients of animal origin, the TSE/BSE-Free Certificate should be submitted for the imported batches/lots.

Appendix 5

JFDA Adverse Incident Report Form

REPORT

Reporting body .... hospital .... health care center .... pharmacy .... others ....

Address ....

Report name ....

Position ....

Telephone number ....

Consultant-in-charge (if known) ....

This report confirms a telephone report ☐ a fax report ☐ neither ☐

Type of device: (tick one only)

☐ Active implantable devices
☐ Administration & giving sets
☐ Anaesthetic machines & monitors
☐ Anaesthetic & breathing masks
☐ Autoclaves
☐ External defibrillators & pacemakers
☐ Feeding tubes
☐ Gloves
☐ Guidewires
☐ Hearing aids
☐ Physiotherapy equipment
☐ Radiotherapy equipment
☐ Radionuclide equipment
☐ Resuscitators
☐ Staples & staple guns

☐ Bath aids	☐ Hypodermic syringes & needles	☐ Stretchers
☐ Beds & mattresses	☐ Implant materials	☐ Surgical instruments
☐ Blood pressure measurement	☐ Infant incubators	☐ Surgical power tools
☐ Breast implants	☐ Infusion pumps, syringe drivers	☐ Sutures
☐ Cardiovascular implants & device	☐ Insulin syringes	☐ Thermometers
☐ Commodes	☐ Intravenous catheters & cannulae	☐ Ultrasound equipment
☐ Contact lenses & care products	☐ Joint prostheses	☐ Urinary catheters
☐ CT systems	☐ Lasers & accessories	☐ Ventilators
☐ Dental materials & appliances	☐ Magnetic resonance equipment & accessories	☐ Walking sticks / frames
☐ Dialysis equipment	☐ Mobile x-ray systems	☐ Wound drains
☐ Diathermy equipment & accessories	☐ Monitors & electrodes	☐ X-ray equipment, systems & accessories
☐ Dressings	☐ Non-active implants	☐ Other (please specify)
☐ Dressings	☐ Non-active implants	☐ Other (please specify)
☐ Endoscopes & accessories	☐ Ophthalmic equipment	....
☐ Endotracheal tubes & airways	☐ Patient hoists	

Further details can be given on additional sheets if necessary

(*Continued*)

Appendix 5 (*Continued*)

MEDICAL DEVICES

Details of device:	Invoice No.		
Product		Catalogue No.	
Model		Serial No.	
Manufacture	Telephone No.		
Supplier			
Batch No.		Expiry date	
Date if mfr		Quantity defective	
Location of device now			
Is there a CE-mark/or FDA? YES ☐ NO ☐		If YES, was the manufacturer or supplier contacted? YES ☐ NO ☐	
Was there a fatality? YES ☐ NO ☐		Was an injury caused? YES ☐ NO ☐	

Consequences of Product problem (s).

Serious: Yes No. If serious please indicate the seriousness of reaction (s).

Death (Date of death .... Cause of death ....)

Life threatening   Hospitalization – initial or prolonged   Leading to congenital anomaly

Persistent disability   Required intervention to prevent impairment/damage (Device)

Other serious consequences (important Medical events ....)

Nature of defect/details of incident:	
Contact name for further details	
Telephone number	
Action taken by staff / manufacturer / supplier:	
.... Signed .... Date	

Please send completed form to JORDAN FOOD AND DRUG ADMNISTRATION **AMMAN-JORDAN TEL. 4602000**
TELEFAX : + 962 – 6- 4

Chapter 31

Republic of Korea (South Korea): Medical Device Regulatory System

Peter Lee
Korea Testing Laboratory
kmlee1452@hanmail.net

Disclaimer

The regulatory information contained in this report is intended for market planning and is subject to change frequently. Translations of laws and regulations are unofficial.

31.1 Market Overview

31.1.1 Facts about South Korea

The Republic of Korea, commonly known as South Korea, is a sovereign state in East Asia, located in the southern portion of the Korean Peninsula. It is neighboured by the People's Republic of China (Mainland China) to the west, Japan to the east, North Korea

Handbook of Medical Device Regulatory Affairs in Asia
Edited by Jack Wong and Raymond K. Y. Tong

ISBN 978-981-4411-21-9 (Hardcover), 978-981-4411-22-6 (eBook)
www.panstanford.com

to the north, and the East China Sea and Republic of China (Taiwan) to the south. South Korea lies in the North Temperate Zone with a predominantly mountainous terrain. Its territory covers a total area of 99,392 square kilometres and has a population of 50,515,000 (in 2010). The capital and largest city is Seoul, with a population of 10,421,782.

South Korea has the highest healthcare expenditure of all the "Asian Tigers", with an estimated 55% funded by the public sector. The government has been forced to implement cost-cutting measures in recent years, owing to a large deficit faced by the healthcare system. Healthcare costs continue to rise, with the country's rapidly aging population adding upward pressure to total spending. In the first half of 2009, for example, senior citizens accounted for 31.7% of costs covered by the National Health Insurance Corporation [18].

31.1.2 Medical Device Market Scale in South Korea

The medical device market scale in South Korea was $3.4 billion in 2010 as shown in Table 31.1, and the market scale has shown average annual growth rate of 9.0% after 2005. Also, the scale has occupied 1.3% of global market scale, ranking 14th in the world [17].

Table 31.1 Market scale

Divisions	Status in 2006	Status in 2008	Status in 2010
Manufacturers	1,624	1,726	1,857
Manufacturing	$1,772,962,000	$2,295,639,000	$2,563,822,000
Exports	$710,039,000	$1,234,670,000	$1,454,360,000
Importers	1,281	1,456	1,496
Imports	$1,563,020,000	$2,128,000,000	$2,265,035,000

Source: Korea Medical Device Industrial Association Bulletin (November 2011).

31.1.3 Definition of Medical Device

According to South Korea's regulation, medical devices are classified as medical instruments, medical supplies, dental materials, and *in vitro* diagnostic (IVD) device reagents and are identified as the products used to diagnose, cure, alleviate and treat illness, injuries or disabilities; to prevent illness or to complement injuries or disabilities; to test, replace or alter structures or functions of the bodies; or for birth control [1, 2].

Also, medical devices are grouped into four classes according to the risk level associated with their intended use. IVD Devices are classified as Class I products mostly. But IVD Device reagents are classified as Class I to IV according to their risk level (Table 31.2).

Table 31.2 Classification

Classification	Risk level	Examples of medical devices
I	Low	Tongue depressor, bandage, dressing, splints
II	Medium–low	Suction pump, gastroscope, transdermal stimulator, X-ray machine
III	Medium–high	Lung ventilator, orthopaedic implant, defibrillator, medical laser
IV	High	Prosthetics heart valve, implantable cardiac pacemaker, heparin-coated catheter

Source: KFDA Notice (December 2010).

31.1.4 Detail of Key Regulator

The Ministry of Health and Welfare (MOHW) is the primary healthcare agency in Korea and regulates the Law and Enforcement decrees. However, the KFDA, an agency under the MOHW, independently regulates all medical devices according to the Medical Device Act; only when the KFDA asks the legislation to fulfil its mission, the agreement with the MOHW is required. Details can be found at KFDA home page: http://www.kfda.go.kr/eng/index.do?nMenuCode=12.

The working level organization of KFDA is the Medical Device Safety Bureau, which consists of one department and seven divisions, including two task forces (Fig. 31.1 and 31.2) [11].

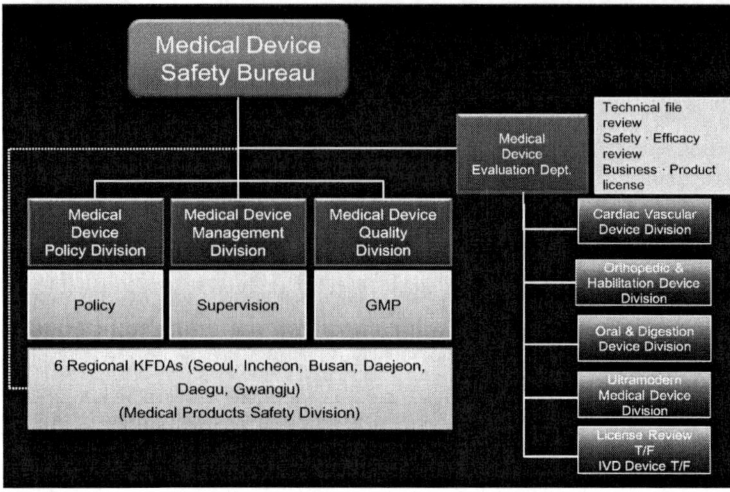

Figure 31.1 KFDA Medical Device Safety Bureau structure (KFDA Web site, November 2011).

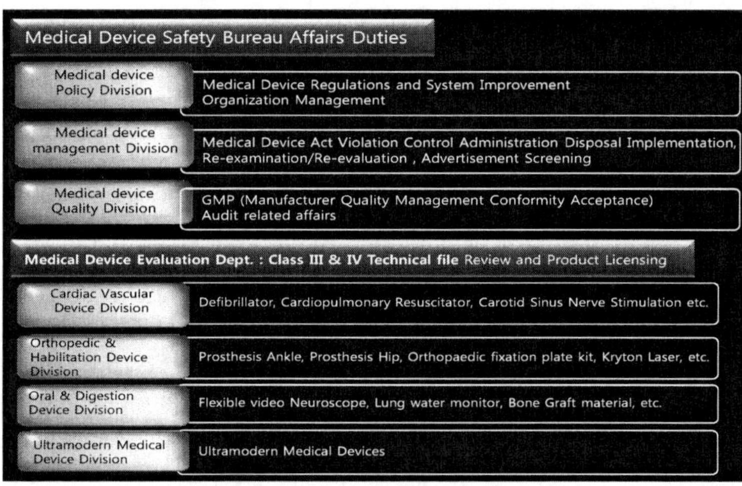

Figure 31.2 Medical Device Safety Bureau Affairs duties (KFDA Web site, November 2011).

31.2 Introduction to Korea Medical Device Regulatory System

31.2.1 History

Since 1997, medical devices have been regulated by the KFDA, which is an independent agency under the supervision of the

MOHW. Previously, the governing law for medical devices was the Pharmaceutical Affairs Act, which also had mainly covered drugs since 1953. However, to better cover medical devices and speed international harmonization, the new Medical Device Act was announced on 29 May 2003. It went into implementation and full enforcement began on May 30, 2004 with the requirement that all medical devices to be sold in South Korea meet the requirements of Korea Good Manufacturing Practices (KGMP), mostly identical with ISO 13485:2003 standard [9, 10].

31.2.2 Procedures

All foreign suppliers of medical devices must apply for either a manufacturing or import business license in order to enter the South Korean market. To obtain an import business license, an importer must provide a copy of KFDA-recommended format to one of the regional KFDAs with a health certificate of the company representative (not for a corporation), a copy of the registered legal entity (only for a corporation) and a list of facilities (in case of conditional application). An importer can have more than one distributor, but each distributor must either register as an importer or have an independent consultant holding the product approval so each importer has equal access to it.

Under Korean regulations, a foreign manufacturer without an office in Korea cannot directly submit a device registration application to the KFDA; therefore, the company may allow its importer to do the registration. The foreign manufacturer also may hire an independent third party based in Korea to make the registration in its own name.

All medical devices require the pre-market registration from the KFDA before they can be manufactured locally or imported into Korea. There are two types of pre-market licenses. One is the pre-market approval for Class II, III and IV devices and the other is the pre-market notification for Class I devices except those that have sterile and/or measurement function.

Pre-market approval for Class II, III and IV devices requires a Technical File Review, Safety and Efficacy Review (SER may be required for devices with new to market features) and Type Testing, while pre-market notification requires only an upload the to KFDA Electronic Filing System (KiFDA system, only Korean version) with product information (no testing is required).

A Technical File Review is a general technical file review, similar to the common submission dossier template (CSDT) or summary technical documentation (STED), for those products that are basically the same as an already approved product, whereas a Safety and Effectiveness Review (SER) is required for devices unlike those currently available on the market. The KFDA now conducts a Technical File Review on all Class II, III and IV products and excludes Class I devices. However, the KFDA authorized the rights to conduct a Technical File Review to six reviewing agencies — Korea Testing Laboratory (KTL), Korea Testing Certification (KTC), Korea Conformity Laboratories (KCL), Korea Testing & Research Institute (KTR), TÜV SÜD Korea and SGS Korea — for all Class II devices from 8 April 2012.

Also, the KFDA has registered 13 domestic laboratories, including KTL, to perform "Type Testing" on medical devices for electrical and mechanical tests, electromagnetic compatibility (EMC) test and/or bio-compatibility tests (*in vivo, in vitro*). However, they have limitations regarding the scope of medical devices they can test; so identifying laboratories appropriate for testing specific devices is essential. The 13 laboratories are listed in Section 31.2.11. Furthermore, the KFDA may accept other laboratories' type test reports if the test has been carried out at the laboratory accredited by International Laboratory Accredition Cooperation (ILAC), Asia Pacific Laboratory Accredition Cooperation (APLAC), Korea Laboratory Accreditation Scheme (KOLAS) and similar schemes under ISO/IEC 17025 Standard from 8 April 2012 [10].

Details can be found at the KFDA English home page: http://www.kfda.go.kr/eng/index.do?nMenuCode=7.

31.2.3 KGMP: Quality Management System

The KFDA had operated KGMP audit system, almost identical to the ISO 13485:2003 requirements, utilizing four audit agencies, including the KTL and the Medical Device Quality Division of the KFDA, to oversee the medical device manufacturer's quality management system for manufacturers of all classes of products, and the Korea Good Importing Practices (KGIP) had been applied to the importer using limited requirements of ISO 13485 up to now. However, to fulfil the requirements of Medical Device Act, the KFDA conducted the pilot KGMP audit at sites of foreign manufacturers in 2010 to 2011 and started the expansion of the KGMP audit to foreign manufacturing sites except those manufacturing Class I devices. Then, the audit began for Class IV device manufacturing sites on 8 April 2012. It will be extended to Class II and III devices subsequently. However, 66 Class I devices, including single-use urine flow meter, shall fall under KGMP, and KGIP for importers has included in the instructions for importer obedience.

An Asian company that wants to obtain KGMP certification shall apply to the one of the four third-party quality system audit agencies. These agencies do not solely perform the entire audit but accompany the KFDA medical device surveillance officer during much of their work. The GMP Certificate is issued by official seals of the audit agency president and KFDA commissioner. The process takes about one month from application and costs approximately $500/man-day, depending on the size of the manufacturing site. The certificate is valid for three years. Expenses for overseas travel and interpreters for KGMP auditors will be borne by the beneficiary (manufacturer or importer).

Three documents are required to get a device registered in Korea:

1. A product license;
2. KGMP certification;
3. Business license (manufacturing and/or importing),

Of these, the KGMP certification must be renewed every three years, and the other two are valid permanently, although major changes may require re-registration. But, the KFDA is considering the induction of license renewal system according to the Medical Device Act. Despite this, it is still a matter of dispute between the KFDA and industries.

As of December 2011, KGMP requirements have been changed. The program features include a requirement that manufacturers need KGMP certification for each product group shown in Table 31.3, and the certification will be in effect for three years. Importers should apply for GMP certification on behalf of overseas manufacturers if they have new development devices or new manufacturing site or if there were quality issues. The audit agency expects to take one month from the date of initial application to coordinate and schedule an audit, accompanied by a medical device surveillance officer from the KFDA. The KGMP audit is carried out on the following 25 product groups [1]:

Table 31.3 Product groups for which KGMP certification is required

1	General treatment device	6	Diagnostic device	11	*In vitro* diagnostic device	16	Sight corrective lens	21	*In vitro* medical supplies
2	Surgical device	7	Stimulating device for medical use	12	Speculums for medical use	17	Hearing aid	22	Contraceptive device
3	Medical chamber	8	Operational device	13	Treatment device for medical use	18	Medicinal sub-stance producing equipment	23	Alloy for dental use
4	Life-sustaining device	9	Patient transport	14	Syringe and puncture	19	Implants	24	Treatment material for dental use
5	Artificial internal organ apparatus	10	Measuring equipment for biological phenomena	15	Treatment device for dental use	20	Human tissue or organ substitute	25	Analyzing products (reagents) for *in vitro* diagnosis

Source: KFDA Notice, December 2011.

Medical devices are divided into four classes, with Class I being lowest risk and Class IV being highest risk, a strict system of 2,139 classifications segments devices, including 64 IVD device reagents and 16 U-healthcare. If a product is not listed in the Korean system, the company should contact the Medical Device Evaluation Department of the KFDA and ask for a classification determination via the website or phone. KFDA may take up to 10 days to process the request (http://emed.kfda.go.kr) [16].

Table 31.4 Treatment days for the services performed by KFDA

Services	Treatment days
Manufacture (import) business license	25
Technical file review	55
Technical file change review	32
Safety-efficacy review	70
Manufacture (import) product license	10
Manufacture (import) product notification	10
Clinical trial plan recognition	30

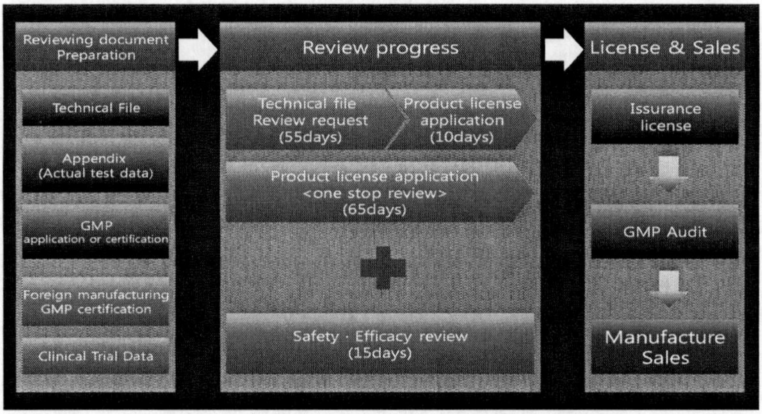

Figure 31.3 Flow chart of medical device-related affairs [11].

31.2.4 Product Notification: Class I Devices

The procedure for Class I devices is relatively simple: only notification is required, not approval. The applicant simply submits a standard notification to the one of the six regional KFDAs, depending on the applicant's residential district. This notification includes information on the product, its manufacturer or importer, its classification, purpose of use, instructions for use, raw materials and specifications, dimensional drawings, precautions and the labelling to be used. Once it is submitted, the regional KFDA will issue an acceptance letter, which is equivalent to a product license in this case [2].

(Processing time: 10 days, fee: approximately $35)

31.2.5 Product License: Class II, III, and IV Devices

Class II, III, and IV devices need to go through a full review and approval process. Approval in the country of origin can speed up the process somewhat but is not sufficient for product registration in Korea. On the other hand, some progress in efficiency has been made by the admission of third-party review organizations into the process. The two main requirements for a product license are a technical file and type testing. In case of Class II devices, the six regional KFDAs can issue the product license beginning 17 June 2011 [9, 10].

31.2.6 Technical File

The first requirement for a product license in case of Class II, III, and IV devices is the submission of a technical file, which falls into two categories:

- The general technical file's requirements are broadly similar to the CSDT or STED requirements. It is used when a similar device already has been approved. There is a one-page application form that contains much of the same material as in the notification form for Class I devices, but others require additional attachments detailing further information. These attachments include information on physical and chemical characteristics, electrical safety and performance, among others, all supported by test reports.
- The SER technical file is required for more novel devices. Besides the general file requirements, it includes information on the development process, stability reports and comparative analysis with other devices. In addition, it requires clinical study reports [16].

31.2.7 Clinical Trials

The KFDA accepts foreign clinical trials for approval, perhaps not necessarily needing local ones, but there are criteria for consideration of these trials. They must be published in a prominent medical journal (the Science Citation Index is one arbiter of prominence), or else they must have been accepted by the government of the country of manufacture for its own approval procedure. In the latter case, documentation of that acceptance in the foreign country should be attached [16].

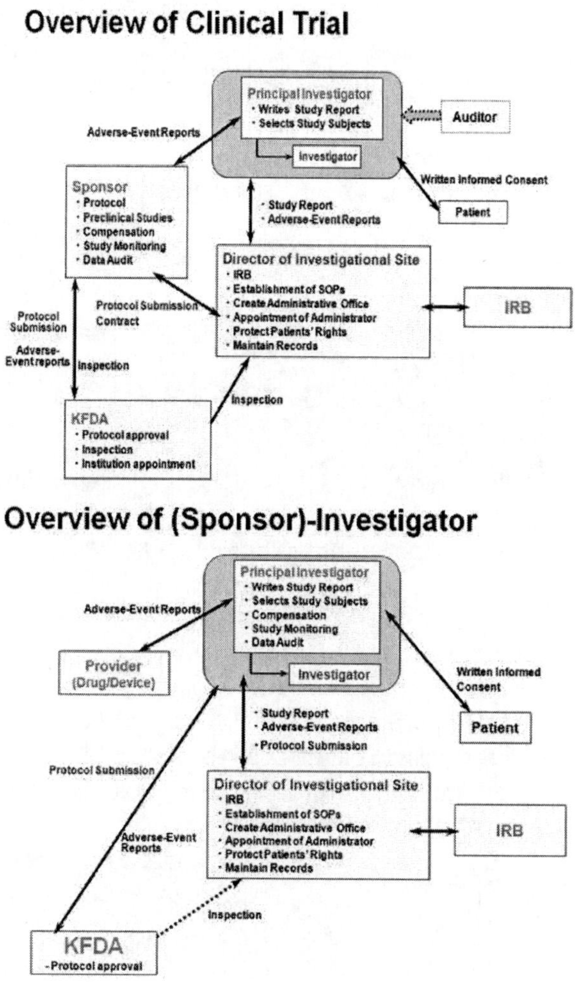

Figure 31.4 Clinical trial process.

Clinical trials are only required as a rule for SER technical files, but the KFDA also may require them at its discretion for general technical files.

31.2.8 Device Notification/License

The technical file must be reviewed and approved before go through. If it is a Class II device and does not require an SER file, a third-party organization can do this. A review by the third-party organization takes only about one month (about $1,200/item). However, the technical file of Class III and IV devices shall be reviewed by the KFDA, not any third-party organization (about $150/item).

Following are general requirements for registering all medical devices in Korea:

- local distributor (Korean importers or Korea registered subsidiary of the foreign supplier rather than the foreign manufacturer/supplier) shall apply for and serve as legal holders of the registration
- technical file
- notarized GMP certificates for the time being (sooner and later KGMP needed)
- raw material specifications and standards
- catalogues/brochures

Additional requirements, according to product class, are as follows:

Class I medical devices require only pre-market notification, which involves

- classifying the device
- the submission of form (to be completed by Korean importer) including
  - local importer information (company name, address and device business license number)
  - local company representative and his/her resident registration number
  - trade name, product name and classification name of device
  - raw materials
  - manufacturing methods
  - dimensional drawings

- specifications of finished product
- packaging unit
- instructions and precautions for use
- labelling
- foreign manufacturers' company name

The notification process would be completed easily if the above information is uploaded to KiFDA online system on the KFDA home page (no English information service currently) (http://emed.kfda.go.kr).

Class II, III, and IV medical devices require pre-market approval, which involves

- classifying the devices
- refer to following items

31.2.9 Technical File Review

- Prepare a Form of Medical Device Technical File Review Request including
    - local importer's company name, address and device business license number; local company representative and his/her resident registration number
    - foreign manufacturer's company name, address and country of manufacture
    - product, model, and classification names of devices
    - external appearance, internal structure, size
    - manufacturing methods
    - effectiveness, performance and purpose of use
    - packaging units
    - storage conditions, validity period
    - standard and test standard
    - labelling

In addition to submitting the form to the KFDA for Class III and IV devices and to one of the six technical file review (TFR) agencies, including the KTL for Class II device, a cover page and an attachment with a description of each supporting document are required. These documents include

- bench test reports
- clinical trial reports

- reference photocopies
- relevant literature
- information on physical/chemical characteristics
- information on electric/mechanical safety
- information on biological safety
- information on radiation safety
- information on electromagnetic compatibility
- rationales and test reports to confirm safety and product performance

During the technical file review, the KFDA may require a Safety and Efficacy Review (SER) for products with new-to-market features in terms of materials, mechanisms of action, usage or effectiveness.

An SER application includes the following additional information:

- information on origin, discovery, and background of development
- characteristics of devices
- stability data
- information on use in foreign countries
- comparative analysis with similar products previously approved in the market
- clinical study report (most important part of SER)

Other items:

- The local clinical study is not important if foreign clinical data is strong enough to demonstrate safety and efficacy.
- The KFDA will accept foreign clinical data if published in a Science Citation Index (SCI) listed journal of if the foreign government regulator has approved the clinical report, and documentation is provided [6].

31.2.10 Type Testing (Mandatory for Class II, III, and IV Devices)

Besides the technical file, the other important requirement for a product license is type testing. Only third-party laboratories do this, not the KFDA. It requires submission of samples and the technical file. Although the technical file has not yet been officially approved, a draft technical file can be submitted instead. Type testing takes from one to three months, with fees ranging from $3,000 to $10,000, all depending on the type of device. At the completion of testing, the laboratory issues a test report to show its compliance with the requirements of the technical file to the applicant.

To lower fees and review time, it also is possible to submit equivalent test reports done abroad and have them validated for a fee of approximately $800. However, the foreign testing must meet certain international standards and should come from the laboratory accredited by ISO/IEC 17025 standard according to ILAC, APLAC or IECEE/CB Scheme [2].

Once the product passes the technical file review, the technical review phase, it must undergo type testing (i.e. a KFDA-registered laboratory tests the product or makes a determination that, based on acceptable foreign data, the product does not require local testing in Korea):

- A firm can initiate type testing before or during the technical file review process.
- The testing must be done by a KFDA-registered third-party laboratory or accredited laboratories.
- Generally it takes one to three months, depending on the nature of type testing done.
- The Company must submit a copy of the draft or approved technical file, foreign test results (if available) and test sample(s) to the laboratory.
- Importers must file Form to receive exemption to import unapproved devices for testing.

Required information includes

- candidate importer and manufacturer
- product name
- necessary quantity
- name of test laboratory asked to carry out testing

Type test reports requested

- **bio-compatibility tests**
    - Tests conducted must be carried out to meet ISO, ASTM and GLP standards.
- **electrical and mechanical safety tests**
    - All testing must meet IEC standards.

- To be exempted from local testing, IEC test reports must be submitted in the "IECEE-CB Scheme" TRF.
- CB certificate and test reports must be certified by a national certification Body and CB testing laboratory.

- **EMC tests**
  - All testing must meet IEC/CISPR standards.
  - To be exempt from local testing, IEC test reports must be submitted in the "IECEE-CB Scheme" TRF.
  - CB certificate and test reports must be certified by a national certification body and CB testing laboratory.
- **performance tests**
  - A full description of test protocols, acceptance criteria, etc., is required.
  - Raw data may be required on a case-by-case basis.
  - Signatures of laboratory technicians and supervisors are required.
  - Notarized test reports are required.

31.2.11 KFDA-Registered 13 Laboratories

Table 31.5 List of KFDA-registered laboratories

No.	Registered laboratory	Areas of expertise
1	Korea Testing Laboratory (KTL)	All medical devices
2	Korea Testing Certification (KTC)	34 product groups, including implants and supplies
3	Korea Testing & Research Institute (KTR)	39 product groups, Except EMC test for only X-ray equipment
4	Korea Conformity Laboratories (KCL)	13 product groups, including medical supplies
5	Seoul National University Hospital Clinical Research Institute	13 product groups, including implanted medical devices and supplies
6	Yonsei University Hospital Medical Technology Evaluation Center	11 product groups, including implanted medical devices and supplies
7	Yonsei University Dental College Dental Devices Testing & Evaluation Center	Dental materials only

8	Kyung-Hee University, Testing & Development Center for Dental Materials.	Dental materials only
9	Kyungpook National University Institute for Bio Materials Research and Development Dental Materials Testing & Evaluation Center (KDMTEC)	Dental materials only
10	Seoul National University, Dental Hospital, Clinic Dental Research Institute	Dental materials only
11	Korea Workers' Compensation & Welfare Service	6 product group, including wheelchairs
12	Korea Institute of Medical Technology (KIMT)	19 product group, including medical instruments
13	Korea Institute of Medical Device Assessment (KIMDA)	13 product group, including medical instruments

Source: KFDA Web site, November 2011.

31.2.12 Applying for a Product License

Once both technical file review and type testing are complete, the approved technical file and a certificate of KGMP or application copy of KGMP must be submitted to the KFDA or regional KFDA using Appendix No. 3 KFDA form. After reviewing all of these, the KFDA issues a product license, which does not expire. The submittal is available to use the KFDA Internet, KiFDA system (Korean version) (http://emed.kfda.go.kr)

(Duration of processing: 10 to 80 days; fee: about $42 to $400: depending on the case) [2]

31.2.13 Business License

There are two types of product license for the manufacturer and the importer, and this business license can be obtained by submitting one product license and other information on the company (business registration and health certificate for its representative) to one of the six regional KFDAs beginning 17 June 2011. The form is required to receive a certificate of product approval from the KFDA. It does not expire. Of course, an importer typically would have such a license already for other products.

(Processing time: 25 days; fee: approximately $140) [2]

31.2.14 Audit of Quality Management System (KGMP Certification)

Manufacturers of Classes II, III, and IV devices must be audited and certified by category for their quality management system according to KGMP requirements, mostly identical with ISO 13485, before entering into the Korean market. Class I device manufacturers are excluded from the KGMP certification, with effect from 8 April 2012, except 66 products. Instead of that, foreign manufacturers of Classes II, III, and IV devices should be audited on site by Korean auditors for their quality systems from 2012. Then, the manufacturers must be re-certified every three years.

Twenty-five KGMP product groups are listed in Section 31.2.3. Firms apply for KGMP certification using one of the KFDA-designated quality system audit agencies (KTL, KCL, KTC, and KTR). The third-party organization coordinates with the KFDA and sets audit dates. The agency normally takes one month from the application date to audit a firm [1, 3, 8].

31.2.15 Post-Market Surveillance System

The regulatory areas of post-market surveillance currently being performed by the officials of the Medical Device Management Division of the KFDA include plans for periodic re-testing, re-evaluation, re-call, control of advertisement contents and adverse events caused by a certain device in the market.

The KFDA is operating the PMS connect with the GMP audit basically, which is called the regular monitoring system. The GMP auditor may can pick up the sample, if it is doubtful, at the manufacturing site and then request that it be tested at one of the registered laboratories.

As the tracking and the management criteria, a person who intends to report matters concerning adverse side effects of the a medical device under Paragraph 1 and 2 of Article 31 of the Medical Device Act shall report within seven days, if the medical device caused death or a life-threatening adverse event. In this case, details shall be additionally reported within eight days from the date of initial reporting. Also, according to criteria and procedure for the recall of harmful medical devices requiring recall, the required recaller shall may submit a recall plan to the KFDA within 5–15 days. The expected end date of the recall shall be within 30 days from the start of recall [5].

31.3 Importer's Note

31.3.1 Import Labelling

Key information that must appear on the device container in Korean includes

- business name and address of a manufacturer or importer
- source of origin (name of manufacturer(s) and the country of manufacture) in case of an imported device
- product name, type name (model name), product license or notification number
- manufacturing (lot or batch) number and date of manufacture
- weight or packing unit

31.3.2 Import Packaging

Key information that should appear on the outside packaging is the same as on the product label; packaging inserts should have the following information:

- directions and precautions for use
- information on technical maintenance
- information required by the KFDA commissioner
- other information required in the Ministerial Decree of the MOHW

31.3.3 Import Documentation

All application forms submitted to the KFDA and to testing laboratories must be written in **Korean**.

In addition, developing a constructive relationship with an experienced Korean importer is also important, as most responsible Korean officials do not understand English well. It is also necessary to cultivate solid relationships with experienced regulatory professionals and government officials during the approval process.

All medical device classes require the following:

- device business license (either for local manufacturer or import distributor)
- KGMP certification except for Class I device

Class I medical devices also are required the notification to the regional KFDA and the submission of a form via KiFDA online system of the KFDA home page (see Section 31.2.8). Once product approval is received and a business license is obtained, the device can be introduced into the Korean market. If an importer has already obtained a business license for a company, it does not have to go through the process again for subsequent medical devices brought into Korea.

Class II, III, and IV devices must go through the following additional steps:

- Technical file review; two types are possible:
    - Technical file review, when a device is basically same as previously approved products
    - Safety and efficacy review, when a device significantly different from previously approved products
- Type testing, by KFDA-registered laboratories; test reports by accredited laboratories may also be accepted

Once these things are completed, a product license is issued, either a manufacturer license or an importer license.

31.3.4 Other Agencies

- The Health Insurance Reimbursement & Assessment Service (**HIRA**), which accepts and reviews applications for reimbursement approvals submitted by device manufacturers (http://www.hira.or.kr/cms/rb/rbb_english/12/12_01/social.html)
- The National Health Insurance Corporation (**NHIC**), which collects premiums and pays hospitals and pharmacies (http://www.nhic.or.kr/english/main.html)
- The Korea Testing Laboratory, which is the only accredited laboratory performing type testing for all 39 categories of

medical devices available in the marketplace (http://www.ktl.re.kr/eng/team/medical.asp)

31.3.5 Medical Device Advertisements

The Korea Medical Device Industry Association (KMDIA) has conducted the screening of medical device advertisements on behalf of the KFDA according to Article 25 of the Medical Device Act and Article 29 of the Enforcement Regulation from April 2007. The Screening Committee of medical device advertisement reviews and deliberates on the advertisement contents, if in general, they are accessible by the general public through newspapers, the Internet, magazines, TV and radio on every 10 days according to the request of clients. The review fee is approximately $88/item (http://eng.kmdia.or.kr/) [17].

31.3.6 Contacts

Asian firms wishing to learn more about regulatory issues related to medical devices in Korea are encouraged to contact the following agencies for additional information:

Korea Food and Drug Administration

Policy part: Medical Device Policy Division
Medical Device Safety Bureau
Korea Food and Drug Administration
Osong Health technology Administration Complex,
187 Osong saengmyeong 2-ro, Gangoe-myeon, Cheongwon-gun, Chungcheongbuk-do, 363-951, Republic of Korea
http://www.kfda.go.kr/eng/index.do
Phone: +82 43 719 3704/Fax: +82 43 719 3700

Technical part: Cardiac Vascular Device Division
Medical Device Evaluation Department
Medical Device Safety Bureau
Korea Food and Drug Administration
Osong Health technology Administration Complex,

187 Osong saengmyeong 2-ro, Gangoe-myeon,
Cheongwon-gun, Chungcheongbuk-do, 363-951,
Republic of Korea
http://www.kfda.go.kr/eng/index.do
Phone: +82 43 719 3902/Fax: +82 43 719 3900

Once the Device Business License, Product License and KGMP Certification have been obtained, it is finally legal to market a medical device in South Korea. Beyond the regulatory permission, there are other important processes as well, such as obtaining reimbursement from Korea's national health insurance system, as well as post-market surveillance requirements.

Dealing with the Korean regulatory structure can be tricky and requires expertise on the ground. Communication and consultation with officials is necessary at many processing stages, and officials will not well discuss applications in English directly. However, these are not reasons to stay away — but reasons to be deliberate and patient in entering this active market.

Also, Asian applicants can find the Korean laws and regulations (English version) at http://www.kfda.go.kr/medicaldevice/index.do?nMenuCode=104.

Asian companies also may contact to following address for the regulations-related policies and technical parts:

Medical Device Evaluation Center
Medical Device Group
Korea Testing Laboratory (KTL)
87, Digital 26-gil, Guro-gu, Seoul, 152-718, Korea
http://www.ktl.re.kr/eng/
Phone: + 82 2 8601 620/Fax: +82 2 8601 619

References

1. KFDA (2012.1), Training textbook for newly changed Medical Device Regulations, KFDA.
2. KFDA (2012.1), Commentary for KFDA Notice of Medical Device License, Notification and Audit.
3. KFDA (2011.12), Revised Notice for Medical Device Manufacturing, Importing and Quality System Requirements, KFDA.
4. KFDA (2011.4), Medical Device Act, KFDA.
5. KFDA (2011.4), Enforcement Regulation of the Medical Device, KFDA.

6. KFDA (2010.12), KFDA Notice for Medical Device Product and Classification, KFDA.
7. Dal-Ho Lim (2011.12), Principal Researcher of KHIDI, The analysis report of medical device industry on 2011, Korea Health Industry Development Institute (KHIDI)/Korea.
8. Peter Lee (2011.12), KTL, The understanding for the global GMP system, Korea Testing Laboratory.
9. Sang-Soo Park and Peter Lee (2011.12), Eulji University/KTL, Korea Medical Device Regulations learning by English, Publisher A-Chim/ Korea.
10. Sang-Soo Park and Peter Lee (2009.8), KTL, Korea Medical Device Regulations, Jungmungak/Korea.
11. Yang-Ha Cho (2010.11), KFDA, Medical Device License Review & Improvement status in Korea.
12. Ji-Un Choi (2010.11), KFDA, 2010 Medical Device Safety Policy in Korea.
13. Ames Gross and John Minot, Medical Device Registration in Korea: An Overview. Retrieved December 2011, from http://www.mpo-mag.com/articles/2007/05/medical-device-registration-in-korea-an-overview.
14. Emergo Group, Retrieved: December 2011, from: www.emergogroup.com.
15. International Trade Administration, Medical Device Regulatory Requirements for South Korea. Retrieved December 2011, from http://www.ita.doc.gov/td/health/korearegs.htm.
16. KFDA, Retrieved December 2011, from http://www.kfda.go.kr/medicaldevice/index.do.
17. Korea Medical Device Industry Association. Retrieved December 2011, from http://eng.kmdia.or.kr.
18. Wikipedia. Retrieved December 2011, from http://en.wikipedia.org/wiki/Korea.

Chapter 32

Malaysia: Medical Device Regulatory System

Yean Ting Ong

Johnson & Johnson Sdn Bhd, G.01, Block B, 10 Jalan Bersatu 13/4, 46200 Petaling Jaya, Malaysia

yong1@its.jnj.com

Disclaimer

The regulatory information contained in this chapter is intended for market planning and is subject to change frequently. Translations of laws and regulations are unofficial.

32.1 Market Overview[1]

Malaysia's medical devices and supplies are mainly imported, especially the more technologically advanced items. The Malaysian

[1] Information for this section was generously provided by Johnson & Johnson Medical, Malaysia.

Handbook of Medical Device Regulatory Affairs in Asia
Edited by Jack Wong and Raymond K. Y. Tong

ISBN 978-981-4411-21-9 (Hardcover), 978-981-4411-22-6 (eBook)
www.panstanford.com

market for medical equipment and supplies was estimated to be worth US$ 1,089 million in 2010. Malaysia spends 11.6% of total health expenditure on medical equipment and supplies — around 0.5% of GDP.

Malaysia's major natural resource is rubber, and the country's exports are dominated by latex products such as surgical gloves and catheters, which together accounted for around 47.0% of the export total in 2008. The share of these two sub-categories have slowly started to diminish with the steady growth of diagnostic imaging exports in recent years, particularly electrocardiographs and other electrodiagnostic apparatus.

There is currently no mandatory registration for medical devices, but this is expected to change by end of 2012, along with the other related regulations involving production and importation of medical devices, including surveillance and monitoring with the gazettement of the Medical Device Act 2012 (Act 737) and the Medical Device Authority Act 2012 (Act 738) on February 9, 2012. Accordingly, this act will come into operation on a date to be appointed by the Minister of Health Malaysia as provided under Section 1 (2) of the Medical Device Act 2012 by way of a notification in the Gazette.

32.2 Regulating Authority

The Medical Device Authority Act 2011 provides for the establishment of the Medical Device Authority to control and regulate medical devices and the medical device industry and its activities and to enforce the medical device laws, and for related matters.

The authority shall consist of the following members:

(a) the Director General of Health as the chairman
(b) the chief executive
(c) a representative of the Ministry of Finance
(d) a representative of the Ministry of Health
(e) not more than five persons with expertise and experience in medical device-related matters to be appointed by the Minister

32.3 Definition of Medical Device

A "medical device" means

(a) any instrument, apparatus, implement, machine, appliance, implant, *in vitro* reagent or calibrator, software, material or other similar or related article intended by the manufacturer to be used, alone or in combination, for human beings for the purpose of

  (i) diagnosis, prevention, monitoring, treatment or alleviation of disease

  (ii) diagnosis, monitoring, treatment, alleviation of or compensation for an injury

  (iii) investigation, replacement or modification, or support of the anatomy or of a physiological process

  (iv) support or sustaining life

  (v) control of conception

  (vi) disinfection of medical device

  (vii) providing information for medical or diagnostic purpose by means of *in vitro* examination of specimens derived from the human body,

which does not achieve its primary intended action in or on the human body by pharmacological, immunological or metabolic means, but that may be assisted in its intended function by such means and

(b) any instrument, apparatus, implement, machine, appliance, implant, *in vitro* reagent or calibrator, software, material or other similar or related article, to be used on the human body, which the Minister may, after taking into consideration issues of public safety, public health or public risk, declare to be a medical device by order published in the Gazette.

32.4 Classification of Medical Devices

Medical Devices are classified into four classes based on risk. The classification is aligned with the Global Harmonization Task Force (GHTF) classification system and is determined from

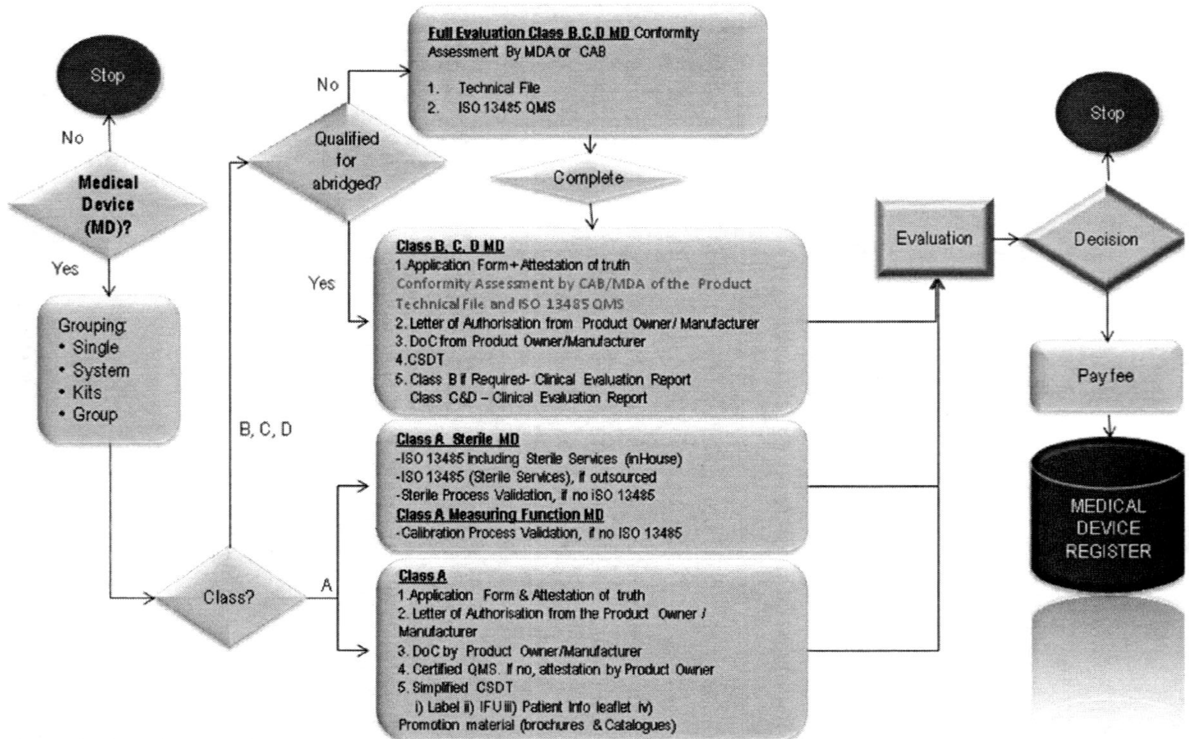

Figure 32.1 Registration route.

- the manufacturer's intended purpose for the medical device
- a set of classification rules; these rules will classify medical devices into one the four classes of medical devices

Table 32.1 General classification system for medical devices for the four risk classes of devices

GHTF	Malaysia class	Risk level	Device examples
I	A	Low risk	Surgical retractors/tongue depressors
II	B	Low-moderate risk	Hypodermic needle/suction equipment
III	C	Moderate-high risk	Lung ventilator/orthopedic implants
IV	D	High risk	Heart valves/implantable defibrillator

Note: The examples given are for illustration only and the manufacturer must apply the classification rules to each medical device according to its intended purpose.

32.5 Registration of Medical Devices

An abridged process is available for devices that have been approved by recognized regulatory bodies such as US Food and Drug Administration, European Union, Therapeutic Goods Administration (Australia), Therapeutic Products (Canada), and Japanese authorities. These devices will still need to go through the local registration process via the abridge evaluation route. Registration is online; however, hardcopies of documents may have to be provided if requested. Time to approval has not been determined.

Medical devices that have not been approved by the recognized authorities/regulators have to go through a conformity assessment process. The risk level of the device determines the stringency of the conformity assessment.

32.5.1 Market Environment

There is a wide range of medical devices, from a simple medical device to a highly complex and sophisticated medical device. The various components can be sold as a separate component, individual customized pack, or group and can be categorized as SINGLE, FAMILY, IVD TEST KIT, SYSTEM, and SET. Each of the categories mentioned can be submitted in the medical device registration application.

Medical devices that can be grouped into one of the following five categories can be submitted in one application for product registration and listing in the Malaysia Medical Device Register (MMDR):

- SINGLE
- FAMILY
- IVD TEST KIT
- SYSTEM
- SET

Three basic rules must all be fulfilled for the grouping to apply:

- one generic proprietary name
- one manufacturer
- one common intended purpose

For the purpose of grouping, the corporate headquarters may be regarded as the manufacturer for its subsidiaries and regional manufacturing sites.

For example, TRS MDB ORTHOPAEDIC SYSTEM consists of the following constituent components (see Fig. 32.2):

- Instruments from ABC Bhd (a subsidiary of TRS MDB Malaysia)
- Instruments from XYZ Bhd (a subsidiary of TRS MDB Mexico),
- Plates from TRS MDB Mexico; and
- Screws from TRS MDB China

For the purpose of grouping, the manufacturer of TRS ORTHOPAEDIC SYSTEM will be TRS MDB Malaysia (Headquarters).

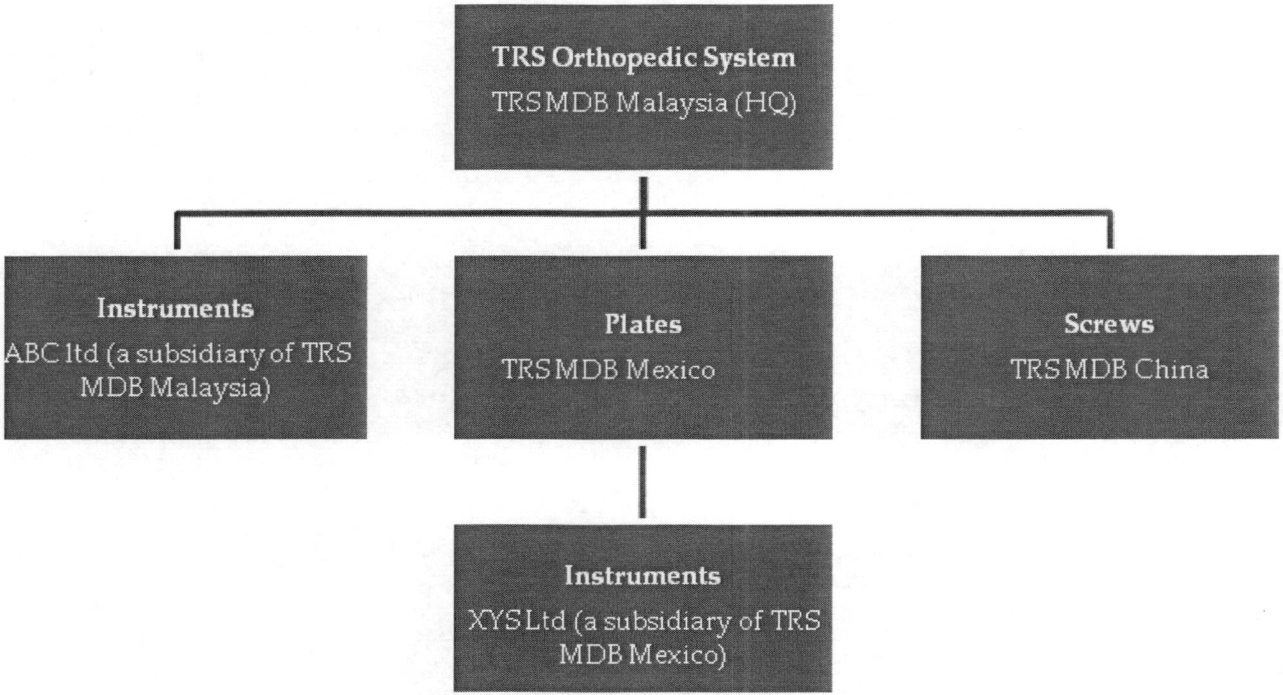

Figure 32.2 Example of referencing the headquarters as the manufacturer for the purpose of grouping.

32.5.2 Conformity Assessment Process

Table 32.2 Requirements

Class	(Full QMS or QMS-design + PMS system) or (Full QMS + PMS system)	Product verification	Technical documentation	Declaration of conformity	Registration and licensing
Class A	Establish and maintain		Prepare and make available upon request	Prepare (and sign) and submit for review/verification	Perform according to requirements
Class A (S)	Establish and maintain	Prepare and make available upon request	Prepare and make available upon request	Prepare (and sign) and submit for review/verification	Perform according to requirements
Class A (M)	Establish and maintain	Prepare and make available upon request	Prepare and make available upon request	Prepare (and sign) and submit for review/verification	Perform according to requirements
Class B	Establish and maintain		Prepare (and sign) and submit for review/verification	Prepare (and sign) and submit for review/verification	Perform according to requirements
Class C	Establish, maintain, and make available for audit		Prepare (and sign) and submit for review/verification	Prepare (and sign) and submit for review/verification	Perform according to requirements
Class D	Establish, maintain, and make available for audit		Prepare (and sign) and submit for review/verification	Prepare (and sign) and submit for review/verification	Perform according to requirements

32.5.3 Combination Products

Definition: A combination product includes

- a product comprising two or more regulated components, i.e., drug/device, biological/device, drug/biological, or drug/device/biological, that are physically, chemically, or otherwise combined or mixed and produced as a single entity
- two or more separate products packaged together in a single package or as a unit and comprising drug and device products, device and biological products, or biological and drug products
- a drug, device or biological product packaged separately that according to its investigational plan or proposed labeling is intended for use only with an approved individually specified drug, device, or biological product where both are required to achieve the intended use, indication, or effect and where upon approval of the proposed product the labeling of the approved product would need to be changed, e.g., to reflect a change in intended use, dosage form, strength, route of administration, or significant change in dose
- any investigational drug, device, or biological product packaged separately that according to its proposed labeling is for use only with another individually specified investigational drug, device, or biological product where both are required to achieve the intended use, indication, or effect

For combination products, both the National Pharmaceutical Control Bureau and the Medical Device Authority will evaluate the relevant sections.

32.6 Post-Market Surveillance and Vigilance

32.6.1 Mandatory Reporting

An establishment shall report to the Authority any incident that comes to the establishment's attention occurring inside or outside Malaysia that

(a) is related to the failure of the medical device or a deterioration in its effectiveness, or any inadequacy in its labeling or in its instructions for use and such report shall be made within thirty days from the discovery

(b) has led to the death or serious deterioration in the state of health of a patient, user or other person, or could do so were the incident to recur and such report shall be made within 10 days from the discovery

(c) is a serious threat to public health and such report shall be made within 48 hours from the discovery.

Any person who contravenes subsection (1) commits an offence and shall, on conviction, be liable to a fine not exceeding 200000 ringgit or to imprisonment for a term not exceeding two years or to both.

32.6.2 Field Corrective Action

An establishment shall undertake corrective or preventive action in relation to a medical device imported and placed in the market which may include

(a) the return of the medical device to the establishment
(b) modification of the medical device
(c) exchange of the medical device
(d) destruction of the medical device
(e) specific advice on the use of the medical device

32.6.3 Recall

An establishment may recall any defective medical device at any time. The establishment shall, on or before undertaking a recall of the medical device, provide information as may be specified by the Authority. The establishment shall, as soon as possible after the completion of a recall, report to the Authority the results of the recall and any action taken to prevent a recurrence of the problem. Notwithstanding the above, the Authority may order the establishment to recall any medical device at any time due to patient safety and public health.

32.6.4 Labeling

No guidelines have been announced for labeling requirements as yet.

32.7 Regulatory Action for Changes and Device Modifications

No guidelines have been announced for changes and device modifications as yet.

References

1. Laws of Malaysia Act 737 Medical Device act 2012.
2. Espicom Business Intelligence (Quarter II 2010) *A World Medical Device Market Report, Malaysia Medical Device Market Intelligence Report*, ISSN 2043–9792.
3. Medical Device Bureau, retrieved January 2012, from http://www.mdb.gov.my/mdb/.

Chapter 33

Philippines: Medical Device Regulatory and Licensing

Mary Claire Cacanindin[a] **and Jennifer Cheah**[b]

[a]*Johnson & Johnson Medical Philippines*
[b]*Johnson & Johnson Medical Singapore*

Ccacani1@its.jnj.com

Disclaimer

The information contained in this chapter is derived from public sources and is current to the best of our knowledge. For detailed and definitive information about a country's laws and policies, the government of the country concerned should be consulted.

33.1 Market Overview

Currently, the Philippines medical device market is valued at approximately $200 million. The Philippines's medical device market is predicted to increase at about 8–10% over the next several years. This growth will be mainly driven by imports,

Handbook of Medical Device Regulatory Affairs in Asia
Edited by Jack Wong and Raymond K. Y. Tong

ISBN 978-981-4411-21-9 (Hardcover), 978-981-4411-22-6 (eBook)
www.panstanford.com

healthcare expenditures, medical tourism, and the private sector. The largest buyers of medical devices are private hospitals.

While the country has some capacity to produce domestic products, imports account for 97% of the medical device market in the Philippines. Almost all sophisticated medical equipment is imported.

Industry sources indicate that the most popular products in the Philippines medical device market are in the diagnosis and treatment of heart and lung diseases, strokes, and kidney failures.

33.2 Regulatory Overview

By virtue of the Republic Act 3720 of 1963, known as the Food, Drug and Cosmetic Act, the Bureau of Food and Drugs was mandated to regulate the manufacture and distribution of food, drugs and cosmetics. In 1987, the President of the Philippines issued Executive Order No. 175, which amended RA3720, to include the regulation of medical devices in the mandated function of the Bureau of Food and Drug Administration (BFAD).

To provide more focus and attention to Medical device regulation, it was in 1999 when the Bureau of Health Devices and Technology (BHDT) was created to regulate medical devices upon issuance of Executive Order No. 102. However, the order has not fully given the BHDT the authority to accept and process registration applications and issue administrative orders relating to medical device registration.

When Republic Act No. 9711 was enacted into law in August 2009, the Philippine Food and Drug Administration (FDA) was created. It introduced a new FDA structure within the Department of Health (DOH) to strengthen the regulatory authority over food, drug, cosmetics, medical devices and other health devices.

The FDA Act created four centers:

(i) Centers for Drug Regulation and Research (to include Veterinary medicine, vaccines and biological)

(ii) Center for Food Regulation and Research

(iii) Center for Cosmetics Regulation and Research (to include household hazardous/urban substances)

(iv) Center for Device Regulation, Radiation Health, and Research

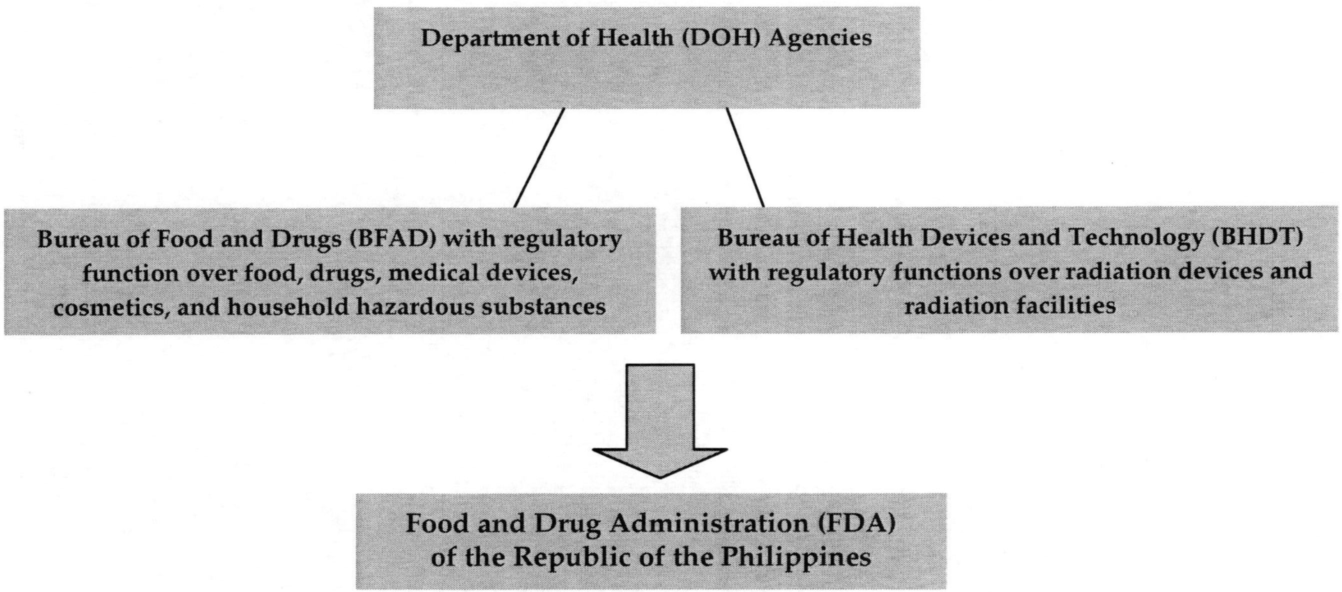

Figure 33.1 The FDA Act affects two existing DOH agencies.

In the Philippines, all foreign medical devices are required to undergo the same registration procedure, regardless of whether they have been previously registered in other countries. Medical equipment does not require pre-registration with BFAD, except for radiation-emitting equipment, which must first undergo local testing and is regulated by the BHDT within DOH. The BHDT will issue a pre-registration certification for radiation-emitting devices. However, distributors that market sterile or invasive medical devices are required to hold a license to operate in the Philippines and a Certificate of Product Registration (CPR) for all registrable products.

33.3 History of Medical Device Regulation

The original provision of Republic Act 3720 did not prohibit the manufacture or distribution, among others, of devices that are not registered in BFAD. With the promulgation, however, of Executive Order 175 on May 22, 1987, the said RA 3720 was amended making it unlawful to manufacture, import, export, sell, offer for sale, distribute or transfer devices that are not registered with the BFAD.

Because of the E.O. 1975 amendment, the registration of devices has become mandatory. Using the standards and requirements and requirements in the registration of drug producզts and in the licensing of drug establishments/outlets, establishments engaged in the manufacture, distribution, etc., of medical devices are issued license to operate and medical devices are given certificates of product registration.

The checklists of requirements for registration of medical devices and *in vitro* diagnostic products appear on 33.6 easy reference. The registration of devices or reagents is generally made subject to the following conditions.

- The device/reagent shall be made available only at drugstores and hospitals and in other medical devices to be used or sold only upon the written order of a practitioner licensed by law to use said device/reagent.
- The labeling of the immediate container of such device/ reagent shall state
    - the date (month and year) within which the device or reagent may be used,

- the lot or batch number of the device or reagent,
- BFAD registration number, and
- name and address of local agent.

There was yet, however, no specific rules or regulations governing medical devices. On January 3, 1991, the Bureau of Food and Drugs issued Memorandum Circular No. 1 series of 1991 to establish what devices should first be registered in BFAD before manufacture or distribution and what devices may not be registered. Any device that was not either in the list of registrable medical devices or in the list of medical devices will be deliberated upon by BFAD for inclusion in either of the two afore-stated lists on a case-to-case basis.

Although there had been efforts to define the coverage, scope, and extent of device regulation over medical devices, the formal issuance of these rules had been put on hold until the mandate to regulate medical devices had been fully transferred to the BHDT. By virtue of the Implementing Rules and Regulations of RA 9711, the definition of the medical device had been adopted based on the ACCSQ definition. To date, the following draft guidelines are being reviewed:

- Registration of Medical Devices
- Registration of IVDs
- Licensing of Distributor/Wholesaler/Importer/Exporter/Retailer
- Licensing of Manufacturer/Repacker/Trader
- Labeling Guidelines
- Advertisement
- Post-market Reporting
- Import Permit
- List of Registrable Products

33.4 Regional Medical Device Harmonization under Development through ASEAN

The Philippines is one of 10 members of the Association of Southeast Asian Nations (ASEAN). The BHDT is representing the Philippine medical device sector at meetings of the ASEAN Consultative Committee on Standards and Quality-Medical Device Product Working Group (ACCSQ-MDPWG — hereafter ACCSQ) (created in 2004), which has met 15 times over the past eight years, most recently in Phuket in April 2012. The working group is focusing on three main activities:

- a comparative study of medical device regulation across all ASEAN countries
- developing an ASEAN Common Submission Dossier Template (more on this initiative below)
- formulating a Post Market Alert System for unsafe and defective devices

The objective of the ACCSQ is to facilitate efforts to remove technical barriers to trade and implement the Common Effective Preferred Tariff to create an ASEAN-wide FTA in the next few years. The ACCSQ is making efforts for fast-track integration within 11 priority areas, including pharmaceutical products and medical devices, over the next few years.

Both the ACCSQ and the Asian Harmonization Working Party (AHWP — a subgroup of the Global Harmonization Task Force [GHTF]) intend to introduce a Common Submission Technical Dossier for application and approval of medical device products in each member country in the next few years (ACCSQ has implemented the CSDT format by calendar year 2008). The two groups have also separately adopted the GHTF medical device definition and classification system for regulating medical devices.

33.5 Definition of Medical Device in Philippines

The Philippines uses the GHTF Study Group 1 guidance document as the basis for its definition of medical devices

A medical device means any instrument, apparatus, implement, machine, appliance, implant, *in vitro* reagent or calibrator, software, material, or other similar or related article

(i) Intended by the manufacturer to be used, alone or in combination, for human beings for one or more of the specific purpose(s) of

- diagnosis, prevention, monitoring, treatment or alleviation of disease
- diagnosis, monitoring, treatment, alleviation of or compensation for an injury

- investigation, replacement, modification or support of the anatomy or of a physiological process, supporting or sustaining life
- control of conception
- disinfection of medical devices
- providing information for medical or diagnostic purposes by means of *in vitro* examination of specimens derived from the human body; and which does not achieve its primary intended action in or on the human body by pharmacological, immunological or metabolic means, but which may be assisted in its intended function by such means.

To explain further, medical devices range from a simple tongue depressor to a complicated MRI machine. Medical devices also included condoms, cottons, and test tubes. *In vitro* diagnostic devices or self-test tubes are also considered medical devices.

33.6 Registration with BFAD

33.6.1 License to Operate

Companies that are selling registrable medical devices should first apply for the License to Operate (LTO). The requirements for the application of the LTO can be downloaded from the DOH Web site (http://www.doh.gov.ph/node/398).

Only complete documents will be accepted during the application and will be scheduled for inspection.

If the company complies with the requirements and passed the inspection, a LTO will be issued. The company is given 60 days to comply with all the deficiencies. Non-compliance will result in temporary stoppage of the selling of medical devices.

The timeline given for the processing of the LTO is 90 days. This is considering that all the documents submitted are in compliance with the requirements and that the company passed the inspection.

Only complete documents will be accepted during the application. The application will be reviewed and evaluated if it is in accordance with the requirements. All complying applications will be issued a CPR. All non-complying applications will be issued a notice of deficiency. Each company is given a non-extendable 90 day compliance period. All those who will not be able to comply will be disapproved but will be given a period of 60 days to file for re-application and comply with all the deficiencies. In case after this period the application did not satisfactory comply all the requirements, the application will be disapproved and the company needs to file for initial application.

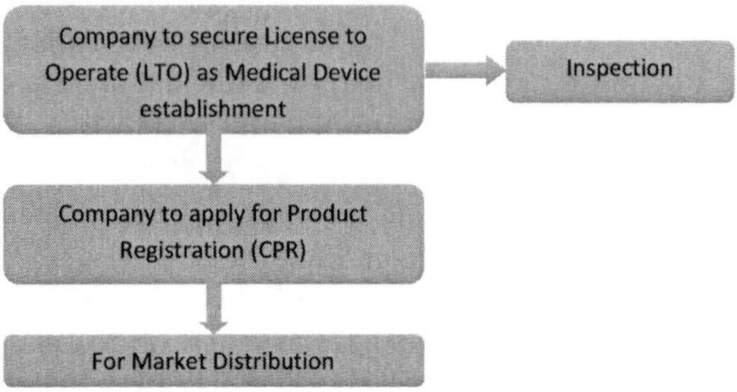

Figure 33.2 Process of registration for registrable products (mandatory).

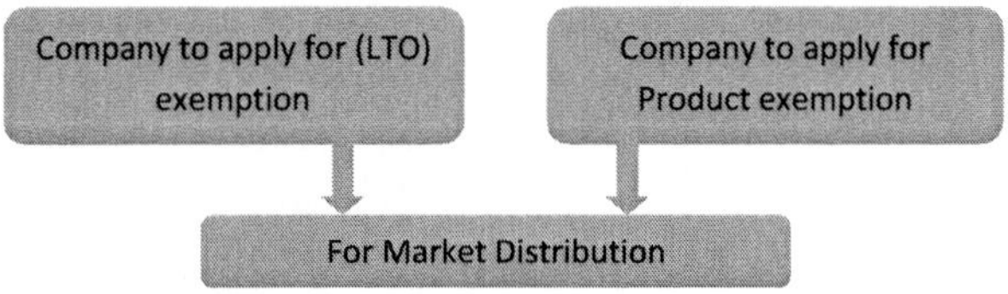

Figure 33.3 Process of registration for non-registrable products (voluntary).

The LTO is valid for one year initially followed by a two-year validity.

33.6.2 License to Operate: Requirements

- Accomplished notarized petition form/joint affidavit of undertaking
- List of medical device products to be imported/distributed
- Copies of Pharmacist's Board of Registration Certificate, PRC ID, valid PTR, ID picture, duties and responsibilities, certificate of attendance of the owner or pharmacist to a BFAD seminar on licensing of establishments
- Location plan and floor plan with dimensions

- For corporations, registration certificate with SEC and articles of incorporation or partnership
- For single proprietor, certificate of Business Name Registration with Bureau of Trade Regulation and Consumer Protection
- Contract of lease for the space of the office and storage to be occupied or any proof of ownership
- FAA duly authenticated by the Philippine Consular Office
- ISO/GMP of manufacturer
- Valid contract with BFAD licensed supplier/manufacturer
- Certification that products to be sold are registered with BFAD
- LTO of local distributor/manufacturer
- Copies of applicable laws
- Batch distribution record, product recall procedure

33.6.3 Certificate of Product Registration

The BFAD has issued the checklist of requirements for medical device registration. Only companies with valid LTO as medical device distributor-importer/wholesaler are qualified to file for product registration application.

The requirements for the application for CPR can be downloaded from the DOH Web site (http://www.doh.gov.ph/node/398).

The timeline given for the processing of a CPR is 90 days. This is considering that all the documents submitted are in compliance with the requirements. In cases there are deficiencies issued to the company, the counting of the timeline stops and will resume only upon submission of the compliance documents.

A Good Manufacturing Practices (GMP) certificate is sufficient to meet a requirement attesting to the status of a manufacturer selling in the Philippines.

A certificate for a Non-Registrable Product may be obtained if the medical device in question falls outside the scope of BHDT regulations. However, companies must submit the product description and brochure to BHDT in order to assess whether the product can be registered at all.

The validity period for initial registration of a medical device is one year. Under BFAD Circular #05, series of 1998, medical device renewal registrations are valid for five years.

33.6.4 Certificate of Product Registration: Technical Requirements

- Specific use and directions for use
- Copy of latest CPR
- List of amount and technical specifications of all raw materials.
- Brief description of the methods used, the facilities and control in the manufacture, processing and packaging of the product; for sterile products, include sterilization procedure
- Technical specification and physical description of the finished product
- Stability studies of the product and physical description of the finished product
- Labeling materials to be used for the product: immediate label, box label and package insert/brochures, if available.
- Representative sample in the market or commercial presentation (at least one of each size)
- Evidence of registration/payment (charge slip/official receipt)

33.6.5 Certificate of Product Registration: Legal Requirements

- Notarized Letter of Application from the manufacturer/trader/distributor
- Valid LTO of manufacturer/trader/importer/distributor/wholesaler
- Government Certificate of Clearance and Free Sale/Registration approval of the product from the country of origin issued by the health authority and duly authenticated by the territorial Philippine Consulate for the imported product
- Government Certificate attesting to the status of the manufacturer, competency and reliability of the personnel and facilities and duly authenticated by the territorial Philippine Consulate and/or valid ISO Certification for the imported product
- Certificate of agreement between the manufacturer and trader/distributor/importer regarding the product involved

33.7 Import Labeling

In addition to the international labeling requirements for medical devices, the BHDT requires that the labeling of the immediate container of such device/reagent states the following:

- the date (month and year) within which the device or reagent may be used
- the lot or batch number of the device or reagent
- BFAD registration number
- name and address of local agent

33.8 Import Documentation

Import documentation requirements are limited to registration of medical device firms and radiation-emitting products; these requirements have been already summarized in the text earlier.

33.9 Summary of Regulatory System

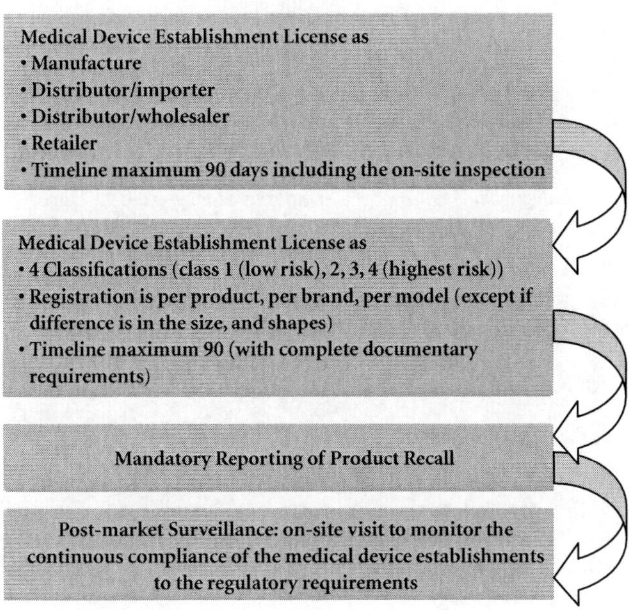

33.10 Contacts

The Republic of Philippines
Department of Health
San Lazaro Compound, Sta Cruz, Manila
Trunkline: +632 651 7800

Department of Health
Bureau of Health Devices and Technology
Building 24, San Lazaro Compound Rizal Avenue, Sta. Cruz, Manila, The Philippines
Telephone: +632 743 8301; local: 3402, 3408
Fax: +632 711 6016; 711 6824

Department of Health
Bureau of Food and Drugs
Civic Drive, Filinvest Corporate City
Alabang, Muntinlupa City 1781, The Philippines
Telephone: +632 807 07 21
Fax: +632 842 56 06

References

1. Medical Device Regulatory Requirements for the Philippines, retrieved May 28, 2012, from http://www.ita.doc.gov/td/health/Philippines%20Reg%20Profile%202006.pdf.
2. Republic of the Philippines, Department of Health, Bureau of Food and Drugs, retrieved May 28, 2012, from http://www.doh.gov.ph/node/1395.
3. Republic of the Philippines, Department of Health, retrieved May 28, 2012, from http://www.doh.gov.ph/faq/350#t350n1432.
4. The New Food and Drug Administration (FDA) of the Republic of the Philippines, retrieved, May 28, 2012, from http://www.who.int/medical_devices/02_agnette_peralta.pdf.
5. Drug-related administrative orders and Memorandum circulars (with summaries and annotations), Republic of the Philippines, Department of Health, Bureau of Food and Drugs DOH Compound, Alabang, Muntinlupa, M.M. Memorandum Circular No. 14 s. from August 19, 1991.

Chapter 34

Saudi Arabia: Medical Device Regulation System

Ali M. Al Dalaan[a,b]

[a]*Asian Harmonization Working Party*
[b]*Saudi Food and Drug Authority, 3292 North Ring Road, Riyadh 13312-6288, Kingdom of Saudi Arabia*

amdalaan@sfda.gov.sa

Disclaimer

The regulatory information contained in this chapter is intended for market planning and is subject to change frequently. Translations of laws and regulations are unofficial.

34.1 Introduction

The Kingdom of Saudi Arabia (KSA) is a leading country in the world economy and an influential market among the Middle East, North Africa, and the Gulf Cooperate Council. It is one of only a few fast-growing countries in the world with a relatively high per capita income of $24,200 (2010); therefore, the Saudi Arabian medical devices market is the biggest market in the middle east, with growth rate of higher than 9%. Saudi Arabia has a highly sophisti-

Handbook of Medical Device Regulatory Affairs in Asia
Edited by Jack Wong and Raymond K. Y. Tong

ISBN 978-981-4411-21-9 (Hardcover), 978-981-4411-22-6 (eBook)
www.panstanford.com

cated healthcare facilities system associated with 390 hospitals occupying more than 54,000 beds, 2037 primary healthcare centers, 175 artificial kidney centers and approximately 217 private medical centers. However, the Saudi Arabia medical device market is expected to grow tremendously in the next few years due to the heavy investment in health care. The Saudi Arabian Government established medical devices regulation to comply with revolution of medical Devices technology and to safe guard the public health of Saudi Arabia.

The Saudi Food and Drug Authority (SFDA) law issued by the royal decree (M/6) on February 13, 2007, gave the SFDA the responsibility to regulate medical devices in Saudi Arabia. The council of ministers' decision no. 181 issued on June 18, 2007, came to stress the importance of regulating medical devices. It was issued specifically for medical devices to address the need of the rapid growth of the Saudi Arabia medical device market to ensure safety, quality, and effectiveness of medical devices throughout their life cycle (pre-market, on-market and post-market).

34.2 Legislative Responsibilities

1. Providing technical support to importers
2. Setting mandatory specifications for medical devices, *in vitro* diagnostics (IVDs), and radiation-emitting electronic devices that affect the human health
3. Setting health and good manufacture practice requirements for all medical device establishments and manufacturers
4. Laying down policies and procedures for medical devices testing
5. Setting requirements for medical devices marketing and distribution and all related issues
6. Laying down regulation for medical devices advertising

34.3 Executive Responsibilities

1. Test medical devices, prescription eye glasses, contact lances, radiation-emitting electronic devices that effect human health to ascertain their quality, safety, effectiveness and compliance with mandatory standard approved by the SFDA

2. Test IVDs medical devices to ascertain of their quality, effectiveness and compliance with the manufacturers standards
3. Register and test of medical devices and all related issues
4. Issue marketing authorization for imported medical devices after doing the necessary validation and testing
5. Permit the marketing of local manufactured medical device, IVDs, prescription eye glasses, contact lenses and their solutions when they have meet the marketing authorization requirements
6. Establishing a central reference laboratory for medical devices in SFDA headquarter, and specialized branched laboratories in the kingdom's provinces
7. Accredit and license the private medical devices laboratories that relate to medical devices work field
8. Establish a medical devices database, and exchange information with local, regional and international bodies
9. Establish a main research center to conduct research and applied study relating to medical devices field
10. Conduct researches, studies and provide consultancy services related to medical devices and cooperate with medical devices establishments, authorities, universities, scientific research centers and other institutions conducting similar activities
11. Conduct training programs that enhance the competency of those working in the medical devices field
12. Promote consumer awareness of medical devices and sector's responsibilities
13. Represent the KSA in regional and international authorities and organizations relating to the sector's activities
14. Establish National Center for Medical Devices Reporting (NCMDR)
15. Establish Medical Devices National Registry (MDNR)

34.4 Surveillance Responsibilities

1. Monitor the implementation of regulations, guidelines and procedures relating to licensing of medical device's manufactures

2. Monitor the market of medical devices, IVDs, prescription eye glasses, contact lenses and their solutions to make sure marketed product have SFDA marketing authorization.
3. Inspection of medical devices establishments to assure their compliance with the SFDA requirements.
4. Monitor the market of medical devices, IVDs, prescription eye glasses, contact lenses and their solutions to ensure the establishment has the establishment license.
5. Follow up medical devices recalls with hospitals, healthcare providers in the kingdom, manufacturers and imports and take appropriate corrective and/ or preventive action.

34.5 Regulation Overview

The Saudi FDA issued medical device interim regulation on December 27, 2008; the interim regulation will be replaced with the medical device main regulation that is being developed.

The medical device interim regulation is based on the GHTF founding member jurisdiction regulatory requirements. Therefore, to obtain marketing authorization, medical devices shall comply with the relevant regulatory requirements applicable in one or more of the jurisdiction of Australia, Japan, the United States and the EU/EFTA, and additionally with provision specific to the KSA concerning labeling and conditions of supply and or use.

The main objectives of the medical devices interim regulation are to protect and maintain public health within the KSA by the implementation of provisions ensuring a high level of safety and health protection of patients, users and third parties with regard to the use of medical devices as it relates to their manufacture, supply and use during their lifecycle and to mandate measures, and allocate responsibilities, to ensure that medical devices placed on the market and/or put into service within the KSA comply with all relevant requirements and provisions of the interim regulation and its implementing rules. Nevertheless, Saudi FDA is working forward the development of framework Regulation to cover all Medical Devices Requirements.

34.6 Registration Requirements

- Each **importer** and **distributor** requires an Establishment National Registry Number issued by the SFDA before it is permitted to apply for a license and import or distribute medical devices within the KSA.
- The application for registration will be made electronically through the Medical Device National Registry (MDNR), which is found on the SFDA Web site and prescribes the information that has to be provided before the SFDA assigns a National Registration Number to the **importer** or **distributor**
- The **importer** and **distributor** shall attest that the information specified in the electronic application is accurate and will be regularly updated
- The same Web site is used to update previously submitted information. In this case the **importer** or **distributor** has 10 calendar days from the occurrence of the change to provide the SFDA with revised information.
- Where an **authorized representative** has also a legal entity involved in importation or distribution activities of medical devices within the KSA, it is subject to all the additional requirements and responsibilities of such an **importer** or **distributor**.
- **Local manufacturers** or **retail pharmacies** are deemed to be **distributors** if they place medical devices on the KSA market.
- The SFDA/MDS may ask the registrant to confirm the registration information it holds remains true and complete

34.7 Information to Be Provided to SFDA

- Each organization involved in the **importation** and/or the **distribution** of medical devices within the KSA requires an establishment license, issued by the SFDA, before it undertakes such activities.

- Such an organization is normally an "**importer**" or "**distributor**" but may be a local manufacturer distributing its own or another manufacturer's medical device, or an authorized representative of an overseas manufacturer involved in the importation or distribution of medical devices, or a **retail pharmacy** distributing medical devices.
- Organizations involved in both importation and distribution will have both activities included on the establishment license.
- Each organization intending to import and/or distribute medical devices in the KSA shall have obtained an Establishment National Registry Number from the SFDA, before it applies for an establishment license.
- Each **importer** shall, in cooperation with the authorized representative(s) of one or more manufacturers, decide which category(ies) or group(s) of medical devices it intend to import into the KSA and establish the contact details of the manufacturer(s) concerned.
- Each **distributor** shall, in cooperation with either the local manufacturer(s) or with the authorized representative(s) of one or more manufacturers, as relevant, shall decide which category(ies) or group(s) of medical devices it distribute within the KSA and establish the contact details of the manufacturer(s) and authorized representative(s) concerned.
- The device category is selected from: active implantable devices; anesthetic and respiratory devices; dental devices; diagnostic electro mechanical medical devices; hospital hardware; *In vitro* diagnostic medical devices; non-active implantable devices; ophthalmic and optical devices; reusable devices instruments; single-use devices; assistive products for persons with disability; diagnostic and therapeutic radiating devices; complementary therapy devices; biologically derived devices; healthcare facility products and adaptations; IVD laboratory equipment.
- The application for establishment licensing will be made electronically through the Medical Device Establishment Licensing (MDEL), which is found on the SFDA Web site and must be completed by each **importer** and **distributor**.

- Once satisfied that the application meets the relevant requirements, the SFDA shall issue the applicant with an establishment license that is renewable annually.
- Licensed organizations shall revise the information provided to the SFDA within 10 days of the change occurring when
  - there is a change in its contact information,
  - there is a change in the category or group of medical device it imports or distributes, and
  - it adds another manufacturer to those it already represents.
- To ensure medical devices placed on the KSA market are suitable and properly supported
  - any organization intending to import medical devices into the KSA or
  - any organization intending to distribute medical devices within the KSA (including **retail pharmacies**) shall do so only with the knowledge of the authorized representative(s) or local manufacturer(s) concerned, as relevant.
- Information for importation and distribution activities will include
  - the name of the overseas manufacturer of the medical devices that the applicant imports or intends to import, together with the name of that manufacturer's licensed authorized representative and its establishment National Registry Number,
  - an attestation that the manufacturer has been informed, through its authorized representative, of the applicant's intention to import its medical devices into the KSA,
  - an attestation that the importer has used its best endeavors to establish that the imported device(s) is/are in compliance with the relevant provisions of the Medical Devices Interim Regulation and its implementing rules,
  - the medical device category and generic device group the applicant intends to import from the manufacturer,
  - the name of the manufacturer of the medical devices that the applicant intends to distribute, together with the Establishment National Registry Number of either the

local manufacturer or, for medical devices manufactured outside the KSA, the authorized representative,
   - an attestation that either the local manufacturer or the authorized representative together with the importer, as applicable, has been informed of the applicant's intention to distribute its medical device(s) within the KSA, and
   - the medical device category or generic device group the applicant intends to distribute within the KSA.

34.8 Medical Device Marketing Authorization (MDMA)

- To obtain marketing authorization, medical devices shall comply with the relevant regulatory requirements applicable in one or more of the jurisdictions of Australia, Canada, Japan, the United States, and the EU/EFTA, and additionally with provisions specific to the KSA concerning labeling and conditions of supply and/or use.
- Marketing authorization is required for
   - all medical devices whatever their classification,
   - contact lenses for cosmetic as well as for medical purposes, and
   - laser surgical equipment intended for cosmetic as well as medical purposes.
- It is not required for medical devices designed and constructed by health facility staff for internal use within that health facility, alone.
- Medical device marketing authorization (MDMA) applications shall be made by either a local manufacturer or, where the manufacturer is established outside the KSA, by its authorized representative.
- Information is submitted to the SFDA using the electronic application forms found on the MDMA section of its Web site. After indicating which of the five GHTF Founding Member jurisdictions will be used as the basis of the MDMA application, the applicant (either a local manufacturer or, where the manufacturer is established outside the KSA, by its authorized representative) will be directed to the appropriate part of

the Web site. Implementing Rule *Marketing Authorization* describes the application procedure and the documentary evidence that has to be provided to support the applicant's claim that the device meets all relevant requirements of the Medical Device Interim Regulation.

- Two categories of information must be provided. The first requires general information (such as the applicant's contact details) and information specific to the KSA. The second requires information specific to the particular GHTF Founding Member jurisdiction the manufacturer has chosen as the basis of the MDMA application. In addition, the manufacturer will hold, and make available to the SFDA upon request, additional documentary evidence to support its MDMA application.
- The documentation provided shall relate to the medical device that is the subject of the MDMA and be sufficient to
  - identify the medical device that is the subject of the application, its manufacturer and the legal entity making the application,
  - demonstrate the device complies with all relevant provisions specific to the KSA, and
  - demonstrate the manufacturer of the device has been authorized to place the device on the market in one of the five GHTF Founding Member jurisdictions.
- MDS-G5 Guidance on Marketing Authorization Procedures/(H)/Comment #13 states, "The end date of the period of validity will be the same as that of the marketing authorization granted in the GHTF Founding Member jurisdiction unless the GHTF Founding Member's authorization is open ended and does not indicate a validity end-date, or where the device has been marketed through a self-declaration process (e.g. Class I devices that are not sterile or having a measuring function under EU regulations), where validity shall be 3 years."
- MDS-G5 Guidance on Marketing Authorization Procedures states, "MDMAs Incorporating More Than One Medical Device Type:
  - Where the applicant's MDMA groups more than one medical device type (referred to as "bundling" in some

jurisdictions) within a single application procedure, the grouped medical device types shall all have been authorized for marketing within the GHTF Founding Member jurisdiction, upon which the MDMA is based, on the same basis.

  - Where the MDMA procedure involves medical device types having different purposes, technical performance and classification, the applicant will have to access the MDMA portion of the SFDA's website on multiple occasions to provide the required information. While some of that information will be common, the KSA national provisions will vary with the different medical device types.

- When the SFDA is satisfied that the medical device meets the provisions of the Medical Devices Interim Regulation, it authorizes the manufacturer to place the device on the KSA market by issuing a numbered Marketing Authorization Certificate and assigning each device to which the certificate applies with a Medical Device Listing National Registry Number.

34.9 Medical Device Listing

To obtain an establishment license, the importer and the distributor have to indicate the categories of medical device they intend to supply to the KSA market but do not have to provide full details of the devices. Before particular medical devices within each category or group are placed on the KSA market for the first time, these devices/must have been authorized by the SFDA and when these devices are imported or distributed within the KSA market, the importers and the distributors must provide listing information to the Medical Device National Registry (MDNR) for the devices concerned.

34.10 Registration Fees

Table 34.1 presents the fee structure for Medical Device Marketing Authorization (MDMA).

Table 34.1 Medical Device Marketing Authorization processing fees

Fee groups	Basis of application for SFDA marketing authorization	Three years or less (SR)	More than three years (SR)	Lead time (working days)
FG(1)	All class I/general IVD (other)/exempt IVD (TGA)	15,000*	N/A	35
FG(2)	All class II/class IIa/self-test IVD, listable IVD	19,000	21,000	35
FG(3)	Class IIb/class III (CA, PAL)/Annex II list B (IVD)	21,000	23,000	35
FG(4)	All other class III/class IV/AIMD/Annex II list A (IVD)/registrable IVD	23,000	25,000	35

*For class I, the Medical Device Marketing Authorization issues by the SFDA will be valid for three years.

Note: For all other classes, the Medical Device Marketing Authorization issues by the SFDA will be valid for the remaining validity of the original license or for three years for license with undefined validity.

Table 34.2 presents the fee structure for the Medical Device Authorized Representative (AR) License.

Table 34.2 Medical Device Authorized Representative License processing fees

Basis of the application for SFDA Authorized representative	Annual fee (SR)	Lead time (working days)
Per manufacturer mandate	5200	20

Table 34.3 presents the fee structure for Medical Device Establishment Licensing (MDEL).

Table 34.3 Medical Device Establishment Licensing processing fees

Establishment class	Annual fees (SR)	Lead time (working days)
(A)	35,000	15
(B)	30,000	15
(C)	25,000	15
(D)	15,000	15

34.11 General Information and Documentary Evidence to Be Provided to SFDA

- Where the applicant is a local manufacturer, he shall provide his company name and contact information, together with the contact details of the person responsible for the medical device MDMA application. Also, he shall provide his Establishment National Registry Number.
- Where the applicant is an authorized representative, he shall provide the same information as in the previous point, together with the contact information of the overseas manufacturer on whose behalf he is acting, and his Authorized Representative License Number.
- The applicant shall provide information that will allow the medical device that is the subject of the application to be identified unambiguously. Where the MDMA application procedure covers more than one medical device type, the requirements in Section 34.6 must be met. If they are not, the MDMA application will be rejected and the applicant must resubmit multiple applications.
- In addition to providing documentary evidence that the medical device that is the subject of the MDMA application complies with the medical devices regulation that applies to it within a selected GHTF Founding Member jurisdiction, the applicant must provide evidence that the device complies with requirements specific to the KSA. These concern labeling, any a/c power supply, environmental factors, handling/ transportation/ storage, and advertising.
- In addition to providing documentary evidence that the medical device that is the subject of the MDMA application complies with requirements specific to the KSA, the applicant must provide evidence that the device complies with the medical devices regulation that applies to it within the particular GHTF Founding Member jurisdiction that has been chosen as the basis of the application. By indicating which GHTF jurisdiction is being used, the applicant will be directed to the relevant part of the Web site.

34.12 Labeling Requirement for Medical Device

- In addition to providing documentary evidence that the medical device that is the subject of the MDMA application complies with the medical devices regulation that applies to it within a selected GHTF Founding Member jurisdiction, the applicant must provide evidence that the device complies with requirements specific to the KSA. These concern labeling, any a/c power supply, environmental factors, handling/ transportation/ storage, and advertising.
- The SFDA requires electronic copies of the labels affixed to the device and its wrappers, as well as a copy of the instructions for use, in the format that will be used when the device is marketed within the KSA. The SFDA will confirm, in particular, they satisfy requirements in respect of product identification, language, and tracking of individual devices through the supply chain.
- Where the device is intended for use by laypersons, the text of labeling shall be written in terms readily understood by such persons.
- All required documents are in English except that labeling has the following requirements:
    - Labeling in English is acceptable where the user(s) of the medical device is likely to be professionally qualified.
    - Where the device is intended to be used by laypersons, the labeling shall be in both Arabic and English. Medical personnel at healthcare facilities are not considered to be laypersons.
    - Instructions for the handling, storage, transportation, installation, maintenance, and disposal of the medical devices shall be in English and, where justified, in Arabic.
    - Advertising and marketing information shall be in English and, where justified, in Arabic.

34.13 Post-Market Surveillance Requirement

- The SFDA shall ensure the appropriate and efficient operation of the necessary medical device vigilance procedures.

It shall, in particular, advise users and persons involved in the provision of healthcare in the KSA to inform without delay the manufacturer concerned of any adverse event and the SFDA of any reportable adverse event they become aware of, involving a specific medical device.

- All parties concerned shall be made aware of the existence and responsibilities of the SFDA being the medical device vigilance authority. Furthermore, the SFDA shall indicate how it may be contacted to notify medical device reportable adverse events.
- Investigate any adverse event of which it becomes aware. If the **manufacturer** confirms a malfunction or deterioration in the characteristics and/or performance of the medical device, as well as any inadequacy in the labeling or the instructions for use, has led, or might have led, to the death of a patient, user or third person, or to a serious deterioration in the state of health of a patient, use or third person, it shall submit an adverse event report to the SFDA and agree a corrective action plan.
- An important aspect of effective post-market surveillance is the need of the SFDA, health authority and/or **overseas manufacturer** to identify an individual medical device so that it may be traced, examined, or recalled after is has been put into service. Therefore, the **manufacturer** is required to label the medical devices it manufactures with an unambiguous identification, such as batch code / lot number, or serial number, preceded by the word LOT or SERIAL NUMBER (or an equivalent symbol) as appropriate. In general, consumable and single-use devices have a batch code, while powered medical devices have individual serial numbers.

References

SFDA, National Provisions & Requirements for Medical Devices, http://www.sfda.gov.sa/NR/rdonlyres/5105459F-B824-4C8A-99BF EE5E0C7519CF/0/NationalProvisionsandRequirementsfor MedicalDevices.pdf.

SFDA, MDS-IR1, Designation and Oversight of Conformity Assessment Bodies, http://www.sfda.gov.sa/NR/rdonlyres/AC5CA167-BDDB-4609-BBE4-9844A0B133AB/0/IR12011.pdf.

SFDA, MDS-IR2, Establishment Registration, http://www.sfda.gov.sa/NR/rdonlyres/B963B4B2-BCEB-4F7C-84D9-74358B4CDF90/0/MDSIR22011.pdf.

SFDA, MDS-IR3, Medical Device Listing, http://www.sfda.gov.sa/NR/rdonlyres/311CDE1B-D150-4483-82F4-6D3C4F211904/0/MDSIR32011.pdf.

SFDA, MDS-IR4, Establishment Licensing, http://www.sfda.gov.sa/NR/rdonlyres/2FAD6767-2C25-410C-A4C0-E06B60ABE64D/0/MDSIR42011.pdf.

SFDA, MDS-IR5, Licensing of Authorized Representatives, http://www.sfda.gov.sa/NR/rdonlyres/75275AAA-6903-431B-83DD-12D4E5B6DEC5/0/MDSIR52011.pdf.

SFDA, MDS-IR6, The Validation of Document to Be Provided to the SFDA by Manufactures for Marketing Authorization, http://www.sfda.gov.sa/NR/rdonlyres/8FB37D1B-C4CD-4B56-BFA0-D9216CE81BEB/0/MDSIR62011.pdf.

SFDA, MDS-IR7, Marketing Surveillance, http://www.sfda.gov.sa/NR/rdonlyres/93ECAE2F-923E-443B-A83C-AFE2E22CE52C/0/MDSIR72011.pdf.

SFDA, MDS-IR8, Safeguard Procedures, http://www.sfda.gov.sa/NR/rdonlyres/51ED1E9D-5E60-42DC-8C5B-B7C332200F98/0/MDSIR82011.pdf.

Appendix: Definitions

KSA: The Kingdom of Saudi Arabia
SFDA: Saudi Food and Drug Authority
The Board: The SFDA board of directors
Party: Any natural or legal person
Medical device: Any instrument, apparatus, implement, machine, appliance, implant, *in vitro* reagent or calibrator, software, material or other similar or related article

(a) intended by the manufacturer to be used, alone or in combination, for human beings for one or more of the specific purpose(s) of
- diagnosis, prevention, monitoring, treatment or alleviation of disease
- diagnosis, monitoring, treatment, alleviation of or compensation for an injury or handicap
- investigation, replacement, modification, or support of the anatomy or of a physiological process,
- supporting or sustaining life
- control of conception
- disinfection of medical devices
- providing information for medical or diagnostic purposes by means of *in vitro* examination of specimens derived from the human body

(b) which does not achieve its primary intended action in or on the human body by pharmacological, immunological or metabolic means, but which may be assisted in its intended function by such means.

Accessory: A product intended specifically by its manufacturer to be used together with a medical device to enable that medical device to achieve its intended purpose

Advertising of medical devices: Any form of information, canvassing activity or inducement intended to promote the supply or use of medical devices

Applicant: Any party established within the KSA required to provide information for establishment licensing purposes

Authorized representative: Any natural or legal person established within the KSA who has received a written mandate from the manufacturer to act on his behalf for specified tasks including the obligation to represent the manufacturer in its dealings with the SFDA

CAB: A conformity assessment body (third party), established within the KSA, independent of both the manufacturer and user of the medical device that is subject to assessment

Distributor: Any natural or legal person in the supply chain who, on his own behalf, furthers the availability of a medical device to the end user

Establishment: Any place of business within the KSA that is involved in the manufacture, and/or placing on the market, and/or distribution of medical devices; or acting on behalf of the manufacturer

Fully refurbished medical device: A used device that has been returned to a state that would allow it to be subject to the same conformity assessment procedures as applied to the original device.

Global Harmonization Task Force (GHTF): Countries working to achieve harmonization in medical device regulation among themselves; these countries are Australia, Canada, Japan, the United States, and the EU/EFTA

Importer: Any natural or legal person in the supply chain who is the first to make a medical device, manufactured in another jurisdiction, available in the KSA

***In vitro* medical device: A** medical device, whether used alone or in combination, intended by the manufacturer for the *in vitro* examination of specimens derived from the human body solely or principally to provide information for diagnostic, monitoring or compatibility purposes; this includes reagents, calibrators, control materials, specimen receptacles, software and related instruments or apparatus or other articles

Labeling: Written, printed or graphic matter

(a) Affixed to a medical device or any of its containers or wrappers
(b) Information accompanying a medical device, related to identification, technical description
(c) Information accompanying a medical device, related to its use, but excluding shipping documents

Manufacturer: Any natural or legal person with responsibility for design and manufacture of a medical device with the intention of making it available for use, under his name; whether or not such a medical device is designed and/or manufactured by that person himself or on his behalf by another person

Medical Devices National Registry (MDNR): The database of registered establishments and the medical devices they manufacture or import or distribute

National Center for Medical Device Reporting (NCMDR): An organization managing a database of information on safety and performance related aspects of medical devices and capable of taking appropriate action on any confirmed problems.

Placing on the market: The first making available in return for payment or free of charge of a medical device, with a view to distribution and/or use within the KSA, regardless of whether it is new or fully refurbished

Putting into service: The stage at which a device has been made available to the final user as being ready for use for the first time in the KSA for its intended purpose

Registrant: Any party established within the KSA required to provide information for establishment registration or medical device listing purposes

Chapter 35

Singapore: Medical Device Regulatory System

Lee Ching Hwee

Johnson & Johnson Medical Singapore,
No. 2 International Business Park, #07-01,
Tower One, The Strategy, 609930 Singapore

Clee14@its.jnj.com

Disclaimer

The regulatory information contained in this chapter is intended for market planning and is subject to change frequently. Translations of laws and regulations are unofficial.

35.1 Market Overview Introduction: An Explanation of the Process and Approach

35.1.1 Market Environment

Singapore, as the region's healthcare hub and center of healthcare excellence, is striving to deliver first-class health care management to its residents as well as serving patient's needs internationally.

Handbook of Medical Device Regulatory Affairs in Asia
Edited by Jack Wong and Raymond K. Y. Tong

ISBN 978-981-4411-21-9 (Hardcover), 978-981-4411-22-6 (eBook)
www.panstanford.com

With improvements in sanitation, medical technology, and public health awareness, life expectancy has risen significantly over years. As of 2011, the resident population of Singapore was 5.18 million. By 2030, elderly people aged 65 and older are expected to make up 19% of the population.* This indirectly signifies the importance of health care delivery and medical care to its nations.

In 2004, Singapore's total market size for medical devices was estimated to be US$ 535 million (Fig. 35.1) The market for medical devices is in the growing trend as a result of Singapore's position as the regional medical and research hub.

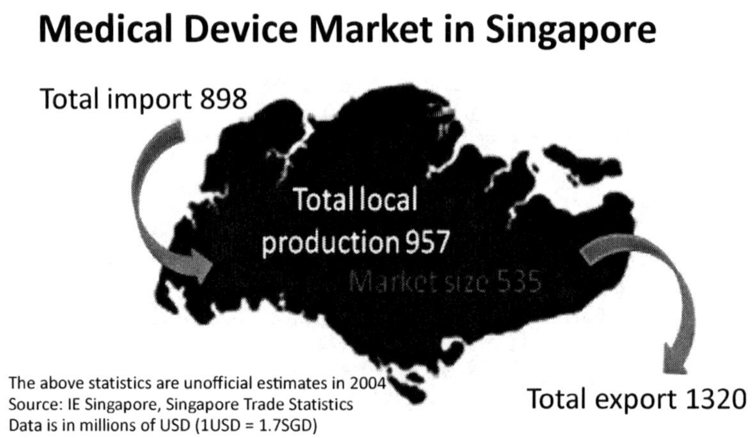

Figure 35.1 Angelique Chan, *Singapore's Changing Structure and the Policy Implications for Financial Security, Employment, Living Arrangements and Health Care.* ASIAN Metacentre Research Paper Series No. 3.

35.1.2 Overview of Regulatory Environment and What Laws/Regulations Govern Medical Devices

Singapore Health Sciences Authority (HSA), Medical Device Branch, is entrusted with regulating medical devices in Singapore. HSA has adopted the new regulatory system based on the principles endorsed by the Global Harmonization Task Force (GHTF) with modification to suit the Singapore context. HSA has also studied the medical device regulatory system in developed country counter parts, including the US Food and Drug Administration (FDA),

* According to the Department of Statistics, Singapore.

European Union, Canada's Medical Devices Bureau (MDB), Japan's Ministry of Health, Labour and Welfare (MHLW), and Australia's Therapeutic Goods Administration (TGA). In general, the regulatory framework for medical devices in Singapore is mapped in order to safeguard public health but without unduly restricting consumer choices and their access to new technologies.

In 2002, HSA introduced the Voluntary Product Registration Scheme and post-market monitoring and surveillance program for medical devices in the Singapore market. With the passage of the Health Products Act 2007 in February 2007, HSA implemented the Health Products (Medical Devices) Regulations to further strengthen the control of medical devices in local market. The regulatory controls were implemented in three phases:

35.1.2.1 Phase I implementation

On November 1, 2007, duties and obligations were imposed on medical device dealers to

- report adverse events to HSA within the stipulated time frame
- notify HSA prior to the initiation of a product recall
- maintenance of product compliant and distribution records

In addition, false or misleading advertisements and promotions of medical devices are prohibited.

35.1.2.2 Phase II implementation

On November 1, 2008, HSA rolled out medical device dealers and registrant licensing, whereby companies dealing with medical device manufacturing, importation, and exportation shall submit application in order to be licensed.

35.1.2.3 Phase III implementation

Since August 10, 2010 (IIIa), unlicensed manufacturing, importation, and wholesaling of medical device have been prohibited. Class C and D medical devices that are imported and supplied must fulfill one of the following criteria:

- listed on Singapore Medical Device register
- listed on the Transition List
- authorized via one of the Authorization Routes

Medical devices licensed under the Radiation Protection Act by the Centre for Radiation Protection and Nuclear Science (CRPNS) of the National Environment Agency (NEA) are exempted from product registration with HSA until August 1, 2011. Post August 1, 2011, the ionizing radiation irradiating medical devices must be registered under HSA Medical Device Branch and separate application should be made to the Centre for Radiation Protection and Nuclear Science (CRPNS) under National Environmental Agency (NEA).

From January 1, 2012 (IIIb), unless exempted from product registration, all medical devices (Class A, B, C, and D) that are imported and supplied must meet one of the criteria listed in Table 35.1:

Table 35.1 Various implementation phases of the regulatory control

November 1, 2007, onward	**November 1, 2008, onward**	**May 1, 2010**	**August 10, 2010**	**January 1, 2012**
Phase 1	**Phase 2**	**Phase 3A**		**Phase 3B**
Imposition of duties and obligations on dealers: • Report product defects and AEs • Recall product upon HSA instructions • Keep distribution records	Acceptance of license application of parties dealing with MD Acceptance of registration of Class C, D MDs (Transition list/ registered)	Transition List is finalized and published (last entry April 30, 2010	Only licensed dealers shall manufacture, import and supply MDs Unless authorized by HSA or listed on the Transition list, all unregistered Class C, D MDs are prohibited from supply	Unless authorized by HSA or listed on the Transition List, all classes of MDs are prohibited from supply (Class A, B, C, D) MDs licensed under Radiation Protection Act, NEA — August 1, 2011
Advertisement and promotion control	Acceptance of registration of Class A, B and MDs currently licensed under CRP, NEA			

35.2 Detail of Key Regulator(s)

The Health Products Regulation Group (HPRG) of HSA is the national regulator for health products. HPRG ensures that drugs, innovative therapeutics, medical devices and health-related products in Singapore are controlled and meet appropriate standards of safety, quality and efficacy.

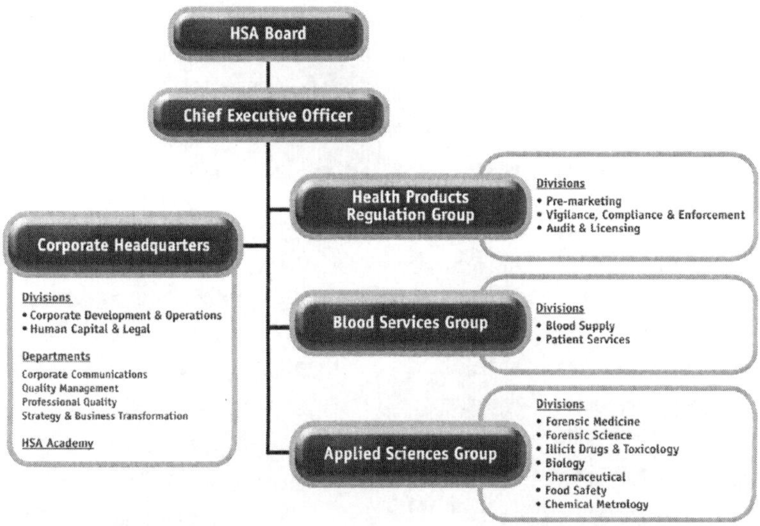

Figure 35.2 The HSA organization chart.

The Medical Device Branch is entrusted with regulating medical devices in Singapore.

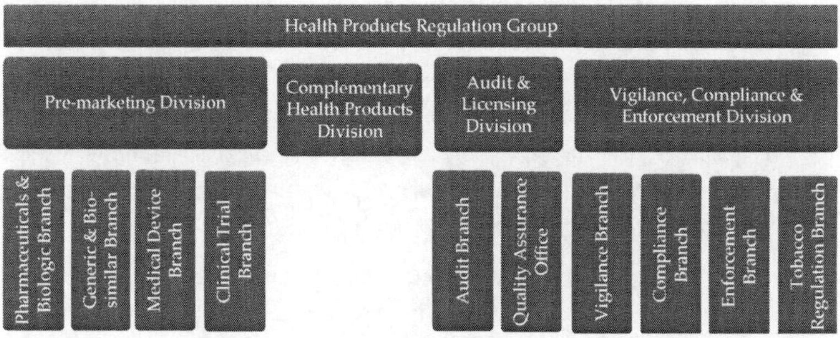

Figure 35.3 The Health Products Regulation Group organization chart.

Contact information

Medical Device Branch — Therapeutic Products Division,
Health Products Regulation Group — Health Sciences Authority,
11 Biopolis Way #11-01 Helios, Singapore 138667
Telephone: +65 6866 3560
Fax: +65 6478 9028
Web site: www.hsa.gov.sg
Email: HSA_MD_Info@hsa.gov.sg

35.3 Regulatory Overview

35.3.1 The Definition of Medical Device

"Medical device" means any instrument, apparatus, implement, machine, appliance, implant, *in vitro* reagent or calibrator, software, material or other similar or related article that is intended by its manufacturer to be used, whether alone or in combination, for humans for one or more of the specific purposes of

- diagnosis, prevention, monitoring, treatment or alleviation of any disease,
- diagnosis, monitoring, treatment, alleviation of or compensation for an injury,
- investigation, replacement, modification, or support of the anatomy or of a physiological process,
- supporting or sustaining life,
- control of conception,
- disinfection of medical devices, or
- providing information for medical or diagnostic purposes by means of *in vitro* examination of specimens derived from the human body, which does not achieve its primary intended action in or on the human body by pharmacological, immunological or metabolic means, but which may be assisted in its intended function by such means.

An *in vitro* diagnostic device includes any medical device that is a reagent product, calibrator, control material kit, instrument, apparatus, equipment, or system, whether used alone or in combination, intended by the manufacturer to be used *in vitro* for the examination of specimens, including blood and tissue donations, derived from human body, solely or principally for the purpose of providing information

- concerning a physiological or pathological state, state of health or disease,
- concerning a congenital abnormality,
- to determine the safety and compatibility with the potential recipients, or
- to monitor therapeutic measures.

Medical devices cover a wide range of products, ranging from simple bandages, walking stick, contact lenses, and wheelchair, through life-maintaining implantable device, equipment to screen and diagnose diseases and health conditions, to the most sophisticated diagnostic imaging and minimal invasive surgery equipment.

Products that are not intended for use in preventing, diagnosing, curing, or alleviating diseases, ailment, defects, or injuries are not medical devices. Examples of products that are not medical devices are body-toning equipment and magnetic accessories.

35.3.2 Classification of Medical Devices (Classes A, B, C, and D)

35.3.2.1 Principle

Regulatory control is proportional to the level of risk associated with a medical device, which increases with higher degree of risk involved. Therefore, medical devices are classified on the basis of their risk to patients and users substantially on its intended purpose and effectiveness of the risk management techniques applied during design, manufacture and use.

35.3.2.2 Classification

Various factors contribute to the risk classification of medical devices, which include

- duration of medical device contact with the body
- degree of invasiveness
- delivery of medicinal products or energy to the user
- intended to have biological effect on the user

Based on the product owner's intended purpose, two or more risk classification rules apply to the medical device, the highest level of risk classification indicated shall be allocated to the medical device.

Table 35.2 The general risk classification system for medical devices

Risk class	Risk level	Medical device examples
A	Low risk	Surgical retractors/tongue depressors
B	Low-moderate risk	Hypodermic needles/suction equipment
C	Moderate-high risk	Lung ventilator/bone fixation plate
D	High risk	Heart valves/implantable defibrillator

35.3.2.3 Determination

The determination of medical device risk class in Singapore uses the rules-based system depending on the claims made by the product owner and on its design and intended purpose.

For more details, please read GN-13-R1 Guidance on the Risk Classification of General Medical Devices and GN-14-R1 Guidance on the Risk Classification of *in vitro* Diagnostic Medical Devices available at the HSA Web site.

35.4 Product Grouping

Diversified medical devices require registration prior to supply to the local market, from simple medical devices, such as syringe and tongue depressor, to highly complex medical devices that comprise myriad components, such as anesthesia monitoring system. These various components can be sold separately, as replacement, in different combinations as a convenient all-in-one kit, or as an individually customized pack. Thus, medical devices can be grouped into one of the following categories, to be submitted as one product registration application — SINGLE, FAMILY, SYSTEM, GROUP, and IVD CLUSTER — and eventually listed in the Singapore Medical Device Register (SMDR).

35.4.1 Single

A SINGLE medical device is a medical device from a product owner identified by a medical device proprietary name with a specific intended purpose. It may be offered in a range of package sizes.

Example: condoms that are sold in packages of 3, 12, and 24 can be registered as a SINGLE medical device.

35.4.2 Family

A medical device FAMILY is a collection of medical devices and each medical device FAMILY member

- is from the same product owner,
- is of the same risk classification class,
- has the same medical device proprietary name,
- has a common intended purpose,
- has the same design and manufacturing process, and
- has variations that are within the scope of the permissible variants, such as concentrations, flavor, color, and diameter.

Example: IV administrative sets that differ in features, such as safety wings and length of tubing, but are manufactured from the same material and manufacturing process and share a common intended purpose.

35.4.3 System

A medical device SYSTEM comprises a number of constituent components that are

- from the same product owner,
- intended to be used in combination to complete a common intended purpose,
- compatible when used as a SYSTEM, and
- sold under single SYSTEM name or the labeling, IFU, brochures, or catalogues for each constituent component states that the constituent component is intended for use with the SYSTEM.

Example: A hip replacement system comprising femoral and acetabular components can be registered as a SYSTEM. The components must be used in combination to achieve a common intended purpose of total hip replacement. The size of the components may vary.

35.4.4 Group

A medical device GROUP is a collection of two or more medical devices, supplied in a single package by a product owner. The medical GROUP has the following:

- a single proprietary GROUP name
- a common intended purpose

Each medical device in the GROUP may have different medical device proprietary name and intended purposes and may be assigned and manufactured by different product owners. When the GROUP is registered, the product owner is able to customize the group for particular hospitals or physicians, while maintaining the same GROUP name and intended purpose. When the GROUP is registered, all other combinations in that GROUP can be supplied on the market.

Example: A first-aid kit consisting of medical devices such as bandages, gauzes, drapes, and thermometers, when assembled together as one package by a product owner.

35.4.5 IVD Cluster

An IVD CLUSTER comprises a number of *in vitro* diagnostic reagents or articles that are

- from the same product owner,
- within risk classification A or B,
- of a common test methodology, and
- of the same IVD CLUSTER category.

The IVD CLUSTER may include analyzers that are designed for use with the reagent in the IVD CLUSTER.

35.5 Product Registration and Time Required

35.5.1 Application Process: Product Registration for Higher Risk Medical Devices (Class B, C, and D)

All product registration applications are to be submitted via the online Medical Device Information and Communication System

(MEDICS). Upon successful submission, the application will be screened before it can be accepted for evaluation to ensure that there are no major deficiencies that would hinder the evaluation.

Along the screening and evaluation processes, the registrant may be requested to provide additional information if any major deficiencies are identified. The input request will be made to the registrant and the registrant will be required to submit the requested material and information within 14 calendar days from the date of request.

The evaluation decision will be made on the basis of the evaluation outcome of the submitted information, i.e., registrable, rejection. For medical devices that receive a "Registrable" evaluation decision, the registrant may submit an application to list the medical device on the SMDR.

35.5.2 Product Registration for Lower Risk Medical Devices (Class A)

Submission in Common Submission Dossier Template (CSDT) is not required for Class A medical devices.

The data requirement for Class A medical devices

- Letter of Authorization
- Singapore Declaration of Conformity
- Copies of product labeling, i.e., instructions for use, brochure, label, etc.
- Name, address, and contact information for all authorized importers
- Quality management system certificate for the manufacturing site and sterilization site (if applicable)
- Sterilization method and sterilization validation standard(s) used (if applicable)

Additional requirement for Class A, *in vitro* Diagnostic (IVD)

- List of all materials and source of animal, human, microbial, and recombinant origin used in the IVD medical device.

- Upon review of its intended purpose/indication and appropriateness in risk classification, the Class A medical devices shall be listed on the SMDR.

35.5.3 Evaluation Routes

For Class B, C, and D medical devices, there are two evaluation routes:

1. Abridged evaluation

   The abridged evaluation route applies to medical device that have been evaluated and approved in at least one of the GHTF founding members (Australia, Canada, European Union, Japan, and the United States).

   All aspects of the medical device's quality, including packaging, labeling, and intended purpose/indication for use, intended for supply in Singapore shall be the same as that approved by the reference agency.

   This route allows submission of summary data sets in certain sections of the submission document.

2. Full evaluation

   All other medical devices without prior approval from the reference agencies are subjected to full evaluation.

Table 35.3 Turn-around-time (TAT) for product registration

Risk classification	TAT for abridged evaluation	TAT for full evaluation
B	100 working days	160 working days
C	160 working days	220 working days
D	220 working days	310 working days
Combination product	310 working days	
A	60 working days	

The product license has a validity of one year.

35.6 Product Registration for Combined Device–Drug Product

A combination product is defined as product that combines a medicinal product and a medical device such that the distinctive nature of the medicinal product component and device component is integrated in a singular product, e.g., heparin-coated catheters, drug-eluting stents.

Guidance on product registration of combination product will be published in the near future. Registrant may consult the Authority for registration requirements.

35.7 Application Fee

The application fee is payable at the time of submission in MEDICS. Evaluation fees are payable upon the acceptance of the application for evaluation.

Table 35.4 Fees for product registration of medical devices

Risk classification	Abridged route (S$)	Full evaluation (S$)
A	25	
Application fee	500	
Combination	10,000	75,000
D	5,700	11,400
C	3,500	5,700
B	1,800	3,500

35.8 Technical Material Requirement

Documents in support of applications submitted to the Authority should be organized according to the ASEAN Common Submission Dossier Template (CSDT) format. The submitted documents in support of product registration must be in English. CSDT requirements are summarized Table 35.5:

General medical devices	***In vitro* diagnostics**
Executive summary	
Essential Principles and Evidence of Conformity	
Device Description	
Summary of Design Verification and Validation • Sterilization validation • Shelf life data • Projected useful life • Metrological requirement Pre-clinical studies • Physical test • Biocompatibility studies • Animal studies • Software validation and verification studies • Biological safety	Summary of Design Verification and Validation • Analytical sensitivity • Analytical specificity • Precision (Repeatability/ Reproducibility) • Linearity/Assay's Measuring • Traceability • Cut-off value • Trueness • Stability of reagent • Stability of specimen type • Devices containing instrument and articles • Sterilization validation for any sterile product • Software verification and validation • Devices containing biological material
Clinical evidence	Clinical evidence • Clinical sensitivity • Clinical specificity • Comparison studies using clinical specimens • Clinical studies/performance evaluation studies involving human specimens • Reference interval • Performance evaluation studies under simulated conditions of use • Batch release • Use of existing bibliography
Device labeling	
Risk analysis	
Manufacturer information	

In addition to a dossier prepared in the CSDT format, the following documents shall also be submitted in the application:

- Name, address and contact information for authorized importers and wholesaler of the medical device
- Declaration of conformity
- Letter of authorization

35.9 Labeling Requirement of Medical Devices

Label, in relation to a medical device, refers to any written, printed or graphic representation that appears on or is attached to the medical device or any part of its packaging, and includes any informational sheet or leaflet that accompanies the health product or active ingredient when it is being supplied.

In general, the labeling for all medical devices should adhere to the following guidelines:

- The information needed to identify and use the device safely should be provided on the device itself, as far as it is practical and appropriate.
- The medium, format, content, readability and location of labeling should be appropriate to the particular device.
- The use of internationally recognized symbols is encouraged.
- The product labeling must be in English.

Content of labeling

Primary and secondary levels of packaging shall contain contact information of the product owner on the labeling, which include the name and contact details, i.e., address, phone number, fax number or Web site. The labeling should bear sufficient information on identification, batch code/lot number, expiry, warning, precautions, side effects, storage and handling where relevant.

The Instructions for Use (IFU) for medical devices shall include detail information informing the users on any contra-indications, warning, and precautions to be taken. It is important to keep the IFU up-to-date with date of issue or identification number where appropriate.

35.10 Post-Marketing Surveillance Requirement

HSA uses a number of post-marketing measures to ensure the continued safe use of medical devices. These measures include reporting from healthcare professionals, mandatory reporting from device dealers, and exchange of regulatory information with other medical device regulatory agencies.

(i) Adverse Events

As a general principle, Adverse Events (AEs), which meet the three basic reporting criteria listed as follows, must be reported to HSA:

- An AE has occurred.
- The medical device is associated with the AE.
- The AE led to one of the following outcomes:
  - a serious threat to public health
  - death of a patient, user or other person
  - serious deterioration in state of health, user or other person
  - no death or serious injury occurred, but the event might lead to death or serious injury of a patient, user or other person if the event recurs

The Adverse Event Report Form can be downloaded from HSA Web site and the completed form is submitted by mail or fax to HSA.

All AEs should be reported immediately and not later than 48 hours for events that represents a serious threat to public health; not later than 10 days for events that has led to the death, or a serious deterioration in the state of health, of a patient, a user of the medical device or any other person; not later than 30 days for events where a recurrence of which might lead to the death, or a serious deterioration in the state of health, of a patient, a user of the medical device or any other person.

Upon submission, the Authority will acknowledge the receipt of the AE report, review it, and enter it into the computer database for tread analysis.

(ii) Field Safety Corrective Actions (FSCA)/Recalls

An FSCA is required when it becomes necessary for the product owner of the medical device to take action (including recall of the device) to eliminate or reduce the risk of, the hazards identified. FSCA may be triggered when information from the product owner's post-market surveillance (including complaints, adverse events etc) indicates an unacceptable increase in risk. On occasions, the Authority may advise product owners or their representative to implement an FSCA in relation to a medical device due to risk of serious injury or death to patients, users or others.

The Authority shall be notified when the product owner or its representative decides to initiate an FSCA. The time frame for notification of an FSCA is within 24 hours of having made the decision to conduct an FSCA. A preliminary report containing full information on the FSCA must be submitted within 24 hours from the commencement of the FSCA. A final report is to be submitted to the Authority within 21 days from the date of commencement of the FSCA.

35.11 Manufacturing-, Importing-, and Wholesaling-Related Regulation

Companies performing manufacturing, importing, and supplying by wholesale medical devices in Singapore have to comply with the licensing conditions and any application legislative requirements. There are three types of licenses for dealing in medical devices:

- Manufacturer's license
- Importer's license
- Wholesaler's license

The supporting documents for application of the licenses are as follows:

- Manufacturer's License — ISO 13485 certificate for finished medical device manufacturing
- Importer's License — GDPMDS of ISO 13485 certificate with scope of storage and distribution
- Wholesaler's License — GDPMDS or ISO 13485 certificate with scope of storage and distribution
- The dealer's license — valid for 12 months

The licensee is obliged to maintain the key regulatory responsibilities, which include product labeling advertising, furnishing information, maintenance of records, reporting of adverse events, conducting field safety corrective action, and verification of quality, safety, and efficacy of health products.

35.12 Good Distribution Practice for Medical Devices

Companies that are involved in wholesaling and/or importing medical devices in Singapore are required to be GDPMDS certified prior to applying for importer or wholesaler's license. In order to be certified by the certification bodies, companies are required to have implemented a quality management system that adheres to current good distribution practices. This ensures medical device products are consistently stored, transported and handled under appropriate condition. In order to demonstrate such assurance, companies are required to set up quality manuals, site master file, and comprehensive procedures as well as to include qualified personnel, credible documentation, and well-maintained facilities and equipment.

35.13 Clinical Trial-Related Regulation

A "Clinical trial" means an investigation in respect of a health product, such as drugs, medical devices, cell, and tissue-based therapeutic products, that involve human subjects and that is intended to

- discover or verify its clinical, pharmacological or pharmacodynamic effects,
- identify any adverse effect that may arise from its use,
- study its absorption, distribution, metabolism and excretion, or
- ascertain its safety or efficacy.

Current regulatory framework for medical devices requires the following:

- Approval from local ethic committee.
- Reporting of defects, adverse events, recalls to authority.
- Labeling requirements "Investigational Device — To be used by Qualified Investigators Only"

- Additional approval of the authority Clinical Trial Test Material (CTM) Medical Devices is required for importation of unregistered medical devices into Singapore for use in clinical trials.

Moving forward to the implementation of the Health Products (Clinical Trials) Regulations in 2012, further regulation will be imposed on the medical devices use in clinical trials. This includes procedures for regulatory submissions, import controls prior to initiation of clinical trials, and safety reporting requirement after the trials have started.

35.14 Special Access

Supply of unregistered medical devices is prohibited under the Health Products Act. However, there exists a possibility where an unregistered medical device is required for a specific treatment modality for a specific patient/patient population, emergency or in a case where all conventional therapies have failed; the special route provides an option to qualify practitioners, licensed laboratories and hospitals to meet special needs arising in the course of his practice. Besides, HSA approval shall be sought for import and re-export as well as supply of unregistered medical device for non-clinical purpose, which includes any form of use other than use or administration on humans, i.e., display of the medical device at an exhibition, training equipment, use on animals or use of *in vitro* diagnostic medical devices for research-use only. The special routes are listed as follows:

- import of unregistered medical devices for supply on named-patient basis
- import of unregistered medical devices for supply to a clinical laboratory, medical clinic, or private hospital licensed under the PHMC Act
- import of unregistered medical devices solely for re-export or for the export of unregistered medical devices
- supply of imported or manufactured unregistered medical devices for non-clinical purpose
- import of medical devices on consignment basis

Companies are required to submit application along with supporting documents to HSA for review. Upon approval, import and supply of medical device may commence. At the end of authorization, the importer shall be required to submit a declaration on the number of devices that have been imported and supplied in Singapore.

35.15 Commercial Aspect

35.15.1 Any Price Control of Medical Device

No, at this moment.

35.15.2 Are Parallel Imports Allowed?

Not allowed.

35.15.3 Any Advertisement Regulation of Medical Device?

Advertisement, for medical devices, means the publication, dissemination, or conveyance of any information for the purpose of promoting, whether directly or indirectly, the sale or use of the medical device. The advertisement may come in any form, including publication in a newspaper, magazine, display of posters, circulars, brochures, letters addressed to individuals, corporate, photographs, sound/visual broadcasting, the Internet, public demonstration, and offer of trials to the member of public. However, it is strictly prohibited to advertise to the general public the medical devices meant for research use only or medical devices intended for professional use only.

The advertisement should truthfully state the nature, quality and properties of the medical device. All claims must be made accurately in moderate terms, substantiated with scientific studies, and should not encourage indiscriminate unnecessary or excessive use. Advertisement also should not contain reference to HSA or language suggesting approval or endorsement of the medical device by HAS.

In addition, all advertisement must also comply with the Singapore Code of Advertising Practice (SCAP) drawn up by the Advertising Standards Authority of Singapore.

35.16 Upcoming Regulatory Implementation

35.16.1 Regulatory Framework for Cell- and Tissue-Based Therapeutic Products

Cell- and tissue-based therapeutic (CTT) products are defined as articles containing or consisting of autologous (the use of tissues and cells removed and applied to the same person) or allogeneic (the use of tissues and cells removed from one person applied to another person) human cells or tissues that are used for or administered to human beings for the diagnosis, treatment, or prevention of human diseases or conditions. Examples of CTT products are bone marrow transplant, embryonic stem cells, and demineralized bone matrix.

The objective of the CTT Regulatory Framework in Singapore is to better regulate the quality, safety and efficacy of CTT products intended for therapeutic use.

CTT products are classified as follows:

- High risk
    - o CTT product had been subject to substantial manipulation
    - o Intended for non-homologous use
    - o Combined with drug, biologic or device
- Low risk
    - o CTT product that is minimally processed and undergoes simple preservation and/or storage steps prior to patient transplantation

The regulatory approach in Singapore is CTT product being jointly regulated by both the Ministry of Health (MOH) and HAS. The MOH will regulate the clinical use of CTT products, while HSA will regulate the quality, safety, and efficacy aspects of high-risk CTT products. The proposed controls include

- pre-market registration for high-risk CTT
- enhanced pharmacovigilance requirements
- patient registry
- good tissue practice
- good manufacturing practice
- clinical trial authorization

References

1. Chan Angelique, ASIAN Metacentre Research Paper Series, *Singapore's Changing Structure and the Policy Implications for Financial Security, Employment, Living Arrangements and Health Care,* No. 3 (Institute for Asian Research National University of Singapore), p. 3.
2. GN-01 *Guidance on the Application of Good Distribution Practice for Medical Devices* (Online), Available (October 2011):

   http://www.hsa.gov.sg/publish/etc/medialib/hsa_library/health_products_regulation/medical_devices/guidance_documents.Par.33419.File.tmp/GN-01-R3%20Guidance%20on%20the%20Application%20of%20Good%20Distribution%20Practice%20for%20Medical%20Devices.pdf.
3. GN-02-R2 *Guidance on Licensing for Manufacturers, Importers and Wholesaler of Medical Devices* (Online), Available (November 2011):

   http://www.hsa.gov.sg/publish/etc/medialib/hsa_library/health_products_regulation/medical_devices/guidance_documents.Par.99323.File.tmp/GN-02-R2_Guidance%20on%20Licensing%20for%20Manufacturers%20Importers%20and%20Wholesalers%20of%20Medical%20Devices.pdf.
4. GN-04 *Guidance on Medical Device Recall* (Online), Available (October 2008):

   http://www.hsa.gov.sg/publish/etc/medialib/hsa_library/health_products_regulation/medical_devices/guidance_documents.Par.11355.File.tmp/GN-04-R1%20Guidance%20on%20Medical%20Device%20Recall.pdf.
5. GN-05-R1 *Guidance on the Reporting of Adverse Events for Medical Devices* (Online), Available (October 2008):

   http://www.hsa.gov.sg/publish/etc/medialib/hsa_library/health_products_regulation/medical_devices/guidance_documents.Par.56812.File.tmp/GN-05-R1%20Guidance%20on%20the%20

Reporting%20of%20Adverse%20Events%20for%20Medical%20Devices.pdf.

6. GN-08 *Guidance on Medical Devices Advertisements and Sales Promotions* (Online), Available (December 2008):

   http://www.hsa.gov.sg/publish/etc/medialib/hsa_library/health_products_regulation/medical_devices/guidance_documents.Par.72207.File.tmp/GN-08%20Guidance%20on%20Medical%20Devices%20Advertisements%20and%20Sales%20Promotions.pdf.

7. GN-10 *Guidance* on Medical Device Field Safety Corrective Action (Online), Available (October 2008):

   http://www.hsa.gov.sg/publish/etc/medialib/hsa_library/health_products_regulation/medical_devices/guidance_documents.Par.81192.File.tmp/GN-10-R1%20Guidance%20on%20Medical%20Device%20Field%20Safety%20Corrective%20Action.pdf.

8. GN-12-R1 *Guidance on Grouping of Medical Devices for Product Registration* (Online), Available (January 2011):

   https://www.hsa.gov.sg/publish/etc/medialib/hsa_library/health_products_regulation/medical_devices/guidance_documents.Par.33271.File.tmp/GN-12-R1_Guidance%20on%20Grouping%20of%20Medical%20Devices%20for%20Product%20Registration.pdf.

9. GN-13-R1 *Guidance on the Risk Classification of General Medical Devices,* Revision 1 (Online), Available (October 2008):

   http://www.hsa.gov.sg/publish/etc/medialib/hsa_library/health_products_regulation/medical_devices/guidance_documents.Par.83962.File.tmp/GN-13-R1%20Guidance%20on%20the%20Risk%20Classification%20of%20General%20Medical%20Devices.pdf.

10. GN-14-R1 *Guidance on the Risk Classification of In Vitro Diagnostic Medical Devices* (Online), Available (October 2008):

    http://www.hsa.gov.sg/publish/etc/medialib/hsa_library/health_products_regulation/medical_devices/guidance_documents.Par.55206.File.tmp/GN-14-R1%20Guidance%20on%20the%20Risk%20Classification%20of%20In%20Vitro%20Diagnostic%20Medical%20Devices.pdf.

11. GN-15-R4.1 *Guidance on Medical Device Product Registration* (Online), Available (November 2011):

    http://www.hsa.gov.sg/publish/etc/medialib/hsa_library/health_products_regulation/medical_devices/guidance_documents.Par.2810.File.tmp/GN-15-R4.1_Guidance%20on%20Medical%20Device%20Product%20Registration.pdf.

12. GN-23 *Guidance on Labeling for Medical Devices* (Online), Available (August 2011):

    http://www.hsa.gov.sg/publish/etc/medialib/hsa_library/health_products_regulation/medical_devices/guidance_documents.Par.12236.File.tmp/GN-23%20Guidance%20on%20Labelling%20for%20Medical%20Devices.pdf.

13. GN-26-R1 *Guidance on the Requirements for Exemption from Product Registration for the Import of an Unregistered Medical Device for Supply on Named-Patient Basis* (Online), Available (June 2010):

    http://www.hsa.gov.sg/publish/etc/medialib/hsa_library/health_products_regulation/medical_devices/guidance_documents.Par.73969.File.tmp/GN-26_Guidance%20on%20Named%20Patient%20Basis.pdf.

14. GN-27-R1 *Guidance on the Requirements for Exemption from Product Registration for the Import of Unregistered Medical Devices for Supply to a Clinical Laboratory, Medical Clinic or Private Hospital licensed under the PHMC Act* (Online), Available (June 2010):

    http://www.hsa.gov.sg/publish/etc/medialib/hsa_library/health_products_regulation/medical_devices/guidance_documents.Par.45595.File.tmp/GN-27_Guidance%20on%20Named%20PHMC%20Licensed%20Clinical%20Diagnostic%20Laboratory%20and%20Hospitals.pdf.

15. GN-28-R1 Guidance on the Requirements for Exemption from Product Registration to Import Unregistered Medical Devices solely for Re-export or for the Export of Unregistered Medical Devices (Online), Available (June 2010):

    http://www.hsa.gov.sg/publish/etc/medialib/hsa_library/health_products_regulation/medical_devices/guidance_documents.Par.27627.File.tmp/GN-28_Guidance%20on%20Authorisation%20Route%20for%20Import%20for%20Re-Export.pdf.

16. GN-29-R1 *Guidance on the Requirements for Exemption from Product Registration to Supply Imported or Manufactured Unregistered Medical Devices for Non-Clinical Purpose* (Online), Available (June 2010):

    http://www.hsa.gov.sg/publish/etc/medialib/hsa_library/health_products_regulation/medical_devices/guidance_documents.Par.81112.File.tmp/GN-29_Guidance%20on%20Authorisation%20Route%20for%20Import%20and%20Supply%20for%20Non-Clinical%20Purpose.pdf.

17. GN-30-R1 *Guidance on the Requirements for Approval to Import Medical Devices on Consignment Basis* (Online), Available (June 2010):

    http://www.hsa.gov.sg/publish/etc/medialib/hsa_library/health_products_regulation/medical_devices/guidance_documents.Par.92544.File.tmp/GN-30-R1_Guidance%20on%20Authorisation%20Route%20for%20Import%20on%20Consignment%20Basis.pdf.

18. *Health Sciences Authority Online* (Online), Available (07 December 2011): www.hsa.gov.sg.

Chapter 36

Taiwan: Medical Device Regulatory System

Li-Ling Liu

Division of Medical Devices and Cosmetics,
Taiwan Food and Drug Administration, Taiwan

LLL@fda.gov.tw

Disclaimer

The regulatory information contained in this chapter is intended for market planning and is subject to change frequently. Translations of laws and regulations are unofficial.

36.1 Market Overview

36.1.1 Overview of Structure and Funding of Local Healthcare System

The population of Taiwan is about 23 million. The Taiwan medical device industry had revenue of NTD 92.86 billion in 2010, which

Handbook of Medical Device Regulatory Affairs in Asia
Edited by Jack Wong and Raymond K. Y. Tong

ISBN 978-981-4411-21-9 (Hardcover), 978-981-4411-22-6 (eBook)
www.panstanford.com

has a 12.5% growth rate compared with that in 2009. The annual revenue of Taiwan is about 1% of the global market. The global market was USD 236 billion in 2010, and the growth rate was 6% per annum (Fig. 36.1). The export value was NTD 40.2 billion and import value was NTD 53.5 billion. The importing dependency of the Taiwan market is 67%. The United States is the largest importing and exporting country (Fig. 36.2).

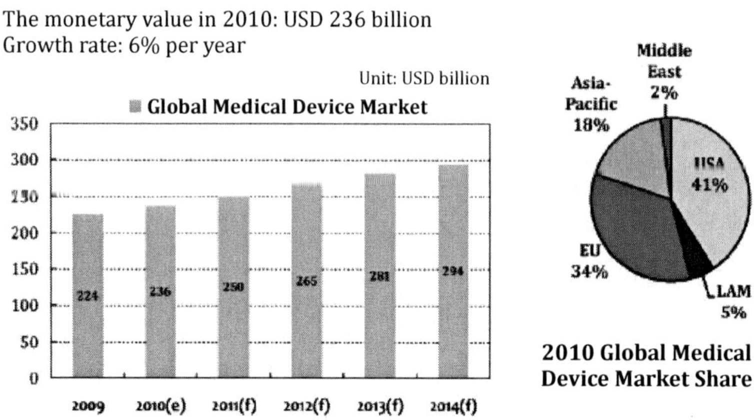

Figure 36.1 Global medical device market (*Sources*: Espicom Business Intelligence (2009); IEK Center (April 2010)).

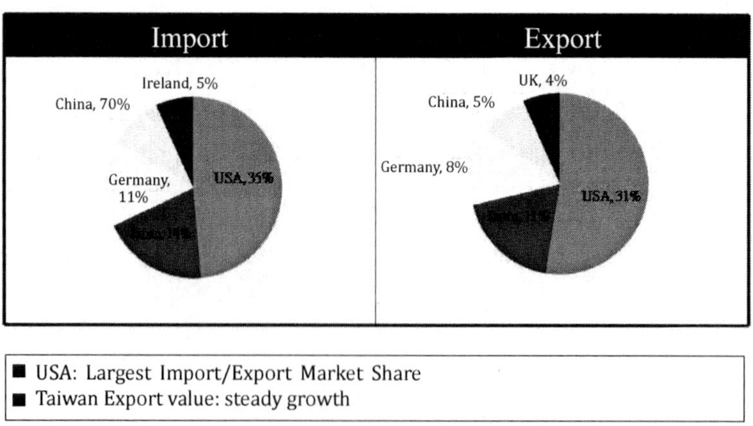

Figure 36.2 Import and export of medical devices in Taiwan (*Sources*: Taiwan Customs (2010); IEK Center (April 2010)).

36.1.2 Overview of Regulatory Environment and Laws/Regulations Governing Medical Devices

Regulation of medical devices in Taiwan dates back to 1970, when the Pharmaceutical Affairs Act was promulgated. Enforcement rules of the act were subsequently enacted in 1973.

Regulatory changes in the premarket approval process and post-market surveillance have continued to take place over the years in order to safeguard public health and harmonize with international regulations. The major ones are as follows:

(1) Pharmaceutical Affairs Act (1993)
(2) Good Manufacturing Practice (1998)
(3) Reclassification of medical devices (2000)
(4) Regulations Governing Management of Medical Devices (2004)
(5) Guidelines for Registration of Medical Devices (2004)
(6) Good Laboratory Practice for Nonclinical Laboratory Studies (2006)
(7) Medical Device Good Clinical Practice (2007)
(8) Guidance of preclinical testing (2009–2011)
(9) Application Guidelines for Registration of *in vitro* Diagnostic Medical Devices (2010)
(10) Medical Device Good Vigilance Practice (2011)

The regulation of medical devices along with product life cycle is shown in Fig. 36.3.

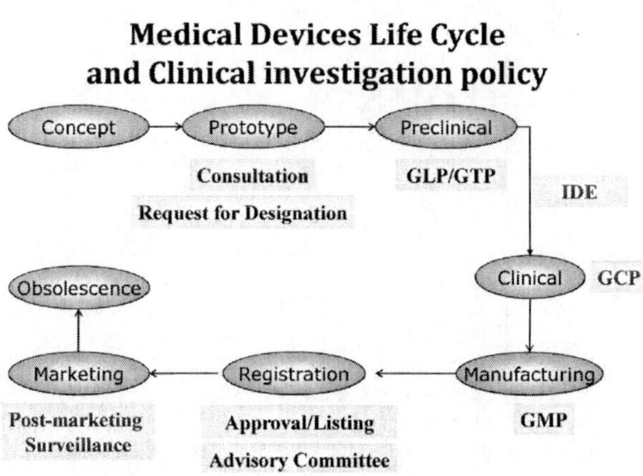

Figure 36.3 Administration of medical device life cycle. (*Source*: Taiwan Food and Drug Administration.)

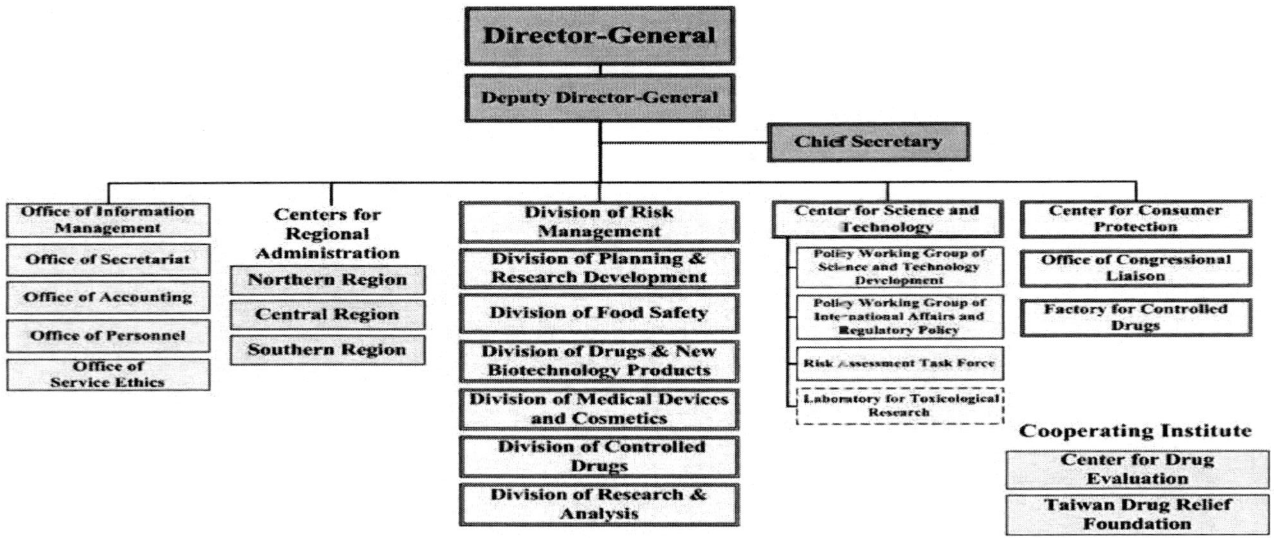

Figure 36.4 TFDA organization chart. (*Source*: Taiwan Food and Drug Administration.)

36.1.3 Detail of Key Regulator(s)

To assure the quality and safety of medical products and to promote industry development, the Taiwan government has strived to reform and renovate the organization of the Department of Health (DOH). By integrating the original Bureau of Food Safety, Bureau of Pharmaceutical Affairs, Bureau of Food and Drug Analysis, and Bureau of Controlled Drugs under the DOH into the newly established Food and Drug Administration (FDA), the Taiwan FDA (TFDA) was inaugurated on January 1, 2010. The organization chart of the TFDA is shown in Fig. 36.4.

The Division of Medical Devices and Cosmetics in the TFDA handles the administration of Medical devices in the public life cycle. All medical devices are required to be registered by TFDA before they can be manufactured domestically or imported from abroad.

36.2 Regulatory Overview

36.2.1 Definition of Medical Device

According to the definition by the law, the term "medical devices" refers to instruments, machines, apparatus, and their accessories, fittings and parts that are used in diagnosing, curing, alleviating, or directly preventing the diseases of human beings, or that may affect the body structure or functions of human beings. *In vitro* diagnostic devices (IVDs) are regulated by Guidelines for registration of medical devices, and include diagnostic reagents, instruments or systems used to collect, prepare, and test specimens from human body in order to diagnose disease or other conditions (such as status of health). Veterinary products are not under the scope of medical devices in Taiwan.

36.2.2 Classification of Medical Device

Medical devices are stratified by risk level and are divided into class I (low risk), class II (medium risk), and class III (high risk). Another parallel classification system emphasizes the intended use and mode of action, listed as follows:

(A) clinical chemistry and clinical toxicology devices
(B) hematology and pathology devices
(C) immunology and microbiology devices
(D) anesthesiology devices

(E) cardiovascular devices
(F) dental devices
(G) ear, nose, and throat devices
(H) gastroenterology-urology devices
(I) general and plastic surgery devices
(J) general hospital and personal use devices
(K) neurological devices
(L) obstetrical and gynecological devices
(M) ophthalmic devices
(N) orthopedic devices
(O) physical medicine devices
(P) radiology devices

For example, a resorbable calcium bone void filler would be under the scope of (N) and class II medical device.

For detailed and updated information, please refer to the TFDA medical device databases Web site (http://www.fda.gov.tw/licnquery/DO8180.asp).

36.2.3 Role of Distributors or Local Subsidiaries

TFDA issues product licenses only to domestic firms, all foreign companies must make submissions through authorized domestic distributors or subsidiaries. These local firms must have licenses for wholesaling, retailing, importing, or exporting medical devices. Also, these local firms are responsible for adverse events reporting, and recalls.

In the future, good distribution practice (GDP) will be implemented for enhancing quality and management of local distributors.

36.2.4 Products Registration, Technical Material Requirement, and Time Required

Device evaluation is based on the risk management concept. For class I products, submission requirements are (1) affidavit (2) GMP/ QSD certificate for sterilized devices or devices with metric function, and (3) medical device dealer license. For class II and III products, technical documents are required for full review, including preclinical testing, quality control, performance testing, sterilization, etc. However, these data can be waivered if the devices belong to class II and have both US and EU free sale certificates. For devices not having substantial equivalent products, clinical evaluation reports are mandated.

Regarding time required, the class I products follow on-site registration. The average review time for new medical devices was around 130 days in 2011; for substantial equivalent products of class II and class III, it was around 80 days in 2011. The statistics does not include the supplemental time for companies. The required documents for registration are clearly depicted in Fig. 36.5.

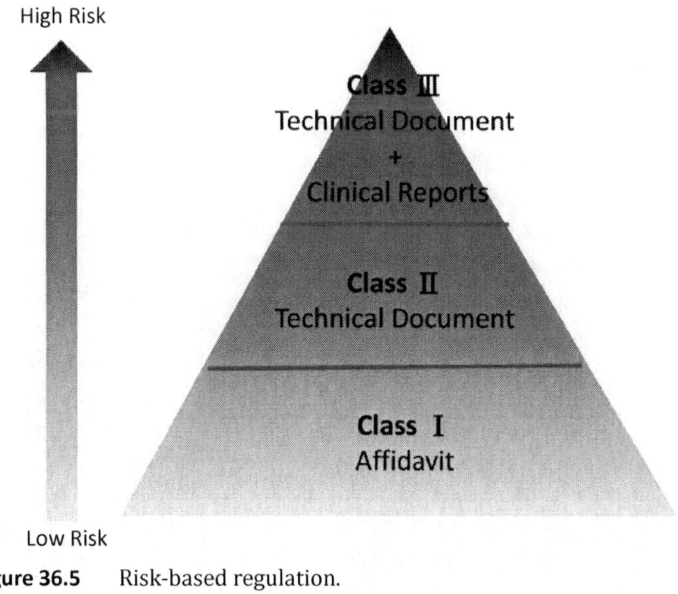

Figure 36.5 Risk-based regulation.

36.3 Quality System Regulation

The quality system of medical device manufacturers is audited to the requirements of GMP using conformity assessment standard based on ISO 13485. Newly established manufacturers and new applications for device registration must comply with GMP beginning on February 10, 1999. Full compliance with GMP for all devices on the market becomes mandatory effective February 10, 2004.

The GMP certificate is valid for three years, so the GMP inspection is done every three years routinely. However, we may go for cause inspection at any time if necessary. GMP Inspection to foreign manufacturers is conducted through the Quality System Documentation review. The foreign manufacturer or its initial importer may apply for on-site inspection as well as domestic manufacturers in Taiwan.

36.4 Combined Device–Drug Product

The registration pathway depends on the primary mode of action. For example, drug-eluting stents are considered a device, because the primary made of action is dilating the blood vessel though the stent. The combination product is jointly reviewed by device and drug experts.

36.5 Registration Fee

For new medical devices, the registration fee is NTD 30,000 (about USD 1000); for medical devices with predicates, the fee is NTD 10,000 (about USD 330); for Class III IVDs without predicates, the fee is NTD 50,000 (about USD 1660), and for those with predicates the fee is NTD 35,000 (about USD 1160).

36.6 Labeling Requirements of Medical Devices

Detailed requirements are listed in the guidelines for the registration of medical devices. For imported products, labeling in standard Mandarin is necessary, including product names, license number, manufacturer and distributor names and addresses, and shelf life.

The labeling, instructions, and packaging of domestically manufactured medical devices shall be in Chinese principally, and the font size for foreign characters shall be relatively smaller.

For imported medical device, in addition to the instruction in Chinese, the labeling and packaging shall also include the product name, license number, and the name and address of the importer pharmaceutical entity in Chinese and shall clearly mark the date of manufacture, expiration date, and storage period in Chinese or in a way easily recognizable. The font size for Chinese characters for the product name shall not be smaller than that for foreign characters.

36.7 Any Post-Marketing Surveillance Requirement

Medical facilities, device firms, and pharmacies are required to report any serious adverse reactions caused by medical devices. For certain devices, TFDA may designate a specific period of time to survey their safety after they have been approved for marketing. Periodic safety update reports (PSUR) from the license holders shall be submitted accordingly in the designated period. Currently, license holders of the devices that have been designated are to submit a PSUR every six months for three years. Taiwan started joining NCAR (National Competent Authority Reporting) program under GHTF (Global Harmonization Task Force) for exchanging ADR reports with other countries in 2010.

36.8 Manufacturing-Related Regulation

The manufacturing of medical devices shall comply with the relevant parts of the Factory Establishment Standards (FES), which is under article 57 of the Pharmaceutical Affairs Act. A manufacturer in compliance with Part 2 of FES, i.e., basic requirements for the establishment of factories, will be issued a factory registration certificate. Such manufacturer may then apply for compliance with FES, which is the requirement for medical device GMP certification.

36.9 Clinical Trial-Related Regulation

Preapproval of clinical trials is required for new medical devices claiming new design, new materials, new combination, etc. The process of submitting clinical trials protocols is illustrated in Fig. 36.6. Both approvals from TFDA and IRB (Institutional Review Board) are required prior to conducting clinical trials.

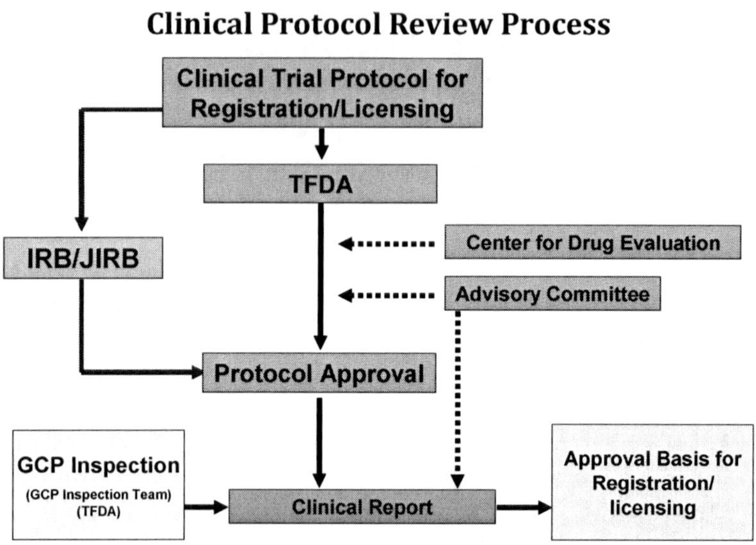

Figure 36.6 Clinical protocol review process.

36.10 International Cooperation

The mutual recognition of marketing approval may be achieved by establishing international agreements. An example is the exchange of letters between the Swissmedic of Switzerland and the Department of Health of Taiwan signed on July 4, 2007, in which both sides recognized that medical devices **manufactured in Taiwan** that legally bear the CE mark require no additional conformity assessment procedure for the Swiss market. Other exchanges of letters, for example, with the United States in 1998 and with the European Union in 2001, have also been signed to expedite the Quality System Documentation (QSD) review process for manufacturers. In an expedited review, QSD is simplified by submitting the following three documents instead: inspection report, Free Sale Certificate, and ISO 13485 certificate.

36.11 Commercial Aspects

36.11.1 Price Control of Medical Device

The national health insurance system is implemented in Taiwan under the National Health Insurance Act. For some diseases, the payment of medical devices is covered in DRG (Diagnosis Related Groups). For those that are not under DRG programs, the insurer should pay the same amount for devices with the same functional type.

36.11.2 Parallel Imports

To ensure the quality of products, only the license holders or consignors can import the devices. The authorization letter to the importer from the foreign original manufacturer is one of the required documents.

36.11.3 Any Advertisement Regulation of Medical Devices?

Persons other than medical devices dealers are not allowed to make advertisements. For publishing or broadcasting advertisement, the dealers shall, before publishing or broadcasting, submit all the written or spoken words and/or drawings or pictures constituting the advertisement to the central or municipal competent health authority for approval. Interviews, news reports, or propaganda-containing information implying or suggesting medical efficacy shall be regarded as advertisements of medicaments.

References

1. Pharmaceutical Affairs Act (1970) (amended 2012), *available as amended at* http://law.moj.gov.tw/LawClass/LawAll. aspx?PCode= L0030001.
2. Medical Care Act (1986) (amended 2012), available in unofficial English translation at http://law.moj.gov.tw/Eng/LawClass/LawAll. aspx?PCode=L0020021.
3. Regulations for Governing the Management of Medical Device (2004) (amended 2012), available in unofficial English translation at http:// www.fda.gov.tw/EN/includes/GetFile.ashx?id=1437&chk=f6a22c5f-0d38-4582-b17 b-40603c41eabb&mid=172&name=fdContent.
4. Regulations for Registration of Medical Device (2004) (amended 2010), available in unofficial English translation at http://www.fda. gov.tw/EN/includes/GetFile.ashx?id=1440&chk=37de015b-86b2-4fa7-ad16-0c133963bc47&mid=172&name=fdContent.

5. Standards for Medicament Factory Establishments (1973) (amended 2012), available in unofficial English translation at http://law.moj.gov.tw/Eng/LawClass/LawAll.aspx?PCode=L0030008.
6. Regulations of Medicament Manufacturer Inspection (1973) (amended 2011), available in unofficial English translation at http://law.moj.gov.tw/Eng/LawClass/LawAll.aspx?PCode=L0030009.
7. Regulations on Human Trials (2009), available in unofficial English translation at http://law.moj.gov.tw/Eng/LawClass/LawAll.aspx?PCode=L0020162.
8. Regulations for Governing the Monitoring of Safety of Pharmaceuticals (2004), available in unofficial English translation at http://www.fda.gov.tw/EN/includes/GetFile.ashx?id=1438&chk=44e02808-072a-4cc3-9d6 d-d65ab39898a3&mid=172&name=fdContent.
9. Regulations for Governing the Reporting of Serious Adverse Event of Pharmaceuticals (2004), available in unofficial English translation at http://www.fda.gov.tw/EN/includes/GetFile.ashx?id=1439&chk=0800b408-a750-4840-92 bf-8ce36951e156&mid=172&name=fdContent.
10. Recognition of Medical Device International Standards (2011), available at http://www.fda.gov.tw/tc/includes/GetFile.ashx?mID=46&id=10960&chk=42484d5f-bf 5b-49d9-baa7-860ed4787740.
11. Guidance for Pre-clinical Testing of Medical Device.
12. Guidance for Medical Device Good Vigilance Practice (2011), available at http://www.fda.gov.tw/tc/includes/GetFile.ashx?mID=19&id=11610&chk=a6edca23-6f ce-4bac-a81d-4b719411e788.
13. Guideline for Medical Device Good Clinical Practice (2007), available at http://www.fda.gov.tw/upload/133/Content/0960300979%e5%85%ac%e5%91%8a%e9%99%84%e4%bb%b6.pdf.
14. Good Laboratory Practice for Nonclinical Laboratory Studies (2006), available at http://www.fda.gov.tw/TC/includes/GetFile.ashx?mID=133&id=1104&chk=a83d8a0b-d6 c9-4502-9048-31b29ad61bf7.
15. Information for Registration of In Vitro Diagnostic Device (2010), available in unofficial English translation at http://www.fda.gov.tw/tc/includes/GetFile.ashx?mID=46&id=11474&chk=0999e953-2ed b-406f-a4c5-d53dd8fdaae6.

Chapter 37

Thailand: Regulatory and Medical Device Control

Patanawong Yuwadee

Thai Food and Drug Administration
Ministry of Public Health, Thailand

puyuwade@fda.moph.go.th

Disclaimer

The regulatory information contained in this chapter is intended for market planning and is subject to change frequently. Translations of laws and regulations are unofficial.

37.1 Market Overview

The health care industry in Thailand continues to grow annually, especially in the area of health care services and medical devices, because of several factors, including the government's universal health care coverage (UC) scheme introduced in 2000, good infrastructure of hospitals and health care personnel, and

Handbook of Medical Device Regulatory Affairs in Asia
Edited by Jack Wong and Raymond K. Y. Tong

ISBN 978-981-4411-21-9 (Hardcover), 978-981-4411-22-6 (eBook)
www.panstanford.com

Thailand's endeavor to become the medical hub of Asia. Thailand's medical device market in 2010 and 2011 was worth US$ 795 million and US$ 900 million, respectively, and it is expected to reach US$ 15 billion in 2015. The majority of the supply of medical devices in Thailand still depends on imports. As of July 5, 2012, 433 medical device local manufacturers and 1911 importers applied for establishment licenses. There are nearly 1400 public and private hospitals serving citizens and foreign patients. The main users of medical devices are public hospitals, while private hospitals play a major role as a hub for medical tourism and medical services for 2 million international visitors each year. It is widely accepted that Thailand is one of the few countries in the world that can provide the best health care for a reasonable cost. Thailand's hospital infrastructure and upgrading drive for the medical-imaging market was US$ 70 million in 2011 and is expected to reach US$ 100 million in 2015 (the year for emerging ASEAN Economic Community: AEC 2015).

37.2 Medical Device Regulations and Regulators

In Thailand, medical devices are regulated under the Medical Device Act 2008 by the Thai Food and Drug Administration (Thai FDA), Ministry of Public Health. The Medical Device Control Division under the Thai FDA is the key body and has main duties and responsibilities for control of manufacture, import, sale and advertisement of medical devices with the goal to ensure safety, effectiveness and quality of medical devices available to consumers. The Medical Device Control Division has performed activities including pre-marketing control, post-marketing control, pre- and post-advertisement control, standard development, and law and regulation development and has worked with the Bureau of Import and Export Control of the Thai FDA to control the import and export of medical devices in Thailand. The import and export of medical devices must undergo an inspection by Thai FDA staff at the port of checkpoint. The previous and first Medical Device Act 1988 was repealed and replaced by the Medical Device Act 2008, which came into force on March 6, 2008. Medical devices regulated under the Medical Device Act 2008 include medical devices for both human and animal use, *in vitro* diagnostic devices and computer software. Any person (natural or legal person) who wishes to manufacture or import medical devices must register for establishment license with the Thai FDA, and the establishment licensee (manufacturer or importer) has to submit for product registration or product approval with the Thai FDA. Once the licensee gets product approval, that medical device can be freely sold throughout the country. At present, sale license is not required except for selling HIV test kits. Thai FDA Good Manufacturing Practice (GMP), which was adapted from the ISO 13485 standard, was introduced in 2005 on a voluntary basis. It is currently compulsory for HIV test kit manufacturers and will be made compulsory for a wider range of devices in future. An establishment license has validity of five years (until December 31 of the fifth year from the year of issuance) and sale license has validity of one year (until December 31 of the year of license issuance). The act also provides some scope for exemption from medical device premise establishment and product registration requirements (with specific condition and procedure), such as importing necessary amount of medical device for personal use or for exhibition or educational purpose.

By law, certain important issues are decided by the Medical Device Committee and Subcommittees. The Medical Device Committee has following powers and duties:

- to give recommendations on policies and measures concerning the control of medical devices so as to ensure compliance with the act.
- to give recommendations on the issuance of Ministerial Notifications,
- to give approvals for suspension and revocation of an establishment license and product registration.

The subcommittees were appointed by the Medical Device Committee, including subcommittee on policy and measure of medical device control, subcommittee on establishment license and sale license, subcommittee on product registration, subcommittee on medical device advertisement, subcommittee on technical issues, subcommittee on standards of manufacture, import and sale of medical devices, and subcommittee on regulation development. Other important rules highlighted from the Medical Device Act 2008 include product liability, technology assessment procedure for announced particular products, and enforcement of Good Importation Practice (GIP), Good Distribution Practice (GDP), and Good Clinical Practice (GCP).

37.3 Definition of a Medical Device

A "medical device" means

(1) any instrument, apparatus, implement, machine, appliance, implant, *in vitro* reagent or calibrator, software, material, or other similar or related article

(a) intended by the manufacturer to be used, alone or in combination, for human beings or animals for one or more of the specific purpose(s) of

- (i) using in medical and health professional practices
- (ii) diagnosis, prevention, monitoring, treatment or alleviation of disease
- (iii) diagnosis, monitoring, treatment, or alleviation of an injury
- (iv) investigation, replacement, modification, or support of the anatomy or of a physiological process
- (v) upporting or sustaining life
- (vi) control of conception or fertility development
- (vii) aids or compensation for disability or handicap of human beings or animals
- (viii) providing information for medical or diagnostic purposes by means of *in vitro* examination of specimens derived from a human or an animal body
- (ix) disinfection of medical devices, and

(b) which does not achieve its primary intended action in or on the human or animal body by pharmacological, immunological or metabolic means, but which may be assisted in its intended function by such means.

(2) apparatus or spare part of instrument, machine, product, or article under (1)

(3) instrument, apparatus, machine, product or any other article as specified to be medical device by the Minister of Public Health.

37.4 Classification of Medical Devices

Currently, medical devices are divided into three classes depending on the level of control as follows:

(1) Licensed Medical Devices

This is the most stringent controlled group consisting of condoms, examination gloves, surgical gloves, HIV test kits for diagnostic purpose, corrective, and cosmetic contact lens.

(2) Notified Medical Devices

The control of this group is less stringent than group (1). It consists of physical therapy products, silicone breast prostheses implants, alcohol detectors, and equipment or instruments topically used for breast enhancement.

(3) General Medical Devices

All other medical devices not classified as group (1) and group (2) are in this class. The control of this group is the least stringent.

This classification is likely to depend only on the risk to public and has not yet followed the GHTF guidelines. However, it is in the process of changing toward a risk-based classification as stipulated in the GHTF and the draft of ASEAN Agreement on Medical Device Directive as well as a concern of the health situation in Thailand.

37.5 Product Registration

37.5.1 Licensed Medical Devices and Notified Medical Devices

For licensed medical devices, the standard requirements of each licensed medical device are normally both adopted and adapted from international standards and announced in the Ministerial Notification. The following details of medical devices are required to be submitted to the Thai FDA by the manufacturer or importer: product name, category and type, product description, packaging, type and quantity of components, details of manufacturing process, intended use or indication, warning, precaution, instruction for use, storage, shelf life (if any), product standard and test report, inspection or analytical procedure, local testing results for most product categories, Certificate of Free Sale and Certificate of Quality System of Manufacture (for imported products), label and leaflet, and the name and address of the manufacturer (manufacturing site/premise) and the importer.

For a notified medical device, the manufacturer or the importer is required to submit to the Thai FDA the same details as required for licensed medical devices except the details of the manufacturing process. Local testing results are required for some products.

It is in the process of changing toward using the ASEAN Common Submission Dossier Template (CSDT) as technical document requirements for submission for product approval of licensed and notified medical devices. At present, the ASEAN CSDT is implemented for contact lens submission.

37.5.2 General Medical Devices

The importer has to submit the Certificate of Free Sale for all kinds of general medical devices and the Certificate of Quality System of Manufacture (in some human use product categories) to get the Thai FDA Letter of Import Approval for product release from the Thai FDA checkpoint at port of customs as indicated and detailed in the Ministerial Notification No. 34 B.E. 2549 (A.D. 2006) on Medical Device Prohibited for Import or Sale, dated July 19, 2006, and Food and Drug Administration Regulation B.E. 2550 on Principles relating to Certification required for Import of Medical Devices and Import Approval under Certification Exemption, dated February 28, 2007. When necessary, additional documents to support the intended use or safety data of medical devices may be required.

Following is the list of medical devices for human use that require the importer to submit a Certificate of Quality System of Manufacture:

(1) implant products
(2) devices derived from tissues or tissue by-product
(3) sterile products
(4) diagnostic or treatment radiation devices

(5) *in vitro* diagnostic products for
  (a) blood group tests: ABO system, Rhesus (C,c,D,E,e) anti-kell
  (b) diagnostic tests: HIV infection (HIV I and II), hepatitis infection (A,B,C, and D), HTLV infection (HTLV I and II), antihumanglobolin (Coombs' reagent), anti-CMV (cytomegalovirus), HPV, HLA typing, biochemical test: glucose, lipid profile, liver function test, uric acid, BUN, creatinine, pregnancy test, drug abuse, hormones (thyroid, fertile), tumor markers (AFP, CEA and PSA) and cardiac markers (CK, CK-MB and troponin)
(6) disinfectant solution for medical devices
(7) restorative and crowning material

37.5.3 Review Period (as Promulgated in 2012)

Type of issuance	Procedure of site inspection or experts/ working group/ subcommitee review	Review period (working days)
Medical device manufacturing/import license	No	25
Medical device manufacturing/import license	Yes	60
Medical device manufacturing/import Notification acceptance	No	15
Medical device manufacturing/import Notification acceptance	Yes	35
Letter of Import Approval: 1 item of device	No	1
Letter of Import Approval: 2–100 items of devices	No	4
Letter of Import Approval: >100 items of devices	No	10
Medical device manufacturing/import license or notification acceptance for new products	Yes	250

37.5.4 Fees and Validity of Granting or Issued Document

Type of granting document	Fees (baht)	Validity (Years)	Remarks
Medical device manufacturing license	10,000	5	until the December 31 of the fifth year from the year of issuance
Medical device import license	20,000	5	until the December 31 of the fifth year from the year of issuance
Medical device manufacturing notification acceptance	5,000	5	until the December 31 of the fifth year from the year of issuance
Medical device import Notification acceptance	10,000	5	until the December 31 of the fifth year from the year of issuance
Letter of import approval: ≤ 10 items of devices	1,000	Align with the validity of the CFS (Certificate of Free Sale), if no validity specified in CFS, Letter of Import Approval will be valid for 5 years	
Letter of import approval: >10 items of devices	2,000		

37.6 Labeling

It is in the process of drafting label requirements under the Medical Device Act 2008. Currently, label requirements follow the Act 1988, which states that medical devices for sale or in possession for sale in Thailand must be labeled in Thai. Other additional languages are also allowed but must correspond with Thai and appear in size not larger than the Thai language.

Labels must include the product name, category and type of medical device, name and address of the manufacturer (manufacturing site/premise) as well as the importer, content, lot number, license number, intended use or indication, instruction for use, storage condition, warning, precaution, expiration date (if any), and the phrase "Single-use only" for single-use devices. The label contents of intended use or indication, instruction for use, and storage condition can be waived if these contents are already in the package insert.

37.7 Advertisement Control

The Medical Device Act 2008 strictly provides the measures on advertisement control for all medical devices, regardless of the class to which they belong. No person is allowed to advertise a medical device for commercial purpose to both the general public and the medical or health professionals unless he/she submits the application to the Thai FDA for advertising license. The objective is to ensure correct and clear dissemination of medical device information, especially to the general public. The act prohibits the following types of advertisement:

(1) to provide false or exaggerated information regarding the benefits, quality, quantity, standard, constituent, or origin of medical devices
(2) to represent any person's endorsement or commendation of the medical device's benefits
(3) to offer a prize conditional upon the taking of chance by any means
(4) to represent benefits of prevention, treatment, relief, or cure of a disease or symptom of a disease, which is prohibited under Ministerial Notification
(5) to issue misleading statement on an essential substance of a medical device

If violation is found, the Thai FDA has the power to issue any of the following orders:

(1) to make changes to the content or means of advertisement
(2) to prohibit the use of certain statements or means of the advertisement
(3) to advertise correct information

References

1. Medical Device Act B.E.2551 (A.D.2008).
2. Ministerial Regulation on the Rules, Procedures and Conditions of the Establishment Registration of Manufacturing Medical Devices, dated November 19, 2009.

3. Ministerial Regulation on the Rules, Procedures and Conditions of the Establishment Registration of Importing Medical devices, dated November 19, 2009.
4. Ministerial Notification No. 34 B.E.2549 (A.D.2006) on Medical Device Prohibited for Import or Sale, dated July 19, 2006.
5. Food and Drug Administration Regulation B.E.2550 on Principles relating to Certification required for Import of Medical Devices and Import Approval under Certification Exemption, dated February 28, 2007.
6. Sasithorn Ongdee. Wind of Change Sweeps Healthcare Industry (Online) (May 4, 2012), available:

   http://www.nationmultimedia.com/business/Wind (July 6, 2012).
7. Oliver Languepin. Medical Device Industry Overview in Thailand (Online) (30 August 2010), available:

   http://thailand-business-news.com/health/2528 (July 5, 2012).

Chapter 38

UAE: Overview of Medical Device/IVD Regulatory System

Amin Al Amiri
Ministry of Health, UAE

Disclaimer

The regulatory information contained in this chapter is intended for market planning and is subject to change frequently. Translations of laws and regulations are unofficial.

38.1 Ministry of Health

38.1.1 Registration and Drug Control Department

The executive Registration and Drug Control Department (RDCD) in the Ministry of Health (MOH) safeguards public health by ensuring

Handbook of Medical Device Regulatory Affairs in Asia
Edited by Jack Wong and Raymond K. Y. Tong

ISBN 978-981-4411-21-9 (Hardcover), 978-981-4411-22-6 (eBook)
www.panstanford.com

that all medicines and medical devices on the UAE market meet appropriate standards of safety, quality and efficacy.

38.1.2 Mission Statement

The mission of the RDCD is to protect and promote high standards of public health through the regulation of the quality, efficacy and safety of medicinal products used for humans and animals, the pharmacy profession and the pharmaceutical industry.

Additionally, the RDCD is required to advise His Excellency the Minister on the pricing of pharmaceutical products and to advise on policy relating to pharmaceuticals and regulatory systems and assist His Excellency in achieving the strategic aims of the UAE MOH.

38.1.3 Medical Device Registration

The regulation of medical devices in the UAE is aimed to maintain a balance between ensuring product safety, quality, and effectiveness and provide the public with timely access to medical devices and prevent the entry of unsafe or ineffective devices into the UAE market. Accordingly, this guideline is constructed to provide safeguard measures for patients, appliers, users, and third parties against possible health and safety hazards they may be exposed to during the use of such devices and their accessories.

The essential requirements for medical devices and their accessories and their implementation were laid down by the guideline to ensure that these devices shall meet the internationally established principles and requirements relating to their design, classification, manufacture, placing on the market, putting into service, and inspection.

Medical device control and regulation in the UAE is supervised and directed by the RDCD, MOH.

Classification, requirements, and evaluation of medical devices in UAE are supported by the UAE Pharmacy Law No. 4 for 1983 and conform to the global trends, rules, and regulations recognized as above.

38.2 Introduction to MD/IVD Regulatory System in UAE

The UAE regulatory system is mostly based on the recommendations of the Global Harmonization Task Force (GHTF) for medical devices (for types of certification, approval, and clearance system according to product class and rules of classification of these systems considered and accepted), and adapting with

(a) EU Medical Device Directives 93/42/EEC, EU *in vitro* Diagnostic Device Directive (IVDD) 98/79/EC and EU Active Implantable Medical Device Directive (AIMDD) 90/385/EEC.
(b) United States Food and Drug Administration (US FDA)
(c) Australia Therapeutic Goods Administration (TGA)
(d) Singapore Health Sciences Authority (HSA)

The regulatory body of medical devices/IVD is the RDCD — Medical Practice and License Sector.

Contact Information:
Key contact persons:
Dr. Amin Al Amiri
Assistant Undersecretary for Medical Practice and License,
Ministry of Health, Abu Dhabi, P.O. Box 848, UAE
Telephone: +971 26117434
Fax: +971 2636742

Dr. Fatima Albraiki
Director of Registration and Drug control Department,
Ministry of Health, Abu Dhabi, P.O. Box 848, UAE
Telephone: +971 26117421
Fax: +971 2636742
www.moh.gov.ae

38.3 Medical Devices Marketing Approval Flow Chart

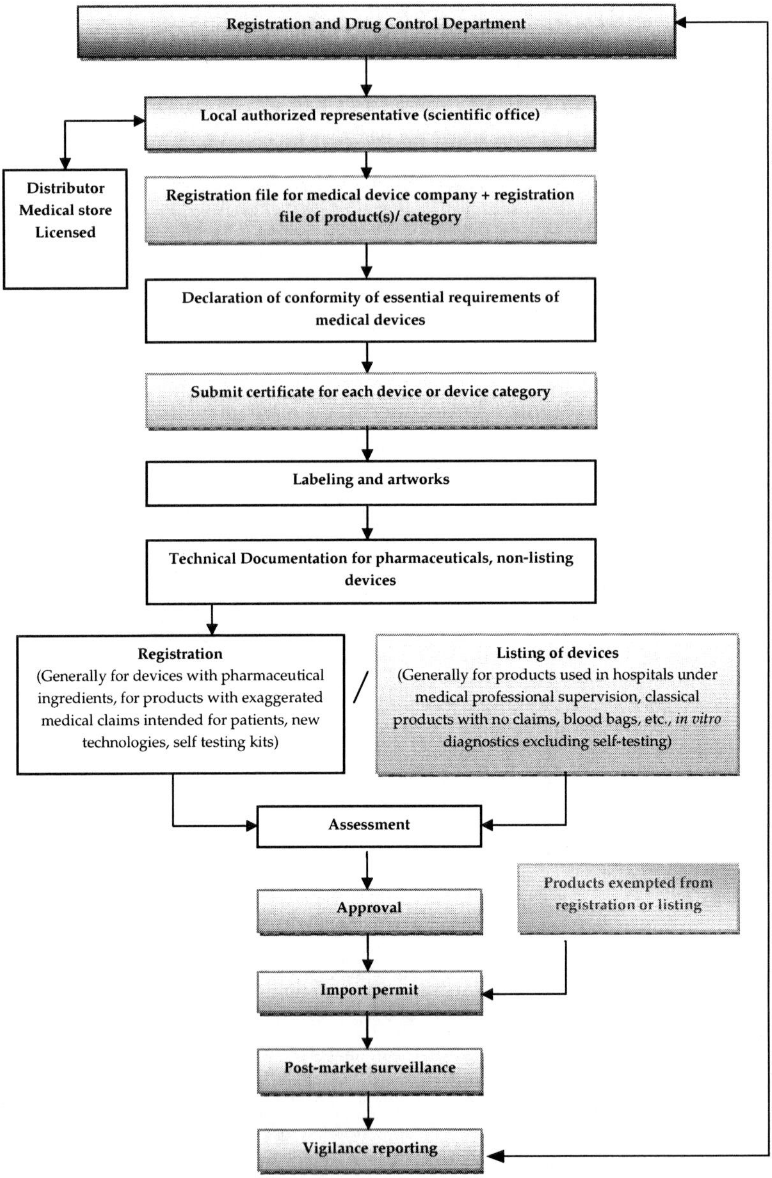

Figure 38.1 Medical device marketing approval flow chart.

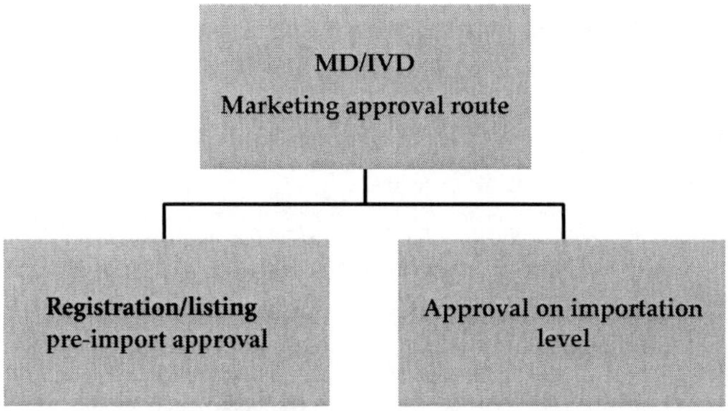

Figure 38.2 Medical device marketing approval flow chart with pre-importation approval for each consignment.

38.4 Approval on Importation Level

Medical devices those are not subject for listing or registration

(a) printing graphing papers
(b) accessories for listed or registered medical devices
(c) medical device instruments operating solvents or liquids that do not contact patients
(d) woven and nonwoven clothing materials and their products (gowns, masks, support bandages, clothes, mattresses, etc.)
(e) hospital and clinic furniture, wheelchairs, walking support devices
(f) *in vitro* diagnostic reagents given that they are not self-testing or high-risk (A or B classes).
(g) optical lenses, except contact lenses
(h) external prosthesis (artificial extension that replaces a missing body part) not intended for implantation.
(i) disposables and their equivalent: not intended for treating disease (tongue pressers, medical trash bins, gloves, diapers, disposable bedsheets, etc.)
(j) casts, plastic casts, collars, or any external devices to support the movement or stabilizing of joints or the body parts
(k) materials and accessories used in manufacturing dental parts, dentures, dental braces, given that they are not intended for implantation within oral cavity and jaws.
(l) hearing aids (nonimplantable)

38.5 Definition of a Medical Device

A medical device is any instrument, apparatus, implement, machine, appliance, implant, *in vitro* reagent or calibrator, software, material or other similar or related article:

(a) intended by the company and its manufacturing site to be used, alone or in combination, for human beings for one or more of the specific purpose(s) of

- diagnosis, prevention, monitoring, treatment or alleviation of disease
- diagnosis, monitoring, treatment, alleviation of or compensation for an injury
- investigation, replacement, modification, or support of the anatomy or of a physiological process
- supporting or sustaining life
- control of conception
- disinfection of medical devices
- Indicate the sterilization process completion
- providing information for medical or diagnostic purposes by means of *in vitro* examination of specimens derived from the human body, and

(b) which does not achieve its primary intended action in or on the human body by pharmacological, immunological or metabolic means, but which may be assisted in its intended function by such means.

38.6 Classification of Medical Device/IVD

(a) The control of medical devices is based on risk assessment and risk management. The level of regulatory control applied to the medical device is proportional to the degree of perceived risk associated with the device.

(b) Medical devices are classified into four classes, based on the GHTF classification: Class I (low risk), II and III (medium risk), and IV (high risk).

- **Class I devices** are those that need the **lowest level of regulation** because of low risk to the patient, except sterile products.

- **Class II devices** are of medium-risk and require assessed quality system according to the ISO 13485 standards. These devices are invasive in their interaction with the human body, but the methods of invasion are limited to natural body orifices.
- **Class III devices** are of a medium risk. They are either partially or totally implantable within the human body and may modify the biological or chemical composition of body fluids.
- **Class IV devices** are of high risk and require design/clinical trial reviews, product certification, and an assessed quality system involving clinical trials. These devices affect the functioning of vital organs and/or life-support systems. They are usually invasive, life-sustaining, life-supporting, or are used "in preventing impairment of human health or if the device presents a potential unreasonable risk of illness or injury."

(c) Classification of *in vitro* diagnostic medical devices is based on the potential risk involved in their use and interpretation clinically:
- Class A (low individual risk and low public health risk), e.g., clinical chemistry analyzer, prepared selective culture media
- Class B (moderate individual risk and/or low public health risk), e.g., pregnancy self-testing, anti-nuclear antibody, urine test strips
- Class C (high individual risk and/or moderate public health risk), e.g., blood glucose self-testing, human leukocyte antigen (HLA) typing, prostate-specific antigen (PSA) screening, rubella.
- Class D (high individual risk and high public health risk), e.g., HIV blood donor screening, HIV blood diagnostics.

38.7 Authorized Representative Concept

(a) Legal manufacturers based outside the UAE **(authorized representative in the country of origin)** have to appoint local representative/s to act on their behalf (MOH licensed medical store or scientific office).

(b) A local representative is the legal entity licensed by the MOH who has received a mandate from the mother company to act on its behalf regarding matters pertaining to placing the product in the UAE Market and all its registration requirements.

(c) A legalized agreement stating the appointment of the local authorized representative by the company should be submitted.

(d) Importation and distribution activities should be performed by an appointed licensed medical Store **(one importer for a product).**

Responsibilities of the Local Representative

(a) Monitor the device on the market and inform the MOH immediately after the detection of any problem related to a registered device.

(b) Handle device recalls.

(c) Provide technical support and services to the users of registered device(s).

(d) Advise on effective implementation of all regulatory procedures, including Adverse and Near Incident Reporting, Advisory Notice Issue (including Product Recall), Post-Market Feedback, Complaint Handling, and Significant Change Notifications.

38.8 Company Registration

38.8.1 Medical Devices Classified as Nonpharmaceutical Dosage Form

For the registration of the authorized representative in country of origin (a legal manufacturer) along with source, the file should include the required documents and information relevant to the main source (manufacturing facility: final releaser/assembly) to be evaluated according to the set regulation.

A declaration from the legal manufacturer should declare the list of their manufacturing sites related to the source/s, along with contract manufacturers, and contract sterilizers, specification developers, packagers or labelers, processors of single-use devices., and manufacturers of components or accessories that are sold or released directly to the end user.

Note: The MOH has the right to ask for certificates for any of the above sites.

38.8.2 Medical Devices Classified as Containing Pharmaceutical Ingredients

For the registration of the manufacturer, the documentation and information relevant to all sites involved in the manufacturing process is required according to the set regulation in case of pharmaceutical dosage forms.

Main Documents to be provided

1. An official application form, which is to be signed by the legal manufacturer and its local authorized representative.
2. Legal manufacturer business license issued by the competent authority in the country of origin, including those for the source/main manufacturing site.

   If the company has multiple manufacturing sites, a flow chart or table should be submitted identifying each manufacturing location with the manufacturing step carried out, as following: design, production, sterilization (if applicable), packaging, labeling, final release.
3. Site Master File for each manufacturing site (if applicable; mainly required for pharmaceutical product manufacturers).
4. Notarized copies of certificates pertaining to quality accreditations from recognized assessment bodies (ISO-13485) or GMP certificate issued by the health authority.
5. Post-marketing surveillance general plan (Global SOP).
6. General profile

38.9 Product Registration

38.9.1 Medical Devices Subject for Listing

(*Must not be of pharmaceutical dosage form*)

- o all class 1, medical devices
- o dressings and blasters intended to be in contact with wounds
- o classical (not new technology) invasive, transient or implantable medical devices used by medical professionals or within hospital use, given that do not carry labels intended for patients or retail sale
- o Blood-collecting tubes and bags

given that all these devices should have no labeling directed for patients with exaggerated medical claims.

38.9.2 Product Registration: Main Documents

Table 38.1 lists the documents required to be provided by the company. The application forms are available in the guide line (published on the MOH Web site) and available for local distributors at the customer service center.

Table 38.1 Main documents needed for product registration

Attachment	Documents required
A	**Application Form** The application to place a medical device on the UAE market must be signed and stamped by the company and local representative
B	**Regulatory Approval** (Free Sale certificate or documentation and letters of regulatory approval) and (certification or FDA clearance, TPP clearance approval clearance, etc.)
C	**Post-market requirement/vigilance system and risk assessment** SOP is required for a specific device
D	**Status of device distribution** List of countries where it is marketed, details of the regulatory status
E	**Device Information** (enclose device description and list of models/codes/ref. no. (if any) intended use, indications, instructions of use, contraindications, warnings, precautions, potential, adverse events, device labeling,* alternative labeling, which include physicians manual, pack labeling, and promotional material, a general description of the device and detailed description of the device attributes
F	**Labeling** • Three copies (artwork) of the each product packaging, labeling. • Labeling and packaging must have: the product name, name and address of the company printed in English and/or Arabic, manufacturing date and/or expiration date (if applicable). • For single use medical devices must be labeled on outer pack label with "SINGLE USE."
G	**Declaration of conformity/evidence of conformity to essential principles + quality certificates issued by assessment bodies**

H	**Safety and effectiveness data (Summary report)** H.1: Safety and effectiveness data H.2: Risk assessment H.3: Pre-clinical and clinical studies H.4: Biocompatibility H.5: Special requirements for devices containing biological material H.6: Literature studies
I	**Manufacturing process (for pharmaceutical forms)**
J	**Special requirements for medical devices manufactured from or incorporating viable or nonviable animal tissue or their derivative(s).**

* Labels are subject to assessment by evaluation committee, and understandable Universal symbols/instructions for professionals and consumers are required on the label such as sterile, single use, storage condition, etc.

38.9.3 Required Attachments per Device Class

Table 38.2 Required attachments per device class

Class I/ general IVD A	Class I (sterile and/ or with measuring function)/general IVD (class A)	Class II/ class B IVD	Class III/ class C IVD/self-testing IVD	Class IV/ class D IVD
A	A	A	A	A
B	B	B	B	B
Not Applicable	*Not Applicable*	C	C	C
Not Applicable	*Not Applicable*	D	D	D
E	E	E	E	E
F	F	F	F	F
G Self-declaration	G F. Self-declaration G. All certificates and documents certifying conformity to the aspects of manufacture relating to sterility and metrology	G	G	G
Not Applicable	*Not Applicable*	*Not Applicable*	H	H
Not Applicable	*Not Applicable*	*Not Applicable*	I (*if required*)	I (*if required*)

38.10 Pricing

- Not applicable unless the device containing ingredient for long term therapeutic use, (e.g., intra-articular hyaluronic acid).
- Registration committee decides for device subject to pricing.

38.11 Parallel Importation

Not allowed.

References

1. Australia TGA (Therapeutic Goods Administration), http://www.tga.gov.au/industry/devices.htm.
2. EU Medical Device Directives 93/42/EEC, EU *in vitro* Diagnostic Device Directive (IVDD) 98/79/EC and EU Active Implantable Medical Device Directive (AIMDD) 90/385/EEC, http://ec.europa.eu/health/medicaldevices/documents/guidelines/index_en.htm.
3. Global Harmonization Task Force (GHTF) for Medical Device Classification, http://www.ghtf.org/documents/sg1/SG1-N15-2006-Classification-FINAL.pdf.
4. Medical Device Registration Guideline/ Registration and Drug Control Department, Ministry of Health, UAE, http://213.42.151.126/admincp/assetsmanager/Files/Pharmacusts/MEDICALDEVICEguidlinesforUAE.pdf.
5. Singapore HSA, http://www.hsa.gov.sg/publish/hsaportal/en/health_products_regulation/medical_devices.html.
6. US FDA, http://www.fda.gov/MedicalDevices/default.htm.

Chapter 39

Vietnam: Medical Device Regulatory System

Thuy Nguyen Thi Thu
Johnson & Johnson Medical Vietnam
17 Ngo Quyen St., Hoan Kiem Dist., Hanoi, Vietnam
thuyntt@its.jnj.com

Disclaimer

The regulatory information contained in this chapter is intended for market planning and is subject to change frequently. Translations of laws and regulations are unofficial.

39.1 Market Overview

(i) Vietnam is a fast-growing country. Its population is about 87 million and is receptive to the use of advanced medical products.

(ii) The main high-technology medical devices are imported from foreign manufacturers. The imported medical devices account for 80% of total medical devices in Vietnam.

(iii) Local manufacture is highly encouraged by the Ministry of Health.

Handbook of Medical Device Regulatory Affairs in Asia
Edited by Jack Wong and Raymond K. Y. Tong

ISBN 978-981-4411-21-9 (Hardcover), 978-981-4411-22-6 (eBook)
www.panstanford.com

39.2 Overview of Regulatory Environment and Laws/Regulations Governing Medical Devices

Medical device regulation is developing in Vietnam. The new regulatory system will be largely based on the ASEAN Medical Device Directives (AMDD), which refer to the Asian Harmonization Working Party (AHWP) and the Global Harmonization Task Force (GHTF) directives. The GHTF is a voluntary consortium with representatives from trade and regulatory authorities from United States, Canada, Australia, Japan, and the European Union, formed in 1992 to harmonize the standards and principles of regulating medical devices.

Currently, Circular 24/2011/TT-BYT dated June, 21, 2011, guides medical device importing, in which imported medical devices belonging to 50 categories need to get import license before importation; other medical devices (except "new medical device") are considered for exemption. However, the requirements for the exempted and non-exempted ones are the same. The only difference is that the documents for exempted ones need not be submitted to the authority to get the import license; instead, the required documents may be inspected by the authority.

All local medical devices need to be registered according to Circular 07/2002/TT-BYT dated May 30, 2002.

39.2.1 Detail of Key Regulator(s)

The regulatory body in Vietnam is the Department of Medical Equipment and Construction (DMEC), the Ministry of Health. Figure 39.1 presents the organizational chart of the DMEC in the Ministry of Health.

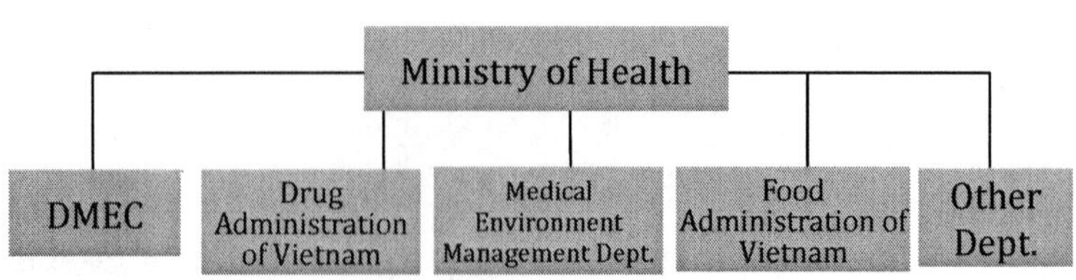

Figure 39.1 DMEC organizational chart.

Contact Information

Department of Medical Equipment and Construction,
Ministry of Health, 138A Giang Vo Street, Badinh District,
Hanoi, Vietnam
Telephone: +844 62732272
Fax: +844 62732279
Web site: http://www.moh.gov.vn

39.3 Regulatory Overview

39.3.1 Definition of Medical Device

Medical devices are equipment, devices, materials, and chemicals, including necessary software, used alone or in combination, for human for the purpose of

(i) preventing, monitoring, diagnosing, treating, or alleviating disease or compensating for an injury
(ii) investigation, replacement, modification, or support of the anatomy or of a physiological process
(iii) supporting and sustaining life
(iv) controlling contraception
(v) disinfecting medical devices (excluding chemicals, insect- and bacterium-killing products for family uses and health)
(vi) specialized transport for health activities

Note:

(i) Disinfection products are not in the scope.
(ii) Accessories/spare parts are listed together with their equipment, if any.
(iii) Combination products will be decided on a case-by-case basis, according to its primary action and reference regulations from the EU and the United States.

Devices designed for the treatment or diagnosis of diseases and injuries in animals are outside the scope of the proposed regulatory framework.

39.4 Classification of Medical Devices (Class A, B, C, D)

The classification of medical devices based on the risk level is being developed in Vietnam. It mainly follows the ASEAN Medical Device Directive (AMDD)/GHTF recommendation.

39.5 Role of Distributors or Local Subsidiaries

The importer is the person who applies and holds the license for the import of a medical device.

They have the following roles under Circular 24/2011/TT-BYT:

(i) effective communication with the manufacturer, distributor, user, and DMEC
(ii) responsible for local labeling activity, if any
(iii) responsible for maintenance and services
(iv) notification and management of safety information to the user and the authority
(v) annual report to the authority about business activity

Details can be found in Circular 24/2011/TT-BYT.

39.6 Product Registration or Conformity Assessment Route and Time Required

The Medical Device Administration Control System is basically divided into two parts: pre-market approval and exemption.

The DMEC is the competent authority and also responsible for conformity assessment. Conformity assessment committee includes DMEC, Medical Service Department, and other experts working within the Ministry of Health.

Pre-market approval is in the form of import license application. The medical device categories are subjects of pre-market approval, including high risk one (e.g., implants) and high-value ones (e.g., MRI, PET). Other medical devices (except new medical device) are exempted. The importer will work directly with the customs for clearance without import license. The documents required for pre-market approval and exemption products are the same.

Suggested license Routes/Steps

The importer collects necessary documents and submits them to the DMEC. Following are the documents required:

(i) CFG/CFS or CE marked
(ii) ISO 9001 or ISO 13485
(iii) Catalogue
(iv) Letter of authorization
(v) Executive summary in Vietnamese

- The DMEC receives the document and carries out assessment (deficiency document will be requested from the importer, if any).
- The conformity assessment committee meeting will be held to approve the document.
- The Ministry of Health issues the import license, which is valid for one year from the date of issue.

The importer pays the fee and receives the license.

According to the regulation, the timeline for evaluation is 15 working days.

39.6.1 Quality System Regulation

Vietnam follows ISO 9001, ISO 13485:2003, and Vietnam's standards (TCVN). It is voluntary to follow them.

39.6.2 Product Registration and Quality System Regulation for Combined Device–Drug Product

There is no specific rule for a combination product. Such a product will follow either the medical device or the pharmaceutical regulation.

39.6.3 Registration Fee

The fee for the import license is about USD 10–150 / product family, depending on the value of the product.

39.6.4 Technical Material Requirement

See Section 39.6 for imported medical devices and Circular 07/2002/TT-BYT dated, May 30, 2002, for local ones.

39.6.5 Labeling Requirements for Medical Devices

The label on a medical device follows Decree No. 89/2006/ND-CP, dated August 30, 2006, of the Prime Minister and Circular 09/2007/TT-BKHCN, dated April 6, 2007, of the Ministry of Science and Technology. The requirements regarding local manufacturing are being developed on the basis of ISO 13485. They are expected to be issued by 2014.

39.6.6 Post-Marketing Surveillance Requirement

The notification and management of safety information to user and the authority must be done by the importer, but there is no specific guideline on this requirement.

39.6.7 Manufacturing-Related Regulation

The requirements regarding local manufacturing are being developed on the basis of ISO 9001 and ISO 13485. They are expected to be issued by 2014.

39.6.8 Clinical Trial-Related Regulation

Clinical trials of medical devices are regulated. They follow Decision 36/2006/QD-BYT, dated November 14, 2006. Clinical trials required in the following cases:

1. Some local products: The Ministry of Health will decide which case requires a clinical trial.
2. Imported products: This applies to medical devices considered "new" products that are used for the application of new diagnosis and therapeutic methods and imported into Vietnam for the first time.

39.6.9 Is There a Procedure for Mutual Recognition of Foreign Marketing Approval or International Standards?

No.

39.7 Commercial Aspects

39.7.1 Any Control over Prices of Medical Devices?

No, at this moment.

39.7.2 Are Parallel Imports Allowed?

Under the current regulation, medical devices are imported via an authorized importer. However, the authority does not always check the authorization letter for exempted products.

39.7.3 Any Regulation Regarding Advertisement of Medical Devices?

The advertisement of medical devices follows the joint-circular 01/2004/TTLT-BVHTT-BYT, dated January 12, 2004.

39.8 Upcoming Events

Revision of the regulation on local clinical trial requirement is being developed and is expected to be issued by 2013.

References

1. Ministry of Health, Vietnam Retrieved (March 2012) from http://www.moh.gov.vn/wps/portal/boyte/trangchu/!ut/p/c5/04_SB8K8xLLM9MSSzPy8xBz9CP0os3hnd0cPE3MfAwMLd3NDA0_XUKdQDy8nQ4NgU_wkA5kFS5uFgZGTqZmnoEGLgYGn-qYQeQMcwNFA388jPzdVvyA7O83RUVERAHJEoy0!/dl3/d3/L2dBISEvZ0FBIS9nQSEh/.

2. Nguyen Minh Tuan, Director of Department of Medical Equipment and Construction, March 2012 (email: ngmtuan@ymail.com; address: 38A Giang Vo, Ba Dinh Dist., Hanoi, Vietnam; phone: + 84 4 62732277).
3. Nguyen Tu Hieu, Expert of Department of Medical Equipment and Construction, March 2012 (email: hieuboyte@yahoo.com; address: 38A Giang Vo, Ba Dinh Dist., Hanoi, Vietnam; phone: + 84 4 62732272).

Appendix:
Regulatory Summary Table

Key dates	Authority/ regulator name	Devices class & particu-larities	Product labeling	Roles & licenses	Registration process	Documen-tation & language	Post-market	Combination products
ASEAN								
First Draft of the Asian Medical Device Directive (AMDD) issued in January 2008 Official Deadline for all ASEAN Member States to comply with AMDD: 2015 ASEAN Consultative Committee on Standards and Quality (**ACCSQ**) Medical Device Product Working Group (**MDPWG**)	Each Authority in each ASEAN Member	A-Low Risk B-Low-moderate C-Moderate-high D-High	Member States may require local languages	Manufacturer/ Authorized Representative shall register or notify the Regulatory Authority of the Member State	Member States must put a system in place to assess Medical Devices MD shall be assessed by the regulatory authority of a Member State, or any appointed bodies recognized by a Member State and should be in conformity and in compliance with the requirements laid down in the AMDD and other relevant statutes of a Member State.	Demonstration of compliance to the Essential Requirements CSDT (Common Submission Dossier Template) Application to be submitted in: English	Member States to take appropriate measures and immediately inform other Member States	AMDD covers the device component of a combination product

(Continued)

Key dates	Authority/ regulator name	Devices class & particularities	Product labeling	Roles & licenses	Registration process	Documentation & language	Post-market	Combination products
AUSTRALIA								
Therapeutic Goods Act 1989 Therapeutic Goods Regulations 1990 Therapeutic Goods (Medical Devices) Regulations 2002 2010: IVDs regulated as subset of Medical Devices	**TGA**: Therapeutic Goods Adminis-tration Office of Devices Authorizat ion<TGA< Australian Government Department of Health and Ageing	**MDD Class:** I- Low Risk Is, Im, IIa -Low - moderate IIb-Moderate-high III-High **AIMD:** All-High Risk	Grouping of MD under one ARTG inclusion if same manufacturer-sponsor-classification-GMDN code For Class III and AIMD: same as above + same Unique Product Identifier (UPI) Product labeling: in English, use of recognized symbols (e.g. ISO 15223-1)	Manufacturer to designate an Australian Sponsor Once MD included in the ARTG (Australian Register of Therapeutic Goods), no expiry date – maintain compliance to Essential Principles and submit changes to TGA for evaluation as required MD supported by a TGA CA (Conformity Assessment) Certificate: validity 5 years	Regulatory System follows EU MD Directive 93/42/EEC 4 processes: 1. For class I(non-sterile, non-measuring) 2. For MD manufactured in AUS (other than Class I) 3. For MD manufactured overseas (other than Class I) 4. For MD containing a medicine or materials of animal, microbial recombinant or human origin **Process 3:** • Device Classification by Manufacturer • Conformity Assessment Procedure by Manufacturer – validated by TGA or EU Notified Body • Australian Declaration of Conformity by Manufacturer • Manufacturer's evidence submitted to TGA by Sponsor • Application lodged on-line by Sponsor to include MD in ARTG **Process 4:** • Device Classification by Manufacturer • TGA Conformity Assessment application by Manufacturer • Australian Declaration of Conformity by Manufacturer • Manufacturer's evidence submitted to TGA by Sponsor • Application lodged on-line by Sponsor to include MD in ARTG	Already CE marked MD: reduced requirements Not CE marked MD: full Conformity Assessment by TGA: • Copy of current conformity assessment evidence • Risk Management File • Clinical evidence • Essential Principles Checklist STED format as reference **Application Audit:** **Level 1: documentation required:** • Australian Declaration of Conformity • Copy of current conformity as-sessment evidence • Information on device (labeling/ IFUs/advertising materials) **Level 2:** • Same as Level 1 • Risk Management Report • Clinical Evaluation Report • Efficacy and performance data Australian-EC Mutual Recognition Agreement (MRA) applicable to all classes and Class III (not containing medicine or material of animal, human, microbial origin): abbreviated approval route	**Adverse Events:** • Serious threat to public health: to be reported or <48h • Led to death: immediately or <10 days • Other events: immediately or <30 days	TGA considers: • the primary intended pur-pose • the mode of action of the product to define if they will be regulated as a medicine or a medical device.

Key dates	Authority/ regulator name	Devices class & particularities	Product labeling	Roles & licenses	Registration process	Documentation & language	Post-market	Combination products
CHINA								
1 April 2000: Regulations for the Supervision and Administration of MD	**SFDA** = State Food and Drug Administration	I-Low Risk II-Moderate III-High	Chinese language required on primary, secondary and IFU **CCC** Mark : issued by China Quality Certification Centre; applies to 8 categories of MD: • rubber condoms • diagnostic x-ray • hemodialysis equipment • hollow fiber dialyzers • extra-corporeal blood circuit • electrocardiographs • pacemakers • artificial heart-lung machines	ISO 13485 recognized Manufacturing site: • complies with Chinese GMPs • Class III and sterile Class II MD: inspected by SFDA	Write product standard following China National Standard (ISO/IEC standard as ref, but to be translated in Chinese) **Product testing** at National Testing centre as per China National Standard **Clinical Trial** if required: • Class III, long-term implantable; CT mandatory in China • Class II domestically produced: exempt from CT (21 MD group qualified for exemption): demonstrate similarity with approved product • Class I: exempt from CT Director Application reviewed by : • SFDA Med Device Technical Evaluation Centre • SFDA Medical Device Registration Department • Director of SFDA Medical devices dept • Director General of SFDA MD Registration Certificate: valid 4 years Recognition of GHTF country approval	Application to be submitted in: Chinese	**Adverse Events:** • Class III MD: severe AE must be reported within 15 days independent of its location in the world	Regulation changing

(*Continued*)

Key dates	Authority/ Regulator name	Devices class & particularities	Product labeling	Roles & licenses	Registration process	Documentation & language	Post-market	Combination products
EUROPE								
1985: New Approach: set up the legislative and technical frame in the European Community (EC) 1989: Global Approach (Conformity Assessment Modules, quality Assurance, Notified Bodies) 1990: **AIMD** 90/385/EEC Directive on Active Implantable Medical Devices 1993: **MDD** 93/42/EEC Medical Device Directive 1998: **IVD** 98/79/EC Directive on In Vitro Diagnostics Medical Devices	**Competent Authority** in each European Member State (27) **NB**: Notified Body **CAB**: Conformity Assessment Body	**MDD Class:** I, Is, Im-Low Risk IIa-Low-moderate IIb-Moderate-high III-High **AIMD:** All-High Risk **IVD:** List A-High List B-Moderate Self-test-Moderate Self-Certifiable-Low Systems and Procedure Packs	National language (23 languages) Use of symbols (EN 980) Add suitable specific label for phthalate-containing devices	Manufacturer: must inform the CA of the Member State in which he has his registered place of business **Foreign Manufacturer** must appoint an **Authorized Representative** located in Europe: Authorized Representative to inform the CA of the Member State in which he has his registered place of business Manufacturer to be ISO 13485 certified Validity of product license (CE Mark): maximum 5 years	**Low risk devices** (MDD: Class I; IVD: Self-tests, Self-certifiable): • Self-Certification by the Legal Manufacturer • CE Declaration of Conformity **Moderate- High risk devices** (MDD: Class Is, Im, IIa, IIb, III; AIMD: High Risk; IVD: list A and B): • NB Selection • Conformity Assessment Procedure • Batch Verification by NB for IVD List A • Technical Documentation review by NB • Quality Management System audit by NB • CE Mark Certificate • Continued Batch Verification by NB for IVD List A • CE Declaration of Conformity	**Low-moderate risk devices** (Class I, Is, Im, IIa and IIb from MDD; List B, Self-test from IVD): Technical File: • Essential Requirements Checklist • Risk Management File • Clinical Evaluation Report **High risk devices** (Class III from MDD; List A from IVD; AIMD): Design File Application to be submitted in: English accepted, unless specified by Member State to submit in local language	<u>**Adverse Events:**</u> • Serious threat to public health: to be reported immediately or <48h • Led to death: immediately or <10 days • Other events: immediately or <30 days Periodic Summary Report **FSCA**: Field Safety Corrective Action **FSN**: Field Safety Notice (= form to be used to notify a FSCA to customers) Guideline MEDDEV 2.12: forms for: • Incident Report to CA • FSCA Report to CA • Template for FSN	Based on **PMOA**: Primary Mode of Action EU Directives do not apply cumulatively Drug/Device combination product: When PMOA physical, classified as MD: • Technical/ Design File submitted to NB • NB assess performance of the device and usefulness of the substance • CA assess the quality, safety, clinical benefit/ risks of the substance • Need the favorable opinion of the CA for NB to deliver CE Mark

Key dates	Authority/ Regulator name	Devices class & particularities	Product labeling	Roles & licenses	Registration process	Documentation & language	Post-market	Combination products
HONG KONG								
MD do not require registration, unless containing pharmaceutical products or emitting ionizing radiation 2004: MDCO established Nov 26th, 2004: Medical Device Administrative Control System MDACS: Voluntary listing of Class IV Nov 14th, 2005: Voluntary listing of Class II and Class III	**MDCO**: Medical Device Control Office **CAB**: Conformity Assessment Body	I-Low Risk II-Low-moderate III-Moderate-high IV-High	English & Chinese	Local responsible Person **LRP** to be assigned (more than one allowed) Validity of product license: 5 years	Regulatory System: follows GHTF **Class II, III, IV:** • Registration of Product, local manufacturer, overseas manufacturer (or its local representative), importer • QMS Certification (ISO 13485) **Class I:** Registration of local manufacturer and importer	**Class II, III, IV:** • STED Application to be submitted in: English	**Adverse Events:** • Serious threat to public health, led to death, serious injury: to be reported <10 days • Other events: <30 days	Drug-Device product: registration and quality system to follow MD requirements
INDIA								
Drugs and Cosmetic Act 1940 Drugs and Cosmetic Rules (1945) October 2005 Gazette notification for 10 categories of MD notified as Drugs	**DCGI**: Drugs Controller General of India under **Central Government** **CDSCO:** Central Drugs Standards Control Organization	Notified MD classified as Drugs: *1. Disposable Hypodermic Syringes* *2. Disposable Hypodermic Needles* *3. Disposable Perfusion Sets*	Add the approval number (Import License No.) Language: English	Foreign Manufacturer/ Importer: local agent, License for sale and distribution Site inspection by CDSCO and FDA; Conformity Assessment Procedures	"Me Too" Route (prior approval): • Abridged Evaluation when already approved in at least one of the GHTF founding members	"Me Too" Route (prior approval): • Application Form 40 → DCGI delivers approval Registration Certificate (Form 41) • Application in Form 8 → DCGI delivers Import License (Form 10)	Complaints & Adverse Reactions for Drugs and New Drugs Clinical Trials No specific requirements for MDs	No definition of combination products as MD regulated as Drugs

(Continued)

Key dates	Authority/ regulator name	Devices class & particularities	Product labeling	Roles & licenses	Registration process	Documentation & language	Post-market	Combination products
INDIA								
	Food and Drug Adminis-tration Drugs Control Depart-ment under State Gover-nment	*3. Disposable Perfusion Sets* *4. In-vitro Diagnostic Devices for HIV, HBsAg and HCV* *5. Cardiac Stents* *6. Drug Eluting Stents* *7. Catheters* *8. Intra Ocular Lenses* *9. I V Cannulae* *10. Bone Cements* *11. Heart Valves* *12. Scalp Vein Sets* *13. Orthopedic Implants* *14. Internal Prosthetic Replacements* *1. Blood Grouping Sera* *2. Ligatures, Sutures and Staplers*		performed by Notified Bodies are acceptable (ISO 13485, USFDA QSRs) Local manufacturer: to comply with GMP; inspection by CDSCO and State FDA; license valid for 5 years Validity of product license (Registration Certificate): 3 years Validity of Form 10 is same as Form 41	New product: • Complete evaluation, clinical trials	New product: • Form 44 application (clinical Data) → Form 45 Cert • Form 40 → Form 41 • Form 8 → Form 10 License Application to be submitted in English at the DCGI office. State FDAs some time may have local language formats along with English as an alternate.		

Key dates	Authority/ regulator name	Devices class & particularities	Product labeling	Roles & licenses	Registration process	Documentation & language	Post-market	Combination products
		3. Intra-Uterine devices (Cu-T) *4. Condoms* *5. Tubal Rings* *6. Surgical Dressings* *7. Umbilical tapes* *8. Blood/Blood Components Bags*						
INDONESIA								
Mandatory registration will be enforced in 2014 based on the ASEAN Medical Device Directive (AMDD)	**Ministry of Health**	I-Low Risk IIa-Low-moderate IIb-Moderate-high III-High	English is acceptable To be provided in Indonesian: • Intended use • Direction for use • Precautions • Warning • Adverse event (can be put in IFU)	Applicant: must hold a distribution license "IPAK", must be officially appointed by source company or legal manufacturer as sole agent – validity of 2 years Validity of product license: 4 years	All manual with hard copies • Pre-registration • Submission • Payment • License	CSDT Application to be submitted in: English or Indonesian	Voluntary reporting Serious adverse health or death: mandatory to report, 24h with corrective action plan	Currently no guideline

(*Continued*)

Key dates	Authority/ regulator name	Devices class & particularities	Product labeling	Roles & licenses	Registration process	Documentation & language	Post-market	Combination products
JAPAN								
Pharma-ceutical Affairs Law (PAL) from 1960	**MHLW:** Ministry of Health, Labour and Welfare **PMDA:** Pharma-ceuticals and Medical Devices Agency **RCB:** Registered Certifi-cation Body	I-Low Risk (= General MD) II-Low-moderate (=Controlled MD) III-Moderate-high (=Highly Controlled MD) IV-High (=Highly Controlled MD) JMDN (Japanese Medical Device Nomenclature) : generic name for single MD and grouping of MD	To be in Japanese: • brand name, generic name, • device category on device itself, wrappers or containers	Regulatory System: follows GHTF **Company**: • License for Marketing Authorization Holder (MAH) (Types 1, 2 and 3) - Validity: 5 years • MAH located in Japan: must comply with GQP (Good Quality Practices) – • Comply with GVP (Good Vigilance Practices) **Manufacturing Site/ Manufacturer**: license for Manufacturer or Foreign Manufacturer Accreditation 4 types of License: Biological, Sterilization, General, Packaging Validity: 5 years Product License: no expiry date	MD: Minister's approval, or 3rd party Certification or Marketing Notification **Class I:** Self-Declaration by MAH **Class II:** • Pre-market certification application reviewed by a Registered Certification Body • QMS inspection (certification valid for 5 years) – similar to ISO 13485 **Class III and IV:** • Application reviewed by the PMDA and MHLW • QMS	STED Application to be submitted in: Japanese	**Adverse Events:** • Serious threat to public health: to be reported <15 days • Led to death: <150 days • Other serious events: <30 days • Non-serious: annual report	No clear definition at this moment

Key dates	Authority/ regulator name	Devices class & particularities	Product labeling	Roles & licenses	Registration process	Documentation & Language	Post-market	Combination products
JORDAN								
Regulations implemented since 2005	**JFDA**: Jordan Food and Drug Adminis-tration	I-Low Risk IIa-Low-moderate IIb-Moderate-high III-High	Country of Origin No specific symbol to be put on the product after approval. Language: English language and/or Arabic.	Distributors & importers should be registered in ministry of trade and industry Validity of product license: 5 years	Evaluation of the importation requests by the Medical Device Committee Analysis test at JFDA Drug Laboratory Control Department Class I follows the same registration process such as II & III	• Notarized FDA Certificate to Foreign Government (CFG) or CE Certificates or Free Sales certificates • Finished product specifications and methods of analysis • For MD containing ingredients of animal origin; TSE/BSE Certificate (Transmissible Spongiform Encephalopathy/ Bovine Spongiform Encephalopathy) Application to be submitted in English	Incidents reporting system to JFDA No timelines	Combination products such as drug containing medical devices should be registered
MALAYSIA								
Dec 2011: Medical Device Bill and Medical Device Authority Bill passed by Parliament MD are registered on a voluntary basis Mandatory registration will be enforced in 2014 based on the ASEAN Medical Device Directive (AMDD)	Medical Device Authority	A-Low Risk B-Low-moderate C-Moderate-high D-High Product grouping: • Single • System • Kits • Group	No labeling requirements at that time	Manufacturer/ Importers/ Distributors would need to apply for establishment licenses: it will be defined in the upcoming regulation Validity of product license not defined yet	**Class B, C, D:** Evaluation routes: • Abridged Evaluation when already approved in at least one of the GHTF founding members • Full Evaluation	**Class B, C & D:** • Abridged Evaluation: CSDT + Doc + Technical File (TF for Class D only) • Full Evaluation: CAB Assessment of CSDT + DoC + Technical File (TF for Class D only) **Class A:** • Simplified CSDT + DoC Application to be submitted in: English acceptable	Voluntary reporting **Adverse Events:** • Serious threat to public health: to be reported <48h • Led to death: <10 days • Other events: <30 days	Evaluated by both National Pharmaceutical Control Bureau and Medical Device Authority

(Continued)

Key dates	Authority/ regulator name	Devices class & particularities	Product labeling	Roles & licenses	Registration process	Documentation & Language	Post-market	Combination products
PHILIPPINES								
BFAD Circular #05-1998	BFAD: Bureau of Food and Drug Adminis-tration	I-Low Risk II-Low-mod-erate III-Mode-rate-high IV-High	No labeling requirements at that time	Regulatory System: follows GHTF Manufacturer/ Importers/ Distributors: local representative to hold a License to Operate (LTO) Validity of product license (Certificate of Product Registration CPR): • initial registration: 1 year • subsequent renewal: 5 years	Sterile and invasive MD must be registered	• GMP Certificate • Government Certificate of clearance and Free Sale from country of origin • ISO Certification for imported product • Certificate of agreement between manufacturer and trader/distributor/importer • Technical specifications of the product/stabilities/labeling Application to be submitted in: English	Voluntary Reporting of Adverse Events Mandatory Reporting of Product Recall	No Combination Product regulation – drug/biologic part registered separately from Device part
REPUBLIC OF KOREA (SOUTH KOREA)								
1997: MD regulated by the KFDA 2003: New	**KFDA**: Korea Food and Drug Adminis-tration	I-Low Risk II-Low-mod-erate	For plastic made MD: label to specify if DEHP was added or used in the	Manufacturer or Importer: Device Business License:	**Class I**: notification to one of the 6 Regional KFDA **Class II, III & IV:** Technical File review:	**Class II, III & IV:** • Technical File (requirements similar to CSDT or STED)	**Adverse Events:** • Serious threat to public health: to	Combination products covered by articles for MD license,

Key dates	Authority/ regulator name	Devices class & particularities	Product labeling	Roles & licenses	Registration process	Documentation & Language	Post-market	Combination products
REPUBLIC OF KOREA (SOUTH KOREA)								
Medical Device Act, fully enforced since May30th, 2004 From April 8th, 2012, foreign manufacturers of Class II, III and IV MD should be audited by Korean auditors for their quality system at the on-site (re-certification every 3 years)	**4 Quality System Audit Agencies:** KTL, KCL, KTC, KTR **6 Technical Files review Agencies "Regional KFDA":** KTL, KTC, KCL, KTR, TUV-SUD, SGS **13 Domestic Labora-tories to perform Type Testing**, including KTL	III-Mode-rate-high IV-High 25 product groups	manu-facturing process Int. recognized symbols accepted Korean language required on both the outer package & IFU	Health certificate of the company representative, registered legal entity, list of facilities Korea Good Manufacturing Practice certification (KGMP) (validity of 3 years) Product License: no expiry date	• Technical File when device basically the same as previously approved ones • Safety and Efficacy review (SER) when significantly different: new-to-market features (new materials, mechanisms of action, usage or effectiveness) Type Testing KGMP Certification (identical to ISO 13485)	• Type Testing: reports to be provided about bio-compatibility, electrical & mechanical safety, electromagnetic compatibility, performance tests • Safety and Efficacy review (SER): requires stability data, clinical study report Local clinical study report not necessary if foreign clinical data strong enough and approved by foreign regulator, if published in Science Citation Index (SCI) Application to be submitted in: Korean preferably	be reported <7 days • Led to death: details shall be additionally reported within 8 days from the date of initial reporting • Recall of harmful medical devices required recall may submit a recall plan to KFDA within 5 to 15 days. • The expected end date of recall shall be within 30 days from the start of recall	notification and technical file review

(*Continued*)

Key dates	Authority/ regulator name	Devices class & particularities	Product labeling	Roles & licenses	Registration process	Documentation & language	Post-market	Combination products
SAUDI ARABIA								
Royal Decree (M/6) issued on Feb 2007 gave the SFDA the responsibility to regulate MD, reinforced by the Council of Ministers decision No. 181 issued on June 2007 MD interim regulation issued by Saudi FDA on Dec 27th, 2008	**SFDA**: Food and Drug Authority	Product group: guidance on MDMA incorporating more than one MD type	When device intended to be used by lay person (i.e. not medical personnel): Arabic & English	**Importer, Distributor & Authorized Represen-tative:** • Register (electro-nically) through the Medical Device national registry (MDNR): National Registration Number issued by |SFDA • Apply through Medical Device Establish-ment Licensing (MDEL) to get an establish-ment License	Regulatory System: follows GHTF Marketing Authorization Certificate and Medical Device Listing national registry Number delivered if: • MD to be already registered in one or more of the 5 GHTF founding countries • MD labeling and conditions of supply to be compliant with provisions from KSA (Kingdom of Saudi Arabia)	Medical Device Marketing Authorization (MDMA) applications: • Electronic form • Electronic copies of labels • Copy of IFUs • Evidence that MD authorized in one of the 5 GHTF founding Member Same registration path for all classes – fees different STED format not applicable Application to be submitted in: English	**Adverse Events:** • Serious injury: to be reported imme-diately, i.d. <10 days • Other events: <30 days National centre of Medical Devices reporting (NCMDR): to report FSCA	Since the MDMA require that the device complies with the regulation of one of the GHTF founding member, the product was fully assessed and the decision was already made to regulate it as medical device or not.

Key dates	Authority/ regulator name	Devices class & particularities	Product labeling	Roles & licenses	Registration process	Documentation & language	Post-market	Combination products
SAUDI ARABIA								
				Validity of license: 1 year Validity of product license: • same as MA granted in GHTF jurisdiction • except when open ended or self-declaration process: 3 years				
SINGAPORE								
2002 • Voluntary Product registration Scheme • Post-Market monitoring • Surveillance program for Medical Devices on market 2007 Health Products act: From Nov 1st, 2007	**HSA**: Singapore Health Sciences Authority - Health Products Regulation Group	A-Low Risk B-Low-moderate C-Moderate-high D-High Product grouping: • Single • Family • System • Group • IVD Cluster	English International Recognized symbols	**Manufac-turers:** ISO 13485 **Importer and Wholesaler:** GDPMDS (Good Distribution Practice for MD) of ISO 13485 with scope of storage and distribution Validity of licenses: 12 months	Regulatory System: follows GHTF **Class B, C, D:** Online Medical Device Information and Communication System (MEDICS) for screening: registrable or rejection Evaluation routes: • Abridged Evaluation when already approved in at least one of the GHTF founding members • Full Evaluation **Class B: Expedited Registration route:** • when approval by at least 2 reference regulatory agencies, or	**Class B, C, D:** Common Submission Dossier template CSDT **Class A:** CSDT not required: • Letter of Authorization • Singapore Declaration of Conformity • Product labeling, IFUs etc • Name, address, contact information of importer • QMS Certificate for manufacturing and sterilization sites Sterilization method and validation standard used	**Adverse Events:** • Serious threat to public health: to be reported immediately and <48h • Led to death: <10 days • Other events: <30 days **FSCA**: • Initiation of FSCA and	Guidance to be published for Drug-Device product

(Continued)

Key dates	Authority/ regulator name	Devices class & particularities	Product labeling	Roles & licenses	Registration process	Documentation & language	Post-market	Combination products
SINGAPORE								
• Report adverse events to HAS within the stipulated time frame • Notify HSA prior to initiation of a product recall • Maintenance of product compliant and distribution records From Nov 1st, 2008: MD dealers and registrants licensing MD licensed under Radiation Protection Act exempted from registration with HSA until Aug 1st, 2011 From Aug 10th, 2010 : Class C and D MD must be licensed From Jan 1st, 2012 : Class A and B MD must be licensed				Validity of product license: 1 year	• Approval by one of independent reference regulatory agency and marketed for at least 3 years without safety concerns. **<u>Class B: Immediate Registration (IBR) Evaluation Route:</u>** • when approved by at least 2 independent reference regulatory agencies (i.e. US FDA, EU/TGA, Health Canada, Japan MHLW) and marketed for at least 3 years without safety concerns.	Application to be submitted in: English	preliminary report to be notified within 24h • Final report to be submitted within 21 days	

Key dates	Authority/ regulator name	Devices class & particularities	Product labeling	Roles & licenses	Registration process	Documentation & language	Post-market	Combination products
TAIWAN								
1970: Pharmaceutical Affairs Act promulgated, enacted in 1973 1998: Good Manufacturing Practices 2000: reclassification of MD 2004: Regulations governing Management of MD 2004: Guidelines for Registration of MD 2006: Good Laboratory Practice for Nonclinical Laboratory Studies 2007 Medical Device Good Clinical Practice	**TFDA**: Taiwan Food and Drug Adminis-tration	I-Low Risk II-Moderate III-High	Mandarin	Authorized domestic &foreign distributors or subsidiaries: must have licensing for wholesaling, retailing, importing or exporting MD No expiration date on the company license Foreign manufacturer: TFDA issue QSD (Quality System Documentation) Certificate (validity: 3 years) Validity of product license: 5 years	**Class II:** Evaluation routes: • Abridged Evaluation (Mutual recognition) when already approved in US and/or EU • Full Evaluation	**Class I:** Affidavit + GMP certificate + MD dealer license **Class II:** Abridged Evaluation: • Technical Documentation without pre-clinical testing • QSD (Quality System Documentation) limited to inspection report, Free Sale Certificate and ISO 13485 Certificate Full Evaluation: full Technical Documentation including pre-clinical testing **Class III:** Full Evaluation: full Technical Documentation including pre-clinical testing (+Clinical Reports when New MD) STED format accepted for Class III Application to be submitted in: English or Mandarin	Periodic safety update reports (PSUR) to be submitted for certain devices every 6 months for 3 years with additional summary report of total of 3 year PSUR.	Drug-Device product: registration and quality system to follow MD requirements

(Continued)

Key dates	Authority/ regulator name	Devices class & particularities	Product labeling	Roles & licenses	Registration process	Documentation & language	Post-market	Combination products
TAIWAN								
2010 Application Guidelines for Registration of In Vitro Diagnostic Medical Devices 2011 Medical Device Good Vigilance Practice								
THAILAND								
Medical Device Act ("the Act") in 1988 Medical Device Act (2008) 2551 B.E.	ThaiFDA	I-Low Risk ("General") II-Moderate ('Higher Risk') III-High (Highest Risk")	In Thai language, product label to contain: • product name, • class, type; • name, address and country of origin of the manufacturer and importer; • license number • lot number; summarized usage instructions • expiration date	Manufacturer or its representative must register in person, through a locally-based legal entity Validity of product license ("letter of importation"): aligned with the validity of CFS/CFG	Manual submission by the importer to the regulator	• Original CFS/CFG • Letter of authorization • Product catalogue • Copy of the establishment for importation license	Mandatory Reporting of Adverse Events and Product Recall	No Guidance Classification based on intended use: either classified and evaluated only as a Device, or as a Drug

Key dates	Authority/ regulator name	Devices class & particularities	Product labeling	Roles & licenses	Registration process	Documentation & language	Post-market	Combination products
UNITED ARAB EMIRATES								
UAE Pharmacy Law No 4 from 1983 MD Regulatory system is already applied and a grace period for importation is granted for non-registered professional use items through a local licensed distributor.	**MOH:** Ministry of Health **RDCR**: Registration and Drug Control department	I-Low Risk II-Low-moderate III-Moderate-high IV-High Follows the GHTF rule-based classification	English and/or Arabic understandable Universal symbols/ instructions for professionals and consumers are required on the label such as Sterile, single use, storage condition,	Regulatory System: follows GHTF Appoint Local Representative: licensed by MOH Local Representative subject to annual renewal Validity of product license: 5 years	**MD classified as non-pharmaceutical dosage form:** Register the Authorized Representative in Country Of Origin (COO) (supported by declaration/certificates from source/manufacturing site) **MD classified containing pharmaceutical ingredients:** Register the manufacturer (supported by documentation from source/ manufacturing site)	**Class I:** • Application form, Free Sale certificate • Device information • Labeling • DoC, evidence of conformity to Essential Principles, Quality certificates **Class II:** Same as Class I + Post-market requirements, risk assessment and Status of device distribution **Class III & IV:** Same as Class II + Safety and effectiveness data and Manufacturing process Application to be submitted in: English	Timeline for Incidents reporting: 15 calendar days. Prior notification to MOH before FSCA is required.	MD classified containing pharmaceutical ingredients Classification according to other international reference bodies is accepted.
USA								
1968 Radiation control of Health and Safety Act (RCHSA) 1976: Medical Device	**USFDA**: United States Food and Drug Administration	I-Low Risk II-Moderate III-High Convenience kits	English required Labeling requirements in 21 CFR Part 801 Additional requirements for:	**Manufacturers (domestic & foreign) & distributors (importers):** • Register establishment	<u>Class I&II:</u> • Premarket Notification (510k) clearance (21 CFR Part 807 Subpart E) • Demonstration of "substantial equivalence": device as safe and effective as a predicate device (=legally marketed device)	<u>Class I:</u> • Unless exempt, require a 510k application • Subject to General Controls (Registration and Listing, labeling, GMP)	**MDR** (medical Device Reporting) (21CFR Part 803): electronic MD reporting program: eMDR (voluntary)	**OCP**: FDA's Office of Combination Products 21 CFR 3.2: physically or

(*Continued*)

Key dates	Authority/ regulator name	Devices class & particularities	Product labeling	Roles & licenses	Registration process	Documentation & language	Post-market	Combination products
USA								
Amendments to the US Federal Food, Drug and Cosmetic Act (FD&C Act) (=Law) Regulations (=Federal Laws) : Title 21 Code of Federal Regulations (CFR) – 9 Volumes: the one containing the MD and electronic product regulations is Part 800-1299	**HHS**: US Department of Health and Human Services (HHS) **CDRH**: Center for Devices and Radiological Health; **CBER**: Center for Biologics Evaluation and Research; **CDER**: Center for Drugs Evaluation and Research		• In-vitro diagnostic device • IDE (Investigational device Exemption) device • Radiation-emitting products • Natural rubber (latex)	• Designate a US Agent (if foreign manufacturer) Establishment registration valid for 1 year Manufacturers to comply with FDA Quality System Regulation (21 CFR Part 820) (=GMP Good Manufacturing Practices) (few substantive differences to ISO 13485, but no conflicting requirements) Product License: no expiry date	**Class III:** • Premarket approval (PMA) process (21 CFR Part 814) • For innovative, non-substantially equivalent MD	**Class I & II:** • Unless exempt, require a 510k application • Subject to General Controls • Subject to Special Controls (special labeling requirements, patient registries, mandatory performance standards, post-market surveillance studies) **Class III:** • Require a PMA application (includes submission of clinical data) • Subject to General Controls • Subject to Special Controls Application to be submitted in: English	**Adverse Events:** • Serious threat to public health: to be reported <5 days • Led to deaths, serious injuries and malfunctions: <30 days • Other events: <30 days • Interim and annual updates required if any baseline information changes after initial submission	chemically combined products; co-packaged products; separately marketed but "cross-labeled" products: • Combination of drug & device • Device & biological product • Biological product & drug • Drug, a device, and a biological product. **PMOA**: Primary Mode of Action **RFD** : Request for Designation submitted to OCP Reviewed by either/or: **CBER, CDRH, CDER**

Key dates	Authority/ regulator name	Devices class & particularities	Product labeling	Roles & licenses	Registration process	Documentation & language	Post-market	Combination products
VIETNAM								
Circulate 24/2011/TT-BYT dated 21st June 2011 guiding MD importing: 50 categories need submission to get import license; others, no need to submit, but documentation may be inspected Local MD need to be registered according to Circular 07/2002/TT-BYT dated 30th may 2002	**DMEC:** Department of Medical Equipment & Construction	Will follow AMDD-GHTF A-Low Risk B-Low-moderate C-Moderate-high D-High	Vietnamese labeling for the outer packaging only (not required for IFU)	**Importer:** applies and holds the import license	**a-Pre-market Approval** = import license application • For high risk MD • Submission to DMEC • Validity of Import License: 1 year **b-Exemption:** importer to work directly with custom for clearance without import license	**a-b: Same documentation needed:** • CFG/CFS or CE mark • ISO 9001 or ISO 13485 • Catalogue • Letter of Authorization Executive summary in Vietnamese	Notification and Management of safety information to user and Authority must be done by importer No specific guideline on timeline	Based on primary mode of action, with reference to EU, US regulations

Index